Neuropediatrics - Recent Advances and Novel Therapeutic Approaches

Edited by Hagit Friedman

Published in London, United Kingdom

Neuropediatrics - Recent Advances and Novel Therapeutic Approaches
http://dx.doi.org/10.5772/intechopen.1000299
Edited by Hagit Friedman

Contributors
Andrea A. García-Contreras, Edgar M. Vásquez-Garibay, Lucila A. Godínez-Méndez, Seema Rohilla, Vikas, Yamini Wadhwa, Deepak Singla, Dhara B. Dhaulakhandi, Aleksei Anurev, Vladimir Gorbachev, Tatiana Pavlova, Alexander Pavlov, Allison Roberto da Silva, Jacqueline Rodrigues da Silva, Maja Kostic, Elizabeth Colvin, Huynh Duy, Sarah Ro, Carolyn Quinsey, Inga Shevtsova, Sriram Machineni, Hanan Demyati, Susan D. Rich, Briana R. Hickey, Elizabeth K. Kaprielian, Hagit Friedman

First published in London, United Kingdom, 2024 by IntechOpen
IntechOpen is the global imprint of INTECHOPEN LIMITED, registered in England and Wales, registration number: 11086078, 5 Princes Gate Court, London, SW7 2QJ, United Kingdom

British Library Cataloguing-in-Publication Data
A catalogue record for this book is available from the British Library

Additional hard and PDF copies can be obtained from orders@intechopen.com

Neuropediatrics - Recent Advances and Novel Therapeutic Approaches
Edited by Hagit Friedman
p. cm.
Print ISBN 978-1-83769-386-3
Online ISBN 978-1-83769-385-6
eBook (PDF) ISBN 978-1-83769-387-0

For EU product safety concerns:
IN TECH d.o.o., Prolaz Marije Krucifikse Kozulić 3, 51000 Rijeka, Croatia,
info@intechopen.com or visit our website at intechopen.com.

Meet the editor

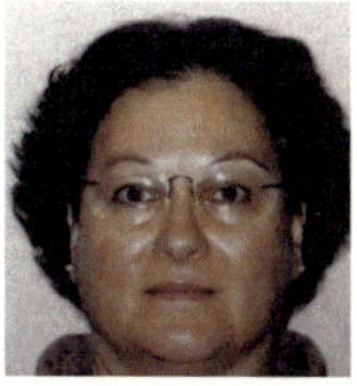

Dr. Hagit Friedman, Ph.D., is an expert in neurodevelopment and neurorehabilitation, researching and developing new scientific-clinical tools for early diagnosis and intervention of neural injuries and developmental disabilities. She has published her scientific clinical work in peer-reviewed scientific international journals and book chapters, as well as top scientific international conferences. Dr. Friedman is certified in 3LT and several clinical-scientific tools for neurodevelopmental assessment of infants and children (USA, England). She is an experienced lecturer in MA, BA, and MD programs in neuroscience, psychology, physiology, and child development. Dr. Friedman is an active member and board member in academic and clinical associations and committees, an invited scientific editor and reviewer in several research foundations and scientific journals, and an active participant in international scientific conferences.

Contents

Preface

Neuropediatrics involves the diagnosis and treatment of congenital and acquired diseases of the central and peripheral nervous system in babies, children, and adolescents, focusing on developmental processes.

Neuropediatrics divides the nervous system, and thus neurological pathologies, into two large classes: the central and the peripheral nervous systems. The central nervous system consists of the brain (controls the body's functions) and the spinal cord (connects the central nervous system with the body). The peripheral nervous system is the network of neural circuits that controls autonomic body functions, carrying hormonal, motor, and sensory information.

Neuropediatric pathologies may manifest in brain function (epilepsy, meningitis), nerve fibers (neuropathy), muscles (myopathy, dystonia), bone marrow (myelitis), and degenerative processes (Creutzfeldt-Jakob syndrome).

Many of the neurological pathologies have a genetic predisposition and ambient epigenetic catalysts. Cellular building blocks of the nervous system—neurons and glial cells—may be injured during their development, causing neural pathologies. Recent studies show that various pathologies, including many neuropediatric pathologies, involve mitochondrial abnormalities.

This book provides a comprehensive overview of neuropediatrics examining the scientific and clinical benefits of rapid advances in brain imaging, neuroscience, and new therapies. It is organized into four sections that present current knowledge about diagnosis, monitoring, intervention, and therapy in neuropediatrics.

The first section of the book includes two chapters about the gut–brain axis in neuropediatric patients. Chapter 1, "Probiotics, Prebiotics, and Synbiotics on Constipation in Children with Cerebral Palsy", by Andrea A. García-Contreras, Edgar M. Vásquez-Garibay, and Lucila A. Godínez-Méndez, describes clinical results in children with cerebral palsy (CP), which is regarded as a severe neural injury. As more very low birth weight (VLBW) premature-born babies survive under advanced Western medicine, the prevalence of severe brain injuries, including CP, increases. The authors give a comprehensive introduction to CP's characteristics, etiology, clinical history, risk factors, and more. An important issue discussed by the authors is the gut microbiota in children with CP, as it is known that gut microbiota and brain development and function have a bidirectional connection/influence. Given the limited scientific research about the effect of pre and probiotic additives on clinical symptoms in CP, the discussion in this chapter leads the way for additional necessary studies. In Chapter 2, "Systematic Approach to Diagnose Inborn Neurometabolic Disorders", Seema Rohilla, Yamini Wadhwa, Deepak Singla, and Dhara B. Dhaulakhandi describe a systemic structural approach to the diagnosis of IEMs and narrow down the list of differentials so that cost-effective yet precise biochemical, genetic, and molecular tests may be performed to arrive at a final diagnosis.

The second section of the book includes two chapters about novel monitoring technologies for optimal outcomes in neuropediatric patients. Chapter 3, "The Role of Monitoring the Electrical Activity of the Diaphragm in a Comprehensive Assessment of the Effectiveness of Intensive Treatment in Premature Infants with Extremely Low Birth Weight", by Aleksei Anurev, Vladimir Gorbachev, Tatiana Pavlova, and Alexander Pavlov, demonstrates the benefits and significance of neural-adjusted ventilatory assist (NAGVA) for the survival and resilience of premature newborns. The authors describe the development of the nervous system in fetuses and newborns, including white matter injuries and neurovascular pathologies and their developmental outcomes. The developmental discussion evolves into the argument about pain sensation and interpretation in newborns and young babies, and the dangerous neurodevelopmental outcomes of chronic interventional pain. The development of the peripheral nervous system and nociception takes the chapter to the phrenic nerve and its control of diaphragm activity and ventilation. The use of NAVA for high-risk patients is painless, noninvasive, and safe for the lungs and shortens the duration of NICU hospitalization.

Chapter 4, "The Role of Surgical Simulation in the Quality of Health Care for Complex Neurosurgical Patients", by Allison Roberto da Silva and Jacqueline Rodrigues da Silva, describes the technological evolution of advanced imaging techniques, which allow surgical teams to perform complex surgeries without exposing the patient in advance. This approach helps improve surgical results and safety, increase precision in operation, and decrease the duration of patient exposure to anesthesia. Altogether this technological advance may improve quality of care and patient quality of life.

The third section of the book includes two chapters about pediatric neurorehabilitation. In Chapter 5, "Application of the International Classification Functioning, Disability, and Health (ICF) as Clinical Reasoning Tool in Pediatric Neurorehabilitation", Hanan Demyati describes his findings on the important clinical issue of the ICF in pediatric neurorehabilitation. The author gives a comprehensive introduction to pediatric neurorehabilitation, and specifically about the ICF tool and its significance as a standard diagnostic language, including components and innovative aspects.

In Chapter 6, "Idiopathic Intracranial Hypertension", Maja Kostic, Elizabeth Colvin, Huynh Duy, Carolyn Quinsey, and Sarah Ro, share their experience and insights about IIH diagnosis and the therapeutic approach in pediatric patients. The authors investigate IIH in pediatric populations, observing demographic issues, clinical characteristics, potential underlying pathophysiologic mechanisms, diagnostic procedures, and the significance of a multidisciplinary therapeutic approach. They find that this approach is the optimal clinical methodology, as it allows patients to receive complete and broad care that will solve more features of IIH while still focusing on longstanding objectives and reduction.

The fourth section of the book comprises two chapters about therapeutic approaches for toddlers and children with early trauma. Chapter 7, "Trauma Informed Farm Animal Assisted Neurotherapy and Green Care Farming for Neurodiverse Conditions" by Susan Rich, Briana Hickey, and Elizabeth Kaprielian, provides a comprehensive and interesting description and analysis of animal-assisted therapeutic approaches. The chapter presents information about neurodevelopmental conditions and mental illness, the various etiologies and traditional therapeutic approaches used in these conditions, and Maslow's hierarchy model and the theory of mind. The authors explain how farm animal-assisted neurotherapy can help neurodiverse children and teens develop a sense of community, meaning, and purpose, as well as adaptive functions for success in life.

Finally, Chapter 8, "Early Trauma, Brain Development, and a Novel Therapeutic Approach", by the editor presents current data on the prevalence, characteristics, etiology, mechanism, and therapy of PTSD. It analyzes the involvement of the HPA axis, neural inflammation, and the neural mitochondrial oxidative stress response in the molecular mechanism of PTSD, reducing neuroplasticity and synapse proliferation. This information serves as the basis for understanding the significance of auricular therapy and the 3LT novel therapeutic tool for early trauma. This chapter is dedicated to the infants and children who grow up in war zones, and those who are victims of violence, terrorism, and cruelty.

Dr. Hagit Friedman
Simaney-Derech Institute,
Tel-Hai Academic College,
Haifa University,
Zichron-Yaakov, Israel

Section 1

Gut Brain Axis in Neuropediatric Pathologies

Chapter 1

Probiotics, Prebiotics, and Synbiotics on Constipation in Children with Cerebral Palsy

Andrea A. García-Contreras, Edgar M. Vásquez-Garibay and Lucila A. Godínez-Méndez

Abstract

Constipation is a common gastrointestinal disorder in children with cerebral palsy, which affects up to 74%. Children with cerebral palsy are at a high risk of gut dysbiosis. Prebiotics and probiotics may modulate gut microbiota and influence brain functions. Probiotics are defined as "live organisms that, when administered in adequate amounts, confer a health benefit on the host." Prebiotics are a substrate that is selectively utilized by host microorganisms that confer a health benefit. Both probiotics and prebiotics have been shown to improve the gut microbiota and confer an improvement in the characteristics of stools such as the history of painful defecation, the presence of fecal mass in the rectum, and stool frequency in children with cerebral palsy. A strong bidirectional communication between the central nervous system and the enteric system exists, which is known as the gut-brain axis, which regulates gastrointestinal motility, gastric secretion, blood flow, gut barrier integrity, immune response, and visceral sensations. The use of probiotics and prebiotics can modulate the production of bioactive compounds that have an impact on the gut-microbiota-brain axis and brain functions in children with cerebral palsy.

Keywords: probiotics, prebiotics, synbiotics, cerebral palsy, constipation, gastrointestinal dysmotility, pediatric neurological impairment, gut microbiota, gut-brain axis

1. Introduction

It has been recognized that cerebral palsy (CP) is a term that encompasses etiologically diverse symptoms, which change with age. The term "cerebral palsy" was first used in the nineteenth century by the English orthopedic surgeon William Little. He observed a dystocia delivery and consequent neonatal hypoxia leading to limb spasticity and musculoskeletal deformities [1]. This disorder occurs in 2–3 out of every 1000 live births and has multiple etiologies resulting in corresponding brain lesions [2, 3].

The risk factors that can cause damage to the central nervous system (CNS) at an early stage of its development are divided into the following categories: before conception, prenatal factors; perinatal factors, and risk factors in the neonatal period and infant stage [4, 5]. In general, CP has a high prevalence of musculoskeletal, gastrointestinal, cardiovascular, and psychiatric diseases. It has been recognized that children with severe motor and intellectual deficiencies, epilepsy, and feeding difficulties have poorer survival.

1.1 Types of cerebral palsy

CP subtypes include spastic, dyskinetic, ataxic, and mixed forms. The Gross Motor Function Classification System (GMFCS) incorporates motor function and is intended to identify differences between CP subtypes in terms of individual abilities. There has been a lot of interest in investigating the function, activity limitations, severity, and quality of life that affect individuals with CP. For this reason, function-based classification groups have been created. The GMFCS is divided into five levels: Level I - ambulation without restriction; Level II - ambulation without assistive devices but with some limitations outside the home; Level III - ambulation with assistance; Level IV – ambulation with assistance with motorized devices or car; level V – little or no ambulation [6]. The mild form of CP is equivalent to levels I and II of the GMFCS, moderate involvement is equivalent to level III, and severe involvement is equivalent to levels IV and V [7]. Spastic CP is the most common form of this movement disorder and affects 80% of children diagnosed with this pathology [8]. Spastic quadriplegia is the most severe form and is often complicated by spinal deformities, speech and feeding disorders, seizures, and muscle contractures. The ataxic type is another form of CP with jerky and uncoordinated movements. This type of cerebral palsy is often associated with speech problems, eye movement dysfunction, and difficulty swallowing [8].

2. Gastrointestinal tract disorders in children with cerebral palsy

Most children with cerebral palsy have feeding difficulties and gastrointestinal (GI) problems such as oropharyngeal dysfunction, gastroesophageal disease, and constipation [1, 9]. In addition, it is known that patients with cerebral palsy may have difficulty swallowing, gastroesophageal reflux, frequent vomiting, and encopresis. During the eating process, food must be chewed, formed into a bolus, and transported to the pharynx, driven primarily by the tongue [10, 11]. Quitadamo et al., [12] have pointed out that almost nine out of ten children with CP experience digestive system alterations, such as difficulty eating, salivation problems, dysphagia, gastroesophageal reflux, and constipation.

2.1 Feeding problems

Children with CP often have difficulty sucking. The inability of an infant to perform safe and successful oral feedings may be an early sign of central nervous system immaturity [13].

Dysphagia in CP is characterized by poor tongue function that makes it difficult to transport the bolus, delaying the start of swallowing with the risk of aspiration, reduced pharyngeal motility, and drooling due to sialorrhea. Feeding problems arise from the prolonged times of this eating process with a delay in the progression of oral feeding skills that can cause growth slowdown due to chronic food insufficiency.

These eating problems can lead to dehydration, malnutrition, aspiration pneumonia, and even death [14]. During this initial phase of swallowing, closing the lips ensures the permanence of the bolus in the oral cavity, while the cyclical movements of the tongue, coordinated with the movements of the jaw, process solid food.

Speyer et al. [15] conducted a systematic review to obtain published data on drooling, swallowing, and feeding problems in people with cerebral palsy throughout life and to estimate the prevalence of drooling, swallowing, and feeding problems by meta-analysis. They obtained 42 articles on the prevalence of drooling, swallowing, and feeding problems in people with cerebral palsy. Estimates in the pediatric population from 0 to 18 years old showed a prevalence of drooling of 44.0% (95% CI 35.6–52.7), of swallowing problems of 50.4% (95% CI 36.0–64.8), and of feeding problems of 53.5. % (95% CI 40.7–65.9).

2.1.1 Feeding problems and malnutrition

Furthermore, feeding difficulties in children with CP play an important role in the pathogenesis of malnutrition and consequently increase the risk of stunting [16]. It even nearly doubled between 2002 and 2015. Minority and economically disadvantaged ethnic groups were more likely to be malnourished. Likewise, gastrointestinal disorders increase the likelihood of malnutrition in hospitalized patients. In this context, physical growth is a fundamental measure of health and well-being in children with CP [17]. However, it must be remembered that patients with CP grow at a slower rate compared to typical developmental milestones, even when medical and nutritional care are optimal. And, also there are feeding schemes that promote rapid weight gain and can cause metabolic syndrome, among other clinical disorders [18–21].

Zhao et al., [22] conducted a multicenter cross-sectional study with children with CP in China. In addition to obtaining the Z score from the anthropometric measurements, they evaluated the GMFCS, the Eating and Drinking Ability Classification System (EDACS), the Subjective Global Nutritional Assessment (SGNA), and the capacity for social life, and they concluded that the degrees of malnutrition in children with CP correlate with the severity of eating and drinking dysfunction and with gross motor impairment.

2.2 Constipation in children with cerebral palsy

Intestinal dysmotility includes various disorders that are characterized by impaired muscle activity in the gastrointestinal tract (GIT) with altered peristalsis [23]. Intestinal motility disorders are common in children with cerebral palsy, which are characterized by abnormal movements of the gut and can result in symptoms such as constipation, diarrhea, reflux, and vomiting [24]. These alterations have a significant impact on the quality of life of the affected population [23]. Constipation would affect 26–74% of children with CP [12, 25]. The etiology is associated with neurological and dietary factors, lifestyle, and decreased mobility [26]. Almost all children with CP and comorbid epilepsy have a gastrointestinal dysfunction, the most troublesome being constipation, followed by abdominal distension, vomiting, and recurrent GIT bleeding [25].

It has been considered important to have a uniform definition of constipation in children with CP [27]. The definition proposed by Veugelers et al. [28], which is, "hard, slimy, scybalous, pebble-like stools in 25% of bowel movements and stool frequency less than three times per week, or large stools palpable on abdominal examination, or use of laxatives or disimpaction faeces manual," appears to be the most comprehensive and is based on three different consensus documents dealing with this issue. Families of children with CP and constipation need to be advised for the effective management of this problem. Parental counseling is necessary for behavior change, positive mental health, problem solving, self-efficacy, and decision making [12].

Rebelo et al. [29] carried out a systematic review with the purpose of synthesizing certain results of randomized clinical trials that evaluated the effect of dietary interventions that improved gastrointestinal problems in children with CP, such as constipation. They only found two clinical trials conducted with the purpose of improving this problem and the characteristics of the stool. One of them evaluated a supplementation for 28 days with probiotics, synbiotics, or prebiotics compared to a placebo. These authors found improvement in the consistency and frequency of bowel movements [30]. In another study conducted by Hassanein et al., [31] they studied supplementation with an oral solution of magnesium sulfate for 1 month compared to a placebo. Although they also reported improvement, the authors of this review considered that both studies were at high risk of bias, and therefore their results would be inconclusive.

2.2.1 Factors associated with constipation in children with cerebral palsy

The mechanisms that produce gut dysmotility are various, and the clinical manifestations are nonspecific [24]. Several factors can influence the stool frequency, consistency, and pH in children with cerebral palsy, such as spasticity [26]. Constipation can be related to reduced mobility, feeding difficulties, or nutritional problems, and it could be a side effect of muscle-relaxing drugs [28]. It has been identified that children with a high degree of motor alterations are the most severely affected. Some alterations such as hypotonia, muscle incoordination, bone deformities (scoliosis, hip dysplasia, etc.), and prolonged immobility exacerbate constipation [28, 32]. Spasticity promotes constipation due to lower mobility of the trunk, lower extremities, abdominal viscera and hypertonia, all these factors contribute to reduce the stool frequency [33]. Moreover, these patients have gut motility alterations, which are related to damage in the brain that affects the entire colon, particularly the proximal colon; another segment commonly affected is the rectum-sigma [26]. A study [34] showed that the production of methane gas contributes to constipation and that the excretion of CH^4 increases due to the reduction of intestinal peristalsis. The normal frequency of defecation in healthy children is variable, usually three times per day to once every 2 days; however, in children with CP, it is reduced to once every seven to 10 days [26, 35]. Other factors associated with constipation in this population are the use of anticonvulsant drugs (phenytoin and valproic acid, among others) [36, 37] and low dietary intake of liquids and fiber [38]. Oral motor dysfunction exacerbates feeding problems, which occurs in more than 90% of children with CP [39]. Caramico-Favero et al., [40] showed that children with CP and constipation had a lower fiber intake compared with the non-constipated group. The study conducted by García-Contreras et al., [30] aimed to identify the association of dietetic factors, use of anticonvulsants, and family history with the stool characteristics of 51 children with cerebral palsy and chronic constipation. There was a positive correlation between stool frequency and the consumption of oilseeds ($r = 0.339$, $p = 0.023$). There was a negative correlation between hard stools and the intake of liquids ($r = -0.335$, $p = 0.026$) and between stool pH and the intake of cereals high in insoluble fiber ($r = -0.339$, $p = 0.030$), vegetables rich in soluble fiber ($r = -0.308$, $p = 0.044$), carrots ($r = -0.336$, $p = 0.027$), and potatoes ($r = -0.307$, $p = 0.045$).

In the same study, an association was identified between the use of human milk substitutes with probiotics/prebiotics with low probability of hard stools [OR = 0.214 (95%CI 0.045–0.98), p = 0.047]; likewise, they increased the probability of a more acid fecal pH [OR = 4.708 (95%CI 1.17–18.91), p = 0.029]. The anticonvulsant polytherapy was associated with hard stools [OR = 14.2 (95%CI 1.16–174), p = 0.038], while the most common polytherapy was the combination of magnesium valproate and vigabatrin (**Table 1**). There was no association between family history and constipation.

Authors concluded that the low consumption of fiber, fluids, and the anticonvulsant polytherapy were associated with harder feces and less frequency of defecation, and they recommend daily intakes of fiber and fluids, especially in children with anticonvulsant polytherapy. High intake of vegetables that contain soluble and insoluble fiber are associated with an improvement in constipation.

2.2.2 Pharmacological treatment for constipation in children with cerebral palsy

Drugs could be necessary to help manage gut dysmotility and constipation, such as laxatives, anticholinergics and prokinetic agents [24]. Mineral oils should be avoided in children with CP since aspiration increases the risk of lipoid pneumonia [41]. Polyethylene glycol (PEG) is a non-poisonous polymer, soluble in water, with high molecular weight, and is not absorbed by GIT. It acts as an osmotic agent and retains water in the lumen of the intestine and colon, softening the stools and stimulating bowel movements by increasing water content, and it is a safe agent without significant side effects in the treatment of chronic constipation in children. It is a safe and effective treatment for constipation in neurologically impaired children [42, 43]. Motilium is a prokinetic drug and is effective in the treatment of gastroesophageal reflux with minimal effect on constipation [44].

A randomized clinical trial in 52 pediatric CP patients with chronic constipation analyzed three therapeutic interventions: (1) PEG, (2) PEG with Motilium, and (3) Motilium for 2 weeks. PEG was administered at 0.5 g/kg/dose three times daily and Motilium at 0.2 mg/kg/dose three times daily. PEG with Motilium showed the highest improvement in chronic constipation symptoms and in stool frequency.

Oral magnesium therapy is accepted as a standard treatment for constipation, and it has been reported to significantly improve spasticity and lower limb movement [45]. A double-blinded randomized control trial was carried out in 100 children with CP (level III-V of the GMCS) and chronic constipation who received oral magnesium sulfate 1 mL/kg/day daily for 1 month. After 1 month of intervention,

Independent variables	Dependent variables	OR	CI 95%	p
Use of formulas with probiotics and prebiotics	Hard Stools	0.214	0.045–0.98	0.047
	Acid pH	4.708	1.17–18.91	0.029
Anticonvulsant polytherapy	Hard Stools	14.250	1.16–174	0.038
Family history of constipation	Frequency of evacuations	0.617	0.11–3.41	0.581

Table 1.
Logistic regression analysis of the factors associated with the stool characteristics.

the constipation score and stool frequency and consistency improved compared to the placebo group ($p < 0.001$). The proportion of painful defecation decreased in the magnesium sulfate group vs. placebo ($p = 0.03$). Oral magnesium sulfate is an effective therapy improving chronic constipation and pain experience in children with CP [31].

3. Probiotics and prebiotics on constipation in children with cerebral palsy

Probiotics are commonly used for both generally healthy consumers and in clinical settings. Probiotics have been defined as "live microorganisms that, when administered in adequate amounts, confer a health benefit on the host;" this definition was grammatically edited from a previous FAO expert consultation [46]. Probiotics contribute to human health after an adequate intake to maintain the balance of the gut microbiota. Some probiotics are capable of producing butyric acid that will maintain the integrity of the intestinal mucosa barrier [47]. In the past 20 years, a class of substances, called prebiotics, were recognized for their ability to modulate the host microbiota [48]. According to the International Scientific Association for Probiotics and Prebiotics (ISAPP) [49], a prebiotic is a 'substrate that is selectively utilized by host microorganisms conferring a health benefit.' This definition also includes non-carbohydrate substances. Beneficial health effects must be documented in order for a substance to be considered a prebiotic. Fructooligosaccharides (FOS) and galactooligosacharides (GOS) currently dominate the prebiotic category as evidenced by various studies [49].

3.1 Types of probiotics and prebiotics used in children with cerebral palsy and constipation

The supplementation with dietary fiber and/or probiotics based on gut microbiota characteristics can effectively improve functional constipation in children with cerebral palsy [50]. Three clinical trials have been carried out to assess the use of probiotics and prebiotics in children with cerebral palsy. Two of them were performed in Mexico and another in China.

Rodríguez-Hernández et al., [51] conducted an intervention of 49 days (7 weeks) with modern kefir on conditions associated with moderate severe spastic quadriparesis cerebral palsy. Milk kefir is a dairy product that includes several microorganisms, which contain bacteria from genera *Bifidobacterium, Lactococcus, Leuconostoc,* and *Lactobacillus,* as well as yeasts from *Saccharomyces,* containing up to 50 probiotic species [52, 53]. In this double-blind randomized clinical trial, 24 children with CP originated due to postnatal causes and GMFCS IV were included. The commercial yogurt contains two species: *Streptococcus thermpophilus* and *Lactobacillus bulgaricus.* The kefir included 12 probiotic species: *Bifidobacterium infantis, Bifidobacterium lactis, Lactobacillus acidophilus, Lactobacillus delbrueckii* spp. *lactis, Lactobacillus fermentum, Lactobacillus paracasei, Lactobacillus rhamnosus, Lactobacillus lactis* spp. *cremoris, L. lactis* spp. *lactis*, *L. lactis* spp. *lactis biovar. Diacetylactis, Leuconostoc mesenteroides,* and *Leuconostoc pseudomensenteroides.* Before the intervention, the most recurrent functional digestive disorder was functional constipation with a prevalence of 90%, followed by functional dyspepsia (27.3%), which was mostly accompanied by aerophagia (9.1%) and pain syndrome in epigastrium (9.1%). There was a decrease in constipation after the intervention to

9.1%. Also, there was a significant difference in stool consistency in the kefir group with a reduction in severity of the hardness of the stool.

A study with *Lactobacillus reuteri* DSM 17938 and agave inulin conducted by García-Contreras et al., [30] in 37 CP children with constipation and level IV-V of the GMFCS showed that the group treated with this probiotic (1×10^8 CFU/day) had significant differences in history of excessive stool retention and history of painful defecation and in the presence of a large fecal mass in the rectum in a period of 28 days. The groups treated with the prebiotic (4 g/day of agave inulin) and the synbiotic (1×10^8 CFU/day and 4 g/day of agave inulin) showed significant differences in excessive stool retention, painful defecation, and large stool diameter and in the presence of voluminous fecal mass in the rectum. The stool frequency increased significantly from 6 to 7.5 stools per week in the probiotic group, and the pH had a significant decrease in the same group ($p = 0.014$). Only the prebiotic group showed a significant improvement in the decrease of frequency of hard stools ($p = 0.008$) and an increase in normal stools ($p = 0.003$) according to Bristol scale. The authors concluded that the therapy with *L. reuteri* DSM 17938 and agave inulin is an effective alternative to improve constipation symptoms in children with CP such as intestinal motility, stool consistency and stool frequency.

The study conducted by Huang et al., [50] aimed to investigate the effect of dietary fiber combined with probiotics on functional constipated children with cerebral palsy with GMFCS level III or above. The average age was 13.48 ± 3.40 years. A group was treated with a general diet ($n = 14$) and another with a liquid diet ($n = 21$); all of them received a compound dietary fiber (CDF) that contained psyllium seed husk (20 g/day) for 1 month and lactic acid-producing and butyric acid-producing probiotics for 6 months. Two types of probiotics were used; one contained $<1.8 \times 10^{10}$ CFU/sachet of *L. paracasei, Lactobacillus plantarum, Bifidobacterium animalis subsp. lactis,* sorbitol, fructose-oligosacharides, and xylose. The other one contained $\geq 1.0 \times 10^7$ CFU/g of *Clostridium butyricum* and $\geq 1.0 \times 10^6$ CFU/g of *Bifidobacterium.* After 1 month, the frequency of spontaneous and manual defecation and Bristol score significantly improved; in addition, CDF combined with probiotics significantly improved constipation symptoms. After 6 months, the spontaneous defecation frequency of all children increased significantly from 2.17 to 3.61 times per week, and manual defecation decreased from 1.77 to 0.28 times per week. The stool consistency significantly increased from 1.68 ± 0.47 to 3.71 ± 0.60 ($p < 0.0001$).

3.2 Gut microbiota in children with cerebral palsy

The gut microbiota is a complex ecosystem of approximately 100 trillion microorganisms that interact with digestion, immune function, and metabolism [54]. The composition of gut microbiota is influenced by many factors, such as gestational age, birth mode, maternal microbiota, exposure to antibiotics, proton pump inhibitors, type of feeding, and "biotics" (probiotics, prebiotics, synbiotics, or postbiotics) [55].

Gut microbiota influences the maturation of the immune system, gut permeability, nutrient absorption, and metabolism; maintains normal GI physiological function; and contributes to cerebral palsy through the gut-brain axis [56]. Several studies have suggested that gut microbiota is associated to neurologic diseases (Autism Spectrum Disorder, Parkinson's Disease, and Alzheimer's Disease) [57].

The dysbiosis in the gut microbiota due to dysmotility of the GI tract can alter the gut-brain axis, exacerbating the neurological symptoms [58]. Moreover, this imbalance results in gastrointestinal diseases including constipation [50]. The modulation by biotics can change the composition of the microbiota and indirectly affect gut motility [24]. Insufficient consumption of dietary fiber induce gut microbiota to use mucus glycoproteins as an alternative, which causes erosion of the colonic mucus barrier, leading to colitis [59]. Also, it can stimulate the production of short-chain fatty acids (SCFAs), which will regulate the immune response of the host [60]. It also provides a nutrient source for gut microbiota contributing to the integrity of the intestinal barrier. Gut microbiota differs between children with CP that receive a liquid diet and a general diet. *Bacteroidetes* ($p = 0.034$) and *Actinobacteria* ($p = 0.013$) differed significantly between the groups.

The microbiota in the general diet group was higher in butyric acid-producing bacteria, which is a characteristic of healthy individuals (*Lachnoclostridium, Dorea, Ruminococcus, Faecalibacterium, Roseburia,* and *Coprococcus*), while the gut microbiota of children in the liquid diet group was high in synbiotic pathogenic bacteria (*Collinsella, Alistipes,* and *Eggerthella*). These differences are associated with the motor function and GI dysfunction symptoms. All children in the liquid diet belonged to level V of the GMFCS, while 47% of children in the general diet group belonged to the same level. GIT dysfunctional symptoms were more common in the liquid diet group. All children in the liquid diet group presented constipation, while only one in the general diet group was constipated [25].

The gut microbiota of children with CP has been compared with the gut microbiota of healthy children. The gut microbiota diversity is higher in the CP children than in healthy children ($p < 0.001$). The most abundant genera in the CP group were *Bifidobacterium, Streptococcus, Akkermansia, Enterococcus, Prevotella, Veillonella, Rothia,* and *Clostridium IV*, and the less genera were represented by *Bacteroides, Faecalibacterium, Blautia, Ruminococcus, Roseburia, Anaerostipes,* and *Parasutterella* [61].

A study conducted by Huang et al., [50] during 6 months with a compound dietary fiber (for 1 month) and a probiotic (for 6 months) in 35 children with cerebral palsy (aged 13.48 ± 3.40 years) and functional constipation showed a significant increase in α-diversity after 1-month and 6-month intervention periods ($p = 0.0025$ and $p = 0.047$, respectively), with higher abundance of butyric acid-producing bacteria (*Bacteroides, Lachnospiracea incertae sedis, Faecalibacterium,* and *Clostridium XIVa)* and a lower abundance of opportunistic pathogens of the gut microbiota (*Alloprevotella, Megasphaera,* and *Collinsella*) after 1 month of intervention. However, the opposite occurred after 6 months; the abundance of butyrate-producing genera decreased, while the opportunistic pathogens increased. At the genus level, before the intervention, the dominant genera were *Bifidobacterium* and *Prevotella*, while *Prevotella, Collinsella, Sutterella,* and *Megamonas* showed lower abundance after the intervention. *Bacteroides, Faecalibacterium,* and *Lachnospiracea incertae sedis* increased at the first month; however, they all decreased at the sixth month of intervention. Opposite trends were observed with *Bifidobacterium, Oscillibacter,* and *Parabacteroides* falling to the lowest points and then rising again. During the 6 months, *Lactobacillus* and *Clostridium* consistently increased; however, *Bifidobacterium* decreased at the first month and then increased at the sixth month of intervention. This finding shows that exogenous *Bifidobacterium* showed less ability to colonize the gut than *Lactobacillus* and *Clostridium* and that a supplement of probiotic alone fails to achieve the expected results in the gut microbiota. Supplementation of a prebiotic with probiotics can improve functional constipation in children with cerebral palsy [28].

4. Gut-microbiota-brain axis: the influence of prebiotics and probiotics

4.1 Introduction to gut-microbiota-brain axis

The gut microbiota plays a crucial role in bidirectional communications with the brain, known as the gut-microbiota-brain axis (GMBA) [62]. This complex network involves various components, including the CNS, which encompasses the brain and spinal cord, as well as the autonomic nervous system, the enteric system, the neuroendocrine system, the hypothalamic-pituitary adrenal axis (HPA), and the neuroimmune system [63, 64]. The GMBA facilitates the change of signals and molecules between the gut microbiota and the brain, influencing various physiological and cognitive processes [65].

The vagus nerve (VN) serves as a crucial communication pathway between the intestine and the brain [66]. Composed by 80% of afferent and 20% efferent fibers, the VN facilitates the transmission of signal in both directions [67]. Afferent fibers carry information from the intestine to the brain, detecting nutrients, chemical or luminal content trough chemoreceptor, and responding to distention or movement trough mechanoreceptor. On the other hand, efferent fibers transmit signal from the brain to the intestine, innervating the striated muscle and forming synapses with the enteric nervous system to regulate motor functions such as motility, secretions, and sphincter relaxation [62, 68].

The gut microbiota employs several mechanisms to transmit the information to CNS [68]. One of these mechanisms involves the production of neurotransmitters and bioactive metabolites that are transported to the brain through afferent vagus nerve fibers [69]. The gut microbiota generates various neurotransmitters, including γ-aminobutyric acid (GABA), dopamine, serotonin, norepinephrine, and histamine [70]. Additionally, bioactive substances with neurological functions, such as SCFAs, amino acids (tryptophan, tyrosine, and phenylalanine), and secondary bile acid, are produced by the gut microbiota [70–72].

Neurotransmitters can be classified into excitatory and inhibitory categories based on their effect in the CNS. Glutamate, histamine, and norepinephrine are examples of excitatory neurotransmitters, while GABA, dopamine, and serotonin are inhibitory neurotransmitters [70]. These molecules play a crucial role in controlling various physiological process such as movement, emotion, memory, learning, and so on [68].

Glutamate (Glu) is the most abundant excitatory neurotransmitter in the brain and plays a crucial role in memory storage and synaptic plasticity [73]. It is released from presynaptic nerve terminals and binds to ionotropic glutamate receptors located on postsynaptic terminals, allowing for signal transmission between nerve cells [70]. Interestingly, enteroendocrine cells in the intestine can synthesize glutamate and use it to transmit signals to the brain [74].

D-glutamate, a component of the peptidoglycan structure in bacterial cell walls, is produced by glutamate racemase, an enzyme that is present in bacteria. Several bacterial species have been identified to possess the ability to convert L-Glu to D-Glu. These bacteria include *Bacillus subtilis, Corynebacterium glutamicum*, *L. lactis*, *L. plantarum*, *Brevibacterium lactofermentum*, and *Brevibacterium avium*. Subsequently, D-Glu can be further converted to GABA by the enzyme glutamate decarboxylase [70, 75]. In the gut microbiota, certain bacteria may contribute to GABA production. *Bacteroides fragilis* is an example that can synthesize GABA. Additionally, other bacterial species such *Parabacteroides*, *Eubacterium*, and

Bifidobacterium have also the ability to produce GABA [74, 76]. Understanding the synthesis, release, and function of GABA is crucial for comprehending its role in the CNS. GABAergic signaling plays a fundamental role in maintaining the balance between excitation and inhibition in the brain, influencing various physiological and cognitive processes [69, 76].

Dopamine, a neurotransmitter, is primarily produced in the substantia nigra, central tegmental area, and hypothalamus. It is released into the nucleus accumbens and prefrontal cortex. Dopamine synthesis occurs in dopaminergic nerve cells and is dependent on the availability of the amino acid tyrosine. Tyrosine, which is obtained from the diet, can be transported across the blood-brain barrier (BBB) to reach the brain [68, 70]. Its synthesis begins with the hydroxylation of tyrosine to L-dihydroxyphenylalanine (L-DOPA), followed by the decarboxylation of L-DOPA to dopamine [77]. The production of dopamine is not exclusive for the brain. Certain bacteria such as *Bacillus*, *Staphylococcus,* and *Serratia* species have been found to produce dopamine in the GIT. In fact, more than 50% of dopamine in the human body is synthesized in the gut [77].

Serotonin also known as 5-hidroxytryptamine (5-HT) is synthesized by serotonergic neurons in the raphe nuclei of the brain [78]. However, it is important to note that a substantial proportion of serotonin, approximately 90%, is produced in the gut by the enterochromaffin cells. This neurotransmitter plays a vital role in regulating sleep, behavior, and various other functions within the CNS and GIT [63, 78]. The production of serotonin in the gut can be influenced by microbial metabolites, including SCFAs, secondary bile acids, a-tocopherol, p-aminobenzoate, and tyramine [62]. Several bacteria have been identified as participants in the production of serotonin. These include *Escherichia coli*, *Hafnia*, *Bacteroides*, *Streptococcus*, *Bifidobacterium*, *Lactococcus*, *Lactobacillus*, *Morganella*, *Klebsiella*, *Propionibacterium*, *Eubacterium*, *Roseburia*, and *Prevotella*. These bacteria are involved in the conversion of tryptophan into serotonin, contributing to the overall serotonin levels in the gut [70, 78].

Histamine plays a crucial role in various homeostatic functions, promoting wakefulness and regulating feeding and motivational behavior [75]. Histamine can also be produced by certain bacteria in the gut, which can activate histamine receptor [79]. A variety of bacterial species are implicated in the synthesis of histamine, comprising *Lactobacillus spp*., *Enterobacter spp*., *Pediococcus parvulus*, *Klebsiella pneumoniae, Streptococcus thermophilus*, and *Hafnia alvei*. These bacteria contribute to the overall histamine levels in the gut and can influence histamine signaling in the body [70]. Histamine receptors are widely distributed throughout the body, including CNS, GIT, and the immune system. Activation of these receptors can have diverse effects, such as regulating neurotransmission, modulating gut motility, and influencing immune response [80].

Norepinephrine (NE) is a catecholamine that serves as a neurotransmitter in both central and peripheral nervous systems. It is produced by neurons in the locus coeruleus, where the precursor molecule tyrosine is converted into dopamine and subsequently into norepinephrine [81]. Bacteria such as *Bacillus mycoides*, *Bacillus subtilis, E. coli K12, Proteus vulgaris,* and *Serratia* have the capacity to synthesize NE with concentration ranging from 0.45 to 2.13 mM [70].

It is important to note that certain neurotransmitters, such as GABA, dopamine, and serotonin, do not penetrate the BBB [74]. Therefore, they must be synthesized within the brain local pools of neurotransmitter precursors [82]. However, the gut microbiota also contributes to the production of these molecules, which in turn can modulate other processes, for example, the enteric nervous system (ENS) [65].

Multiple brain disorders, such as Alzheimer's disease, Parkinson's disease, depression, anxiety, and cerebral palsy, are associated with the dysregulation of the gut microbiota, which can impact neurotransmitter production and disrupt the GMBA [62, 83]. Modulating the gut microbiota through the use of prebiotics and probiotics has emerged as a promising therapeutic approach to improve the GMBA and potentially treat these conditions [67]. However, further research is needed to fully understand the underlying mechanisms involved in the regulation of the GMBA by the gut microbiota.

4.2 Prebiotics and probiotics in the gut-microbiota-brain Axis

The gut microbiota is influenced by various factors including age, antibiotic therapy, diet, and gut microbiology, among others [84]. Diet plays a significant role in modulating the bacterial community and promoting changes in the alpha and beta diversity of the microbial ecosystem [85]. Prebiotics are utilized to selectively increase the abundance of specific beneficial bacteria, such as *Bifidobacterium*, *Lactobacillus,* and butyrate-producer bacteria, thereby fostering a healthy microbial community [49]. Probiotics, on the other hand, are employed to promote colonization of beneficial bacteria that confer intestinal benefits and support host health [49]. Both prebiotics and probiotics have been shown to modulate the gut-brain axis, contributing to improved neurotransmission and amelioration of complications associated with brain disorders [86]. However, the precise mechanism by which these substances function in the gut-brain axis remains unknown.

Ongoing research aims to elucidate the mechanisms through which prebiotics and probiotics modulate the GMBA. Prebiotics, such as FOS, GOS and pectin, are a type of dietary fibers that are utilized by the gut microbiota to produce SCFAs [87]. The production of SCFAs has been implicated in the modulation of GMBA through various mechanisms, including the production of neurotransmitters, modulation of the BBB, development and regulation of the immune system, and modulation of inflammation in both the brain and GIT [71].

The concentration of SCFAs in the cerebrospinal fluid ranges from 0 to 171 uM for acetate, 0–5 uM for propionate, and 0–2.8 uM for butyrate. In the human brain tissue, the reported concentrations are 17 pmol/mg for butyrate and 18.8 pmol/mg for propionate. These concentrations highlight the close relationship between the GIT and brain through GMBA. Furthermore, they indicate that SCFAs have the ability to cross BBB and influence brain function [63].

SCFAs have been found to promote the maturation of glial cells and astrocytes [62]. Butyrate, synthesized by gut microbiota, stimulates memory and synaptic plasticity by inhibiting histone deacetylase [88]. Also, it influences the release of the neurotransmitter serotonin from intestinal enterochromaffin cells. Propionate, on the other hand, has a protective effect on the BBB by mitigating oxidative stress [89]. Acetate can cross the BBB and can be incorporated into the GABA metabolic cycle in the hypothalamus [74]. Additionally, acetate can activate the HPA axis, sending signals to the enteroendocrine cells. SCFAs also can modulate the stress response and mood suppressing the HPA axis, also known as the "stress axis." [69] Furthermore, SCFAs can influence neuroinflammation by modulating the production and recruitment of immune cells such as T cells, neutrophils, and inflammatory cytokines [71, 89]. Propionate and butyrate possess the capability to activate cell signaling systems by modulating potassium levels and regulating key enzymes involved in neurotransmitter synthesis. These SCFAs have been demonstrated to specifically impact the levels of tryptophan 5-hydroxylase 1, an enzyme implicated in the production of serotonin, as well as tyrosine hydroxylase, an enzyme implicated in the synthesis of dopamine, adrenaline, and noradrenaline [63, 71]. These effects highlight the ampliated impact of SCFAs on neurotransmitter regulation and cellular signaling [67].

The use of probiotics modulates the production of bioactive compounds and the GMBA [90]. *Bifidobacterium spp*. *Lactobacillus spp*., and *Enterococcus spp*., are commonly used in human nutrition and extensively studied for their beneficial effects [91]. Numerous studies highlighted the ability of these probiotics to promote the health in both the brain and intestine. For instance, *Lactobacillus spp*. has been found to play a role in the modulation of tryptophan metabolism, leading to the production of serotonin and metabolic products such as kynurenine and indole compounds [82]. These substances improve immune response and brain neurotransmission [92, 93].

The utilization of prebiotics and probiotics has emerged as a strategy to potentially modulate brain functions and behavior in psychiatric diseases such as anxiety and depression, as well as in neurological conditions that may affect brain physiology, such as cerebral palsy [94, 95]. In the following paragraphs, we will explore the potential mechanisms through which prebiotics and probiotics may exert their effects on cerebral palsy.

4.2.1 Role of the gut-microbiota-brain axis in cerebral palsy

The investigation of the GMBA through the modification using prebiotics and probiotics in CP has not been extensively explored. However, a comparative study examined the role of GMBA in CP and epilepsy (CPE). The study evaluates the abundance of gut microbiota and the principal metabolites in children with CP, with and without epilepsy [96]. In children with non-epileptic cerebral palsy (NECP), a reduction in *B. fragilis* and *Dialister invisus* was observed. Moreover, a higher abundance of *phascolarctobacterium faecium* and *Eubacterium limosum* was found in NECP children. In contrast, *Veillonella parvula* has been found to have a higher colonization rate in children with drug resistant epilepsy (DRE) compared to those with drug-sensitive epilepsy (DSE). Functional pathways analysis of the microbiome revealed a decrease in serine degradation, quinolinic acid degradation, glycerol degradation, and sulfate degradation I in patients with CPE. However, pathways related to ethanol production were increased [96].

Metabolomic analysis demonstrated a higher concentration of kynurenic acid, 2-oxindole, dopamine, hydroxyphenyalanie, and 3–4-dihydroxyphenylglycol (3–4-DHPG) in CPE patients. Besides, children with DRE had higher concentrations of indole compared to those with DSE. Notably, a negative correlation was found between *B. fragilis* and kynurenic acid concentration in CPE patients. The co-abundance of *E. limosum* with 3–4-DPHG, which is implicated in the conversion of NE to 3–4-DPHG, may contribute to a proconvulsant effect [96].

4.2.2 Influence of prebiotics and probiotics on the brain and CNS in children with CP

The investigation about prebiotics and probiotics in GMBA in CP is still limited, with only one study exploring the use of *Saccharomyces boulardii* in improving behavior and emotions in spastic CP rats. In this study, CP was induced by destroying the left-brain motor cortex and cingulate cortex, resulting in paralysis, high muscle tension, and neurological deficits in the rats. The administration of *S. boulardii* to the CP group improved the weight, fecal water content, and general state compared to the CP group without *S. boulardii*. On the other hand, there were no significant differences in the evaluation of neurological deficits between the CP and CP+ *S. boulardii* groups. However, it is worth noting that the assessment of muscle tension, adductor angle, grasping test, hind limb suspension test, tail suspension test, and sucrose preference test showed improvement in the CP + *S. boulardii* group.

Furthermore, the administration of *S. boulardii* in CP also improved behavior and emotions, suggesting the involvement of the GMBA in these conditions. To confirm the role of GMBA in CP + *S. boulardii*, the researchers examined aspects related to inflammation, the HPA axis, and gut microbiome.

The levels of proinflammatory cytokine such as IL-6 and TNF-alfa were evaluated, and it was found that the administration of *S. boulardii* in CP group reduced the concentration of these cytokines in the plasma. The HPA axis was assessed by measuring the levels of cortisol and adrenocorticotropic hormone (ACTH). In both the CP and CP+ *S. boulardii* groups, the levels of cortisol and ACTH were increased. However, in the CP + *S. boulardii* group, the levels of these hormones were significantly decreased [95].

Finally, the analysis of gut microbiome showed that the alfa and beta diversity were not significantly different between the groups. However, when the circus diagram is performed, the distribution ratio shows dominant species for each group. At the genus level, the CP+ *S. boulardii* group exhibited a dominance of *Lactobacillus*, whereas the control group was characterized by a prevalence of *Prevotella*. Additionally, the CP group showed a predominant distribution of *Bacteroidetes*. These results highlight the potential importance of using probiotics, as they may be implicated in the improvement of clinical symptoms in CP [95]. Furthermore, it is necessary to promote further investigation into the potential of prebiotics and probiotics in modulating the CNS in children with CP trough the GMBA.

5. Conclusion

Gastrointestinal disorders are common in children with CP such as constipation, which can alter the gut microbiota through the gut-microbiota-brain axis. Therapy with probiotics, prebiotics, and synbiotics can alleviate clinical symptoms and can modulate the gut microbiota. Probiotics that have been studied in children with CP are *L. reuteri* DSM 17938, kefir, *L. paracasei, L. plantarum, B. animalis subsp. lactis, and C. butyricum*. On the other hand, prebiotics that have been studied in this population are fructose-oligosacharides, agave inulin, and psyllium seed husk. More studies that evaluate the effect of probiotics and prebiotics on the gut microbiota, on the CNS and brain, and on clinical variables in children with CP are needed.

Conflict of interest

"The authors declare no conflict of interest."

Abbreviations

3–4-DHPG	3–4-dihydroxyphenylglycol
5-HT	5-hidroxytryptamine

ACTH	adrenocorticotropic hormone
BBB	blood-brain barrier
CDF	compound dietary fiber
CFU	colon-forming unit
CNS	central nervous system
CP	cerebral palsy
CPE	cerebral palsy and epilepsy
DRE	drug resistant epilepsy
DSE	drug-sensitive epilepsy
EDACS	eating and Drinking Ability Classification System
ENS	enteric nervous system
FOS	fructooligosacharides
GABA	γ-aminobutyric acid
GI	gastrointestinal
GIT	gastrointestinal tract
Glu	glutamate
GMBA	gut-microbiota-brain axis
GMFCS	gross Motor Function Classification System
GOS	galactooligosacharides
HPA	hypothalamic-pituitary adrenal axis
ISAPP	International Scientific Association for Probiotics and Prebiotics
L-DOPA	L-dihydroxyphenylalanine
NCPE	non-epileptic cerebral palsy
NE	norepinephrine
PEG	polyethylene glycol
SCFAs	short-chain fatty acids
SGNA	subjective Global Nutritional Assessment
VN	vagus nerve

Author details

Andrea A. García-Contreras[1], Edgar M. Vásquez-Garibay[1*] and
Lucila A. Godínez-Méndez[2]

1 Department of Clinical Human Reproduction, Institute of Human Nutrition, University of Guadalajara, Guadalajara, Jalisco, México

2 Department of Physiology, University of Guadalajara, Guadalajara, Jalisco, México

*Address all correspondence to: edgar.vgaribay@academicos.udg.mx

References

[1] Sadowska M, Sarecka-Hujar B, Kopyta I. Cerebral palsy: Current opinions on definition, epidemiology, risk factors, classification and treatment options. Neuropsychiatric Disease and Treatment. 2020;**16**:1505-1518. DOI: 10.2147/NDT.S235165

[2] Gulati S, Sondhi V. Cerebral palsy: An overview. Indian Journal of Pediatrics. 2018;**85**(11):1006-1016. DOI: 10.1007/s12098-017-2475-1

[3] Paul S, Nahar A, Bhagawati M, Kunwar AJ. A review on recent advances of cerebral palsy. Oxidative Medicine and Cellular Longevity. 2022;**2022**:1-20. DOI: 10.1155/2022/2622310

[4] Linsell L, Malouf R, Morris J, Kurinczuk JJ, Marlow N. Prognostic factors for cerebral palsy and motor impairment in children born very preterm or very low birthweight: A systematic review. Developmental Medicine and Child Neurology. 2016;**58**(6):554-569. DOI: 10.1111/dmcn.12972

[5] McIntyre S, Taitz D, Keogh J, Goldsmith S, Badawi N, Blair E. A systematic review of risk factors for cerebral palsy in children born at term in developed countries. Developmental Medicine and Child Neurology. 2013;**55**(6):499-508. DOI: 10.1111/dmcn.12017

[6] Imms C, Carlin J, Eliasson A-C. Stability of caregiver-reported manual ability and gross motor function classifications of cerebral palsy. Developmental Medicine and Child Neurology. 2010;**52**(2):153-159. DOI: 10.1111/j.1469-8749.2009.03346.x

[7] Palisano RJ, Rosenbaum P, Bartlett D, Livingston MH. Content validity of the expanded and revised gross motor function classification system. Developmental Medicine and Child Neurology. 2008;**50**(10):744-750. DOI: 10.1111/j.1469-8749.2008.03089.x

[8] Ikeudenta BA, Rutkofsky IH. Unmasking the enigma of cerebral palsy: A traditional review. Cureus. 2020;**12**(10):e11004. DOI: 10.7759/cureus.11004

[9] Trivić I, Hojsak I. Evaluation and treatment of malnutrition and associated gastrointestinal complications in children with cerebral palsy. Pediatric Gastroenterology, Hepatology & Nutrition. 2019;**22**(2):122-131. DOI: 10.5223/pghn.2019.22.2.122

[10] Matsuo K, Palmer JB. Anatomy and physiology of feeding and swallowing: Normal and abnormal. Physical Medicine and Rehabilitation Clinics of North America. 2008;**19**(4):691-707. DOI: 10.1016/j.pmr.2008.06.001

[11] Nurek J, Wisniewski OW, Kupsz J, et al. Hormones regulating energy homeostasis in breastfeeding versus formula feeding mothers. Journal of Physiology and Pharmacology. 2021;**72**(5):731-739. DOI: 10.26402/jpp.2021.5.08

[12] Quitadamo P, Thapar N, Staiano ABO. Gastrointestinal and nutritional problems in neurologically impaired children. European Journal of Paediatric Neurology. 2016;**20**(6):810-815. DOI: 10.1016/j.ejpn.2016.05.019

[13] Tamilia E, Taffoni F, Formica D, et al. Technological solutions and main indices for the assessment of newborns' Nutritive Sucking: A review. Sensors (Switzerland). 2014;**14**(1):634-658. DOI: 10.3390/s140100634

[14] Arvedson JC. Feeding children with cerebral palsy and swallowing difficulties. European Journal of Clinical Nutrition. 2013;**67**(S2):S9-S12. DOI: 10.1038/ejcn.2013.224

[15] Speyer R, Cordier R, Kim JH, Cocks N, Michou E, Wilkes-Gillan S. Prevalence of drooling, swallowing, and feeding problems in cerebral palsy across the lifespan: a systematic review and meta-analyses. Developmental Medicine and Child Neurology. 2019;**61**(11):1249-1258. DOI: 10.1111/dmcn.14316

[16] Karim T, Jahan I, Dossetor R, et al. Nutritional status of children with cerebral palsy—findings from prospective hospital-based surveillance in Vietnam indicate a need for action. Nutrients. 2019;**11**(9):2132. DOI: 10.3390/nu11092132

[17] Kuperminc MN, Stevenson RD. Growth and nutrition disorders in children with cerebral palsy. Developmental Disabilities Research Reviews. 2008;**14**(2):137-146. DOI: 10.1002/ddrr.14

[18] Sun D, Wang Q, Hou M, et al. Clinical characteristics and functional status of children with different subtypes of dyskinetic cerebral palsy. Medicine (United States). 2018;**97**(21):e10817. DOI: 10.1097/MD.0000000000010817

[19] Bell KL, Samson-Fang L. Nutritional management of children with cerebral palsy. European Journal of Clinical Nutrition. 2013;**67**(S2):S13-S16. DOI: 10.1038/ejcn.2013.225

[20] Herrera-AnayaE,Angarita-FonsecaA, Herrera-GalindoVM,Martínez-MarínRDP, Rodríguez-Bayona CN. Association between gross motor function and nutritional status in children with cerebral palsy: a cross-sectional study from Colombia. Developmental Medicine and Child Neurology. 2016;**58**(9):936-941. DOI: 10.1111/dmcn.13108

[21] Stanek JL, Emerson JA, Murdock FA, Petroski GF. Growth characteristics in cerebral palsy subtypes: a comparative assessment. Developmental Medicine and Child Neurology. 2016;**58**(9):931-935. DOI: 10.1111/dmcn.13116

[22] Zhao Y, Tang H, Peng T, et al. Relationship between nutritional status and severity of cerebral palsy: A multicentre cross-sectional study. Journal of Rehabilitation Medicine. 2023;**55**. DOI: 10.2340/jrm.v55.4395

[23] Gfroerer S. Pediatric intestinal motility disorders. World Journal of Gastroenterology. 2015;**21**(33):9683. DOI: 10.3748/wjg.v21.i33.9683

[24] Corsello A, Scatigno L, Govoni A, et al. Gut dysmotility in children with neurological impairment: The nutritional management. Frontiers in Neurology. 2023;**14**:1200101. DOI: 10.3389/fneur.2023.1200101

[25] Huang C, Li X, Wu L, et al. The effect of different dietary structure on gastrointestinal dysfunction in children with cerebral palsy and epilepsy based on gut microbiota. Brain & Development. 2021;**43**(2):192-199. DOI: 10.1016/j.braindev.2020.09.013

[26] Park ES, Park C, Cho S-R, Na S, Cho YS. Colonic transit time and constipation in children with spastic cerebral palsy. Archives of Physical Medicine and Rehabilitation. 2004;**85**(3):453-456. DOI: 10.1016/S0003-9993(03)00479-9

[27] Vande Velde S, Van Renterghem K, Van Winkel M, De Bruyne R, Van Biervliet S. Constipation and fecal incontinence in children with cerebral palsy. Overview of literature and

flowchart for a stepwise approach. Acta Gastroenterologica Belgica. 2018;**81**(3):415-418. PMID: 30350531

[28] Veugelers R, Benninga MA, Calis EA, et al. Prevalence and clinical presentation of constipation in children with severe generalized cerebral palsy. Developmental Medicine and Child Neurology. 2010;**52**(9):e216-e221. DOI: 10.1111/j.1469-8749.2010.03701.x

[29] Rebelo F, Mansur IR, Miglioli TC, Meio MDB, Gomes SC. Dietary and nutritional interventions in children with cerebral palsy: A systematic literature review. PLoS One. 2022;**17**(7):1-15. DOI: 10.1371/journal.pone.0271993

[30] García Contreras AA, Vásquez Garibay EM, Sánchez Ramírez CA, Fafutis Morris MDRV. *Lactobacillus reuteri* DSM 17938 and Agave Inulin in Children with Cerebral Palsy and Chronic Constipation: A Double-Blind Randomized Placebo Controlled Clinical Trial. Nutrients. 2020;**12**(10):2971. DOI: 10.3390/nu12102971

[31] Hassanein SMA, Deifallah SM, Bastawy HA. Efficacy of oral magnesium therapy in the treatment of chronic constipation in spastic cerebral palsy children: a randomized controlled trial. World Journal of Pediatrics. 2021;**17**(1):92-98. DOI: 10.1007/s12519-020-00401-0

[32] Del Giudice E, Staiano A, Capano G, et al. Gastrointestinal manifestations in children with cerebral palsy. Brain & Development. 1999;**21**(5):307-311. DOI: 10.1016/S0387-7604(99)00025-X

[33] Wa A. Role of stretching exercises in the management of constipation in spastic cerebral palsy. Journal of Ayub Medical College, Abbottabad. 2016;**28**(4):798-801

[34] Pimentel M, Chatterjee S, Chow EJ, Park S, Kong Y. Neomycin improves constipation-predominant irritable bowel syndrome in a fashion that is dependent on the presence of methane gas: Subanalysis of a double-blind randomized controlled study. Digestive Diseases and Sciences. 2006;**51**(8):1297-1301. DOI: 10.1007/s10620-006-9104-6

[35] Sullivan PB. Gastrointestinal disorders in children with neurodevelopmental disabilities. Developmental Disabilities Research Reviews. 2008;**14**(2):128-136. DOI: 10.1002/ddrr.18

[36] Jahromi SR, Togha M, Fesharaki SH, et al. Gastrointestinal adverse effects of antiepileptic drugs in intractable epileptic patients. Seizure. 2011;**20**(4):343-346. DOI: 10.1016/j.seizure.2010.12.011

[37] González Jiménez D, Díaz Martin JJ, Bousoño García C, Jiménez TS. Patología gastrointestinal en niños con parálisis cerebral infantil y otras discapacidades neurológicas. An Pediatría. 2010;**73**(6):361. DOI: 10.1016/j.anpedi.2010.03.003

[38] Staiano A, Simeone D, Del Giudice E, Miele E, Tozzi A, Toraldo C. Effect of the dietary fiber glucomannan on chronic constipation in neurologically impaired children. The Journal of Pediatrics. 2000;**136**(1):41-45. DOI: 10.1016/S0022-3476(00)90047-7

[39] Reilly S, Skuse D, Poblete X. Prevalence of feeding problems and oral motor dysfunction in children with cerebral palsy: A community survey. The Journal of Pediatrics. 1996;**129**(6):877-882. DOI: 10.1016/S0022-3476(96)70032-X

[40] Caramico-Favero DCO, Guedes ZCF, Morais MB. Food intake, nutritional

status and gastrointestinal symptoms in children with cerebral palsy. Arquivos de Gastroenterologia. 2018;**55**(4):352-357. DOI: 10.1590/s0004-2803.201800000-78

[41] Bandla HPR, Davis SH, Hopkins NE. Lipoid pneumonia: A silent complication of mineral oil aspiration. Pediatrics. 1999;**103**(2):e19-e19. DOI: 10.1542/peds.103.2.e19

[42] Koppen IJN, Lammers LA, Benninga MA, Tabbers MM. Management of functional constipation in children: therapy in practice. Pediatric Drugs. 2015;**17**(5):349-360. DOI: 10.1007/s40272-015-0142-4

[43] Imanieh MH, Golpayegan MR, Sedighi M, et al. Comparison of three therapeutic interventions for chronic constipation in paediatric patients with cerebral palsy: a randomised clinical trial. Gastroenterol Rev. 2019;**14**(4):292-297. DOI: 10.5114/pg.2019.84872

[44] Longo WE, Vernava AM. Prokinetic agents for lower gastrointestinal motility disorders. Diseases of the Colon and Rectum. 1993;**36**(7):696-708. DOI: 10.1007/BF02238599

[45] Rossier P, van Erven S, Wade DT. The effect of magnesium oral therapy on spasticity in a patient with multiple sclerosis. European Journal of Neurology. 2000;**7**(6):741-744. DOI: 10.1046/j.1468-1331.2000.00142.x

[46] Hill C, Guarner F, Reid G, et al. The International Scientific Association for Probiotics and Prebiotics consensus statement on the scope and appropriate use of the term probiotic. Nature Reviews. Gastroenterology & Hepatology. 2014;**11**(8):506-514. DOI: 10.1038/nrgastro.2014.66

[47] Zhang JQ, Zhang LY, Wang X, Xie JY, Wang FY, Tang XD. Effects of mitochondrial dysfunction on gastrointestinal dysmotility in functional dyspepsia. China Journal of Traditional China Medical Pharmacy. 2019;**34**:3637-3639

[48] Gibson GR, Roberfroid MB. Dietary modulation of the human colonic microbiota: Introducing the concept of prebiotics. The Journal of Nutrition. 1995;**125**(6):1401-1412. DOI: 10.1093/jn/125.6.1401

[49] Gibson GR, Hutkins R, Sanders ME, et al. Expert consensus document: The International Scientific Association for Probiotics and Prebiotics (ISAPP) consensus statement on the definition and scope of prebiotics. Nature Reviews. Gastroenterology & Hepatology. 2017;**14**(8):491-502. DOI: 10.1038/nrgastro.2017.75

[50] Huang C, Lyu J, Chu C, et al. Dietary fiber and probiotics based on gut microbiota targeting for functional constipation in children with cerebral palsy. Frontiers in Pediatrics. 2022;**10**:1001789. DOI: 10.3389/fped.2022.1001789

[51] Rodríguez-Hernández AI, Salinas E, Tirado González DN, et al. Effects of a modern kefir on conditions associated with moderate severe spastic quadriparesis cerebral palsy. Microorganisms. 2022;**10**(7):1291. DOI: 10.3390/microorganisms10071291

[52] Altay F, Karbancıoglu-Güler F, Daskaya-Dikmen C, Heperkan D. A review on traditional Turkish fermented non-alcoholic beverages: Microbiota, fermentation process and quality characteristics. International Journal of Food Microbiology. 2013;**167**(1):44-56. DOI: 10.1016/j.ijfoodmicro.2013.06.016

[53] Lopitz-Otsoa F, Rementeria A, Elguezabal N, Garaizar J. Kefir: una comunidad simbiótica de bacterias y

levaduras con propiedades saludables. Revista Iberoamericana de Micología. 2006;**23**(2):67-74. DOI: 10.1016/S1130-1406(06)70016-X

[54] Rinninella E, Raoul P, Cintoni M, et al. What is the healthy gut microbiota composition? A changing ecosystem across age, environment, diet, and diseases. Microorganisms. 2019;**7**(1):14. DOI: 10.3390/microorganisms7010014

[55] Fouhy F, Watkins C, Hill CJ, et al. Perinatal factors affect the gut microbiota up to four years after birth. Nature Communications. 2019;**10**(1):1517. DOI: 10.1038/s41467-019-09252-4

[56] Huang C, Chu C, Peng Y, et al. Correlations between gastrointestinal and oral microbiota in children with cerebral palsy and epilepsy. Frontiers in Pediatrics. 2022;**10**(November):1-7. DOI: 10.3389/fped.2022.988601

[57] Jiang C, Li G, Huang P, Liu Z, Zhao B. The gut microbiota and Alzheimer's disease. Journal of Alzheimer's Disease. 2017;**58**(1):1-15. DOI: 10.3233/JAD-161141

[58] Quigley EMM. Microbiota-brain-gut axis and neurodegenerative diseases. Current Neurology and Neuroscience Reports. 2017;**17**(12):94. DOI: 10.1007/s11910-017-0802-6

[59] Ms D, Am S, Nm K, et al. A dietary fiber-deprived gut microbiota degrades the colonic mucus barrier and enhances pathogen susceptibility. Cell. 2016;**167**(5):1339-1353. DOI: 10.1016/j.cell.10043

[60] Bosch G, Verbrugghe A, et al. The effects of dietary fibre type on satiety-related hormones and voluntary food intake in dogs. The British Journal of Nutrition. 2009;**102**(2):318-325. DOI: 10.1017/s000711450814 9194

[61] Huang C, Li Y, Feng X, et al. Distinct gut microbiota composition and functional category in children with cerebral palsy and epilepsy. Frontiers in Pediatrics. 2019;**7**:394. DOI: 10.3389/fped.2019.00394

[62] Morais LH, Schreiber HL, Mazmanian SK. The gut microbiota–brain axis in behaviour and brain disorders. Nature Reviews. Microbiology. 2021;**19**(4):241-255. DOI: 10.1038/s41579-020-00460-0

[63] O'Riordan KJ, Collins MK, Moloney GM, et al. Short chain fatty acids: Microbial metabolites for gut-brain axis signalling. Molecular and Cellular Endocrinology. 2022;**546**:111572. DOI: 10.1016/j.mce.2022.111572

[64] Appleton J. The gut-brain axis: influence of microbiota on mood and mental health. Integrated Medicine (Encinitas). 2018;**17**(4):28-32

[65] Rhee SH, Pothoulakis C, Mayer EA. Principles and clinical implications of the brain-gut-enteric microbiota axis. Nature Reviews. Gastroenterology & Hepatology. 2009;**6**(5):306-314. DOI: 10.1038/nrgastro.2009.35

[66] Foster JA, Baker GB, Dursun SM. The relationship between the gut microbiome-immune system-brain axis and major depressive disorder. Frontiers in Neurology. 2021;**12**:721126. DOI: 10.3389/fneur.2021.721126

[67] Radford-Smith DE, Anthony DC. Prebiotic and probiotic modulation of the microbiota–gut–brain axis in depression. Nutrients. 2023;**15**(8):1880. DOI: 10.3390/nu15081880

[68] Powell N, Walker MM, Talley NJ. The mucosal immune system: Master regulator of bidirectional gut-brain communications. Nature Reviews. Gastroenterology & Hepatology.

2017;**14**(3):143-159. DOI: 10.1038/nrgastro.2016.191

[69] Parker A, Fonseca S, Carding SR. Gut microbes and metabolites as modulators of blood-brain barrier integrity and brain health. Gut Microbes. 2020;**11**(2):135-157. DOI: 10.1080/19490976.2019.1638722

[70] Dicks LMT. Gut bacteria and neurotransmitters. Microorganisms. 2022;**10**(9):1838. DOI: 10.3390/microorganisms10091838

[71] Dalile B, Van Oudenhove L, Vervliet B, Verbeke K. The role of short-chain fatty acids in microbiota–gut–brain communication. Nature Reviews. Gastroenterology & Hepatology. 2019;**16**(8):461-478. DOI: 10.1038/s41575-019-0157-3

[72] de Wouters A, Huwart SJP, Cani PD, Everard A. Gut microbes and food reward: From the gut to the brain. Frontiers in Neuroscience. 2022;**16**:947240. DOI: 10.3389/fnins.2022.947240

[73] Huang F, Wu X. Brain neurotransmitter modulation by gut microbiota in anxiety and depression. Frontiers in Cell and Development Biology. 2021;**9**:649103. DOI: 10.3389/fcell.2021.649103

[74] Chen Y, Xu J, Chen Y. Regulation of neurotransmitters by the gut microbiota and effects on cognition in neurological disorders. Nutrients. 2021;**13**(6):2099. DOI: 10.3390/nu13062099

[75] Baj A, Moro E, Bistoletti M, Orlandi V, Crema F, Giaroni C. Glutamatergic signaling along the microbiota-gut-brain axis. International Journal of Molecular Sciences. 2019;**20**(6):1482. DOI: 10.3390/ijms20061482

[76] Otaru N, Ye K, Mujezinovic D, et al. GABA production by human intestinal Bacteroides spp.: Prevalence, regulation, and role in acid stress tolerance. Frontier in Microbiology. 2021;**12**:656895. DOI: 10.3389/fmicb.2021.656895

[77] Hamamah S, Aghazarian A, Nazaryan A, Hajnal A, Covasa M. Role of microbiota-gut-brain axis in regulating dopaminergic signaling. Biomedicine. 2022;**10**(2):436. DOI: 10.3390/biomedicines10020436

[78] Layunta E, Buey B, Mesonero JE, Latorre E. Crosstalk between intestinal serotonergic system and pattern recognition receptors on the microbiota–gut–brain axis. Frontier in Endocrinology (Lausanne). 2021;**12**:748254. DOI: 10.3389/fendo.2021.748254

[79] Haas HL, Sergeeva OA, Selbach O. Histamine in the nervous system. Physiological Reviews. 2008;**88**(3):1183-1241. DOI: 10.1152/physrev.00043.2007

[80] Thangam EB, Jemima EA, Singh H, et al. The role of histamine and histamine receptors in mast cell-mediated allergy and inflammation: The hunt for new therapeutic targets. Frontiers in Immunology. 2018;**9**:1873. DOI: 10.3389/fimmu.2018.01873

[81] Sudo N. Biogenic amines: Signals between commensal microbiota and gut physiology. Frontiers in Endocrinology. 2019;**10**:504. DOI: 10.3389/fendo.2019.00504

[82] Bosi A, Banfi D, Bistoletti M, Giaroni C, Baj A. Tryptophan metabolites along the microbiota-gut-brain axis: An interkingdom communication system influencing the gut in health and disease. International Journal of Tryptophan Research. 2020;**13**:1178646920928984. DOI: 10.1177/1178646920928984

[83] Rao M, Gershon MD. The bowel and beyond: The enteric nervous system in neurological disorders. Nature Reviews.

Gastroenterology & Hepatology. 2016;**13**(9):517-528. DOI: 10.1038/nrgastro.2016.107

[84] Liu X, Cao S, Zhang X. Modulation of gut microbiota-brain axis by probiotics, prebiotics, and diet. Journal of Agricultural and Food Chemistry. 2015;**63**(36):7885-7895. DOI: 10.1021/acs.jafc.5b02404

[85] Thompson RS, Vargas F, Dorrestein PC, Chichlowski M, Berg BM, Fleshner M. Dietary prebiotics alter novel microbial dependent fecal metabolites that improve sleep. Scientific Reports. 2020;**10**(1):3848. DOI: 10.1038/s41598-020-60679-y

[86] Cuervo-Zanatta D, Perez-Grijalva B, González-Magaña E, et al. Modulation of the microbiota-gut-brain axis by bioactive food, prebiotics, and probiotics decelerates the course of Alzheimer's disease. In: Studies in Natural Products Chemistry. Vol. 70. Amsterdam, Neththerlands: Elsevier B.V; 2021. pp. 51-86. DOI: 10.1016/B978-0-12-819489-8.00019-3

[87] Godínez-Méndez LA, Gurrola-Díaz CM, Zepeda-Nuño JS, et al. In vivo healthy benefits of galacto-oligosaccharides from lupinus albus (La-gos) in butyrate production through intestinal microbiota. Biomolecules. 2021;**11**(11):1-22. DOI: 10.3390/biom11111658

[88] Cavaliere G, Catapano A, Trinchese G, et al. Butyrate improves neuroinflammation and mitochondrial impairment in cerebral cortex and synaptic fraction in an animal model of diet-induced obesity. Antioxidants. 2023;**12**(1):4. DOI: 10.3390/antiox12010004

[89] Kaur H, Bose C, Mande SS. Tryptophan metabolism by gut microbiome and gut-brain-axis: An in silico analysis. Frontiers in Neuroscience. 2019;**13**:1365. DOI: 10.3389/fnins.2019.01365

[90] Roager HM, Licht TR. Microbial tryptophan catabolites in health and disease. Nature Communications. 2018;**9**(1):3294. DOI: 10.1038/s41467-018-05470-4

[91] Sabit H, Kassab A, Alaa D, et al. The effect of probiotic supplementation on the gut–brain axis in psychiatric patients. Current Issues in Molecular Biology. 2023;**45**(5):4080-4099. DOI: 10.3390/cimb45050260

[92] Cervantes-Barragan L, Chai JN, Tianero MD, et al. *Lactobacillus reuteri* induces gut intraepithelial CD4 $^{+}$ CD8αα $^{+}$ T cells. Science. 2017;**357**(6353):806-810. DOI: 10.1126/science.aah5825

[93] Jenkins TA, Nguyen JCD, Polglaze KE, Bertrand PP. Influence of tryptophan and serotonin on mood and cognition with a possible role of the gut-brain axis. Nutrients. 2016;**8**(1):56. DOI: 10.3390/nu8010056

[94] Yang C, Fujita Y, Ren Q, Ma M, Dong C, Hashimoto K. Bifidobacterium in the gut microbiota confer resilience to chronic social defeat stress in mice. Scientific Reports. 2017;7:45942. DOI: 10.1038/srep45942

[95] Tao D, Zhong T, Pang W, Li X. *Saccharomyces boulardii* improves the behaviour and emotions of spastic cerebral palsy rats through the gut-brain axis pathway. BMC Neuroscience. 2021;**22**(1):76. DOI: 10.1186/s12868-021-00679-4

[96] Peng Y, Chiu ATG, Li VWY, et al. The role of the gut-microbiome-brain axis in metabolic remodeling amongst children with cerebral palsy and epilepsy. Frontiers in Neurology. 2023;**14**:1109469. DOI: 10.3389/fneur.2023.1109469

Chapter 2

Systematic Approach to Diagnose Inborn Neurometabolic Disorders

Seema Rohilla, Vikas, Yamini Wadhwa, Deepak Singla and Dhara B. Dhaulakhandi

Abstract

There is no dearth of literature detailing individual inborn neurometabolic disorders (INMDs), but it is hard to find a systematic approach to precisely diagnose these. Early diagnosis can go a long way in managing them and improving quality of life and cure in some cases. A systematic structured approach taking into account age, type of presentation, clinical features, imaging, biochemical tests, histopathology and molecular diagnostics often helps in arriving at a particular diagnosis, or a broad category of disorders, which helps in further management. Newer treatment options such as bone marrow transplantation, umbilical cord blood stem cell transplantation, enzyme substitution, somatic gene therapy, and fetal neuronal transplants have given a ray of hope, making it imperative to arrive at early diagnosis of these conditions. Even if a child is lost to inborn error of metabolism (IEM), the cord blood of a normal sibling may be frozen as a reservoir for stem cells for an affected sibling in future pregnancies. In this chapter, we would try to evolve a systematic approach for diagnosis of IEMs and to narrow down the list of differentials. This will lead to cost-effective yet precise biochemical, genetic, and molecular tests to arrive at a final diagnosis.

Keywords: inborn errors of metabolism, neurometabolic, MRI, metabolic brain disorders, proteomics, genome sequencing

1. Introduction

Inborn errors of metabolism (IEM) are a group of disorders caused due to defects in a given biochemical pathway or a deficiency or abnormality of an enzyme, its cofactor, or a transporter resulting into an accumulation of a substrate or suppression of formation of a product. Circulating metabolites may have systemic toxic effects. Moreover, metabolites accumulated in a disorder can further inhibit enzymes; an example being methyl malonic acidemia (MMA). In MMA, methylmalonyl coenzyme A inhibits pyruvate carboxylase, and methylmalonic acid inhibits succinate dehydrogenase. Hence, gluconeogenesis is affected and manifests as hypoglycemia and ketosis, which can further affect the brain parenchyma. There may also be activation of alternative metabolic pathways. In urea cycle defects (UCDs), hyperammonemia may increase synthesis of glutamate, leading to excitotoxic injury to the brain parenchyma. INMDs are monogenic and lack genotype-phenotype correlation (evident from the presence of different phenotypes for the same genetic variation in a family). This further adds to their complexity and makes the diagnoses of such disorders difficult. The studies that applied targeted next generation sequencing panels could diagnose 11–51% of IEMs [1]. Navarette et al. using personalized exome sequencing panel, could confirm only 59% of IEMs [2]. Though individual diseases may be rare, as a whole, these group of disorders are not as uncommon as previously thought. Most of these disorders have genetic basis and are autosomal recessive; hence, they are more common in consanguinity. A proper approach to diagnose these disorders is very important. In this chapter, we would try to develop a systematic approach to diagnose INMDs without going into details of individual disorders.

2. Classification

Classification gives an overview and helps simplify approach. There are different ways of classifying inborn errors of metabolism: on the basis of organ systems involved (neurometabolic, systemic or mixed), cell organelles involved (mitochondrial, lysosomal, peroxisomal and golgi complex disorders), biochemical abnormality (organic acidurias, aminoacidemias, carbohydrate metabolism abnormalities, metal metabolism disorders), or the brain substance involved (polio-, leuko- or pandystrophies).

3. Clinical criteria

It is very important to systematically analyze patients' illness based on the following criteria to direct further investigations:

3.1 Age of onset

Neurometabolic disorders can present at different ages (neonatal—birth to 1 month; early infantile—1 to 6 months; late infantile—6 months to 3 years; childhood—3 to 6 years, juvenile—6 to 16 years, adult—more than 16 years) depending on the genetic defect and residual enzyme activity. Even different phenotypes of the same disease can present at different ages. Most organic acidemias (primary lactic acidosis, UCDs, propionic acidemia, methylmalonic aciduria, isovaleric acidemia) present in the neonatal period. Others like glutaric aciduria, lysosomal disorders (Tay-Sachs and Sandhoff diseases), and mucopolysccharidoses (Hurler, Hunter, Maroteaux-Lamy disease) present in infancy. Diseases like Gaucher disease, metachromatic leukodystrophy (MLD), multiple sulfatase deficiency, Krabbe disease, GM1 and GM2 gangliosidoses, neuronal ceroid lipofuscinosis and mitochondrial myopathy, encephalopathy, lactic acidosis, and stroke-like episodes (MELAS) may have all the ages of presentation. Fabry disease, Leber hereditary optic neuropathy (LHON), and Kearns-Sayre syndrome are seen in the juvenile age. Premature birth, though uncommon in IEM, may be seen in glutaric aciduria type II [3].

3.2 Type of onset

The disease may present as acute illness or chronic encephalopathy or have an intermittent course. Ethylmalonic aciduria, 3-hydroxy-3-methylglutaryl (HMG) coenzyme A lyase deficiency, pyroglutamic aciduria, isovaleric acidemia, holocarboxylase synthetase deficiency, β-ketothiolase deficiency, and malonic aciduria mostly present as acute metabolic decompensation. Chronic progressive encephalopathy (with pyramidal or extrapyramidal signs) is seen in L2-hydroxyglutaric aciduria, N-acetylaspartic aciduria (Canavan disease), and 4-hydroxybutyric aciduria. Acute metabolic crises with interval progressive encephalopathy occur in propionic acidemia, methylmalonic acidemia, and glutaric aciduria type I.

3.3 Head circumference

The head circumference of every child suspected of having neurometabolic disorder should be measured and put in percentile by comparing to standard nomograms for that population. A head circumference (HC) between 5th and 95th percentile is considered normal; more than 95th percentile is macrocephaly (Van der knap disease, Canavan disease, Alexander disease, type I glutaric aciduria, L-2-hydroxyglutaric aciduria, GM2 gangliosidosis, vanishing white matter disease, mucopolysaccharidosis), and less than 5th percentile is microcephaly (Zellweger disease, Aicardi-Goutieres syndrome, Cockyne ds, Pelizaeus-Merzbacher disease). In addition to the initial assessment, the HC should be measured at regular intervals to see the progress with time. In Zellweger disease, the HC is normal at birth but progressively lags behind.

3.4 Neurological abnormalities

3.4.1 Pyramidal signs

Stroke-like picture is predominantly seen in leukodystrophies and is often progressive. It may be hemorrhagic or ischemic. Hemorrhagic stroke is seen in organic acidopathies (propionic, isovaleric and methylmalonic acidemias particularly during metabolic crisis [4, 5]). Ischemic stroke is seen in some aminoacidopathies like homocystinuria, ornithine transcarbamylase deficiency, L-carnitine and carbamyl phosphatase synthetase deficiency [6–9]. Rarely, organic acidopathies such as HMG-coenzyme A lyase deficiency, 3-methylcrotonyl-coenzyme A carboxylase deficiency, cystinosis, Menkes disease, sulfite oxidase deficiency (molybdenum cofactor deficiency), and carbohydrate deficient glycoprotein syndrome may also cause ischemic stroke [10–12]. Fabry disease can have both ischemic and hemorrhagic complications. MELAS, myoclonus epilepsy and ragged-red fibers (MERRF), and Kearns-Sayre disease can have stroke-like episodes. Mitochondrial disorders may also show familial hemiplegic migraine and alternating hemiplegia.

3.4.2 Extrapyramidal movement disorders

Dyskinesis, choreoathetosis, and tremor are hallmarks of basal ganglia (BG) disorders [13]. Most IEMs have hyperkinetic movements. Very limited IEMs present with hypokinesia/hypokinetic rigid syndrome (HRS). HRS starting before 2 years of age is found in monoamine neurotransmitter defects, mitochondrial diseases, or neurodegeneration with brain iron accumulation disorders, while that starting in children above 2 years of age can be seen in many IEMs like Wilson disease, GLUT-1 deficiency, Niemann-Pick type C, Gaucher disease, and glutaric aciduria type 1 [14]. Motor symptoms show diurnal variation in monoamine neurotransmitter defects [1]. Status dystonicus may be seen in Wilson disease, pantothenate kinase associated neurodegeneration [15]. The distribution of movement disorders may also point toward particular pathology. Oromandibular dystonia may be seen in creatine deficiency, while dystonic hand syndrome is seen in AFG3L2-spinocerebellar ataxia type 28 [16].

3.4.3 Seizures

Seizures are common but non-specific. They may be missed in neonates and early infants unless specifically sought. This is because tonic clonic seizures are uncommon below 6 months of age, and mostly, the child has subtle signs like fixed glare, myoclonic jerks, particularly in UCDs, nonketotic hyperglycinemia, and organic acidopathies. Hypoglycemia-related seizures may be seen especially in fatty acid oxidation disorders and nesidioblastosis.

3.4.4 Tone abnormalities

Tone abnormalities also give some insight into the type of disease. Hypotonia may be seen in primary lactic acidosis, respiratory chain defects, multiple carboxylase deficiency, propionic acidemia (ketotic hyperglycinemia), 3-methylglutaconic aciduria, combined methylmalonic acidemia and homocystinuria, nonketotic hyperglycinemia, neonatal peroxisomal disorders (Zellweger syndrome), Menkes disease, sulfite oxidase deficiency, and UCDs [17]. Canavan disease and fatty acid oxidation defects may also have hypotonia. Hypertonia is seen in methylmalonic and isovaleric acidemias and Krabbe disease. Alternating hypo- and hypertonia suggests maple syrup urine disease (MSUD).

3.4.5 Peripheral neuropathy

Peripheral neuropathy is peculiar to lysosomal storage disorders (Krabbe disease, MLD, Farber disease), peroxisomal diseases (adrenomyelinoneuropathy), and galactossemia.

3.4.6 Visual disturbances

Visual disturbances are common in adrenoleukodystrophy (ALD), MLD, Krabbe disease, and LHON. It is pertinent to mention that in ALD, MLD, as well as Krabbe disease, there is a predominant involvement of posterior white matter including optic radiations, which well explains visual disturbances.

3.4.7 Psychiatric manifestations

Both acute metabolic crisis and end-stage disease may have psychiatric manifestations. Late onset diseases like acute intermittent porphyria, Wilson disease, and MLD may be missed when psychiatric symptoms are the initial manifestation [18].

3.5 Systemic abnormalities

It is very important to look for systemic manifestations, too. Failure to thrive is frequent in organic acidurias, UCDs, respiratory chain defects, and carbohydrate deficient glycoprotein syndrome. Mitochondrial diseases may show cardiomegaly; storage disorders or peroxisomal diseases mostly have heptosplenomegaly; skeletal abnormalities are seen in mucopolysaccharidoses and peroxisomal diseases. Meningitis and meningoencephalitis are also common in these patients and often trigger a metabolic crisis [19]. Neutropenia and thrombocytopenia are seen in organic acidopathies, while systemic hemorrhagic complications are found in ethylmalonic aciduria [20]. Anemia and thrombocytopenia are seen in Gaucher disease. Hemolytic anemia is seen in 5-oxoprolinuria. Acute pancreatitis may be seen in organic and aminoacidopathies, homocystinuria, MSUD, and cytochrome c oxidase deficiency [21, 22]. Inborn errors of metabolism, in particular, branched chain organic acidemias should be considered in children with pancreatitis of unknown origin.

3.6 Odor

The typical odor betrays some diseases. Isovaleric acidemia and glutaric aciduria type 2 have smelly cheese or sweaty feet odor; urine in MSUD has a sweet syrupy smell; multiple carboxylase deficiency has a cat urine smell; tyrosinemia smells like rotten cabbage. Urine of patients on carnitine treatment smells like rotten fish due to therapy-induced excessive trimethylamine formation and excretion.

3.7 Facies

Typical facies (depressed nasal bridge, epicanthal folds, short or long philtrum) are seen in organic acidopathies (propionic acidemia, methylmalonic aciduria, isovaleric acidemia, 3-methylglutaric aciduria). Facial dysmorphia is also seen in peroxisomal disorders and mucopolysccharidoses.

3.8 Skin stigmata

Patients with D-2-hydroxyglutaric aciduria have alopecia. Alopecia with skin rashes suggests biotinidase deficiency. Methylmalonic acidemia may lead to erosive desquamative dermatitis and hair loss. Skin pigmentation and scleroderma may occur in phenylketonuria. Hypopigmentation and photosensitivity are seen in Cockayne disease. Congenital ichthyosis is seen in Sjogren-Larson syndrome. Nipple abnormalities (inverted, hypoplastic, supernumerary) may be seen in propionic acidemia. Trichorrhexis nodosa, a beaded appearance of fragile hair, suggests arginosuccinic acid lyase deficiency, thus even helping in identifying the type of UCD [23].

3.9 Ophthalmologic abnormalities

Corneal clouding is very common in mucopolysccharidoses (except type II and III), many lysosomal storage disorders, multiple sulfatase deficiency, Fabry disease, Farber disease, some oligosaccharidosis, and cystinosis. Cataract is seen in galactossemia, isovaleric acidemia, 4-hydroxybutyric aciduria, cerebrotendinous xanthomatosis, and Cockayne disease. Kayser-Fleischer ring is pathognomonic of Wilson disease. Lens dislocation suggests homocystinuria and sulfite oxidase deficiency [24].

Cherry red spots help in identifying GM gangliosidoses, Niemann Pick disease, Farber disease, some mucolipidoses, and MLD. Retinitis pigmentosa is seen in many peroxisomal and mitochondrial disorders, neuronal ceroid lipofuscinosis, and abetalipoproteinemia. Electroretinographic abnormalities are seen in poliodystrophies and are exceptionally rare in leukodystrophies.

4. Imaging

MRI is the only radiological investigation relevant in assessing patients with neurometabolic disorders.

4.1 Sequences

The basic MRI sequences (T1W, T2W, TIW/IR) are mostly sufficient, but DWI, MR spectroscopy, and contrast studies add value in some cases. It is important to note that T1W/IR is better than T1W except for the detection of BG hyperintensity in hepatic encephalopathy, Krabbe disease, or GM2 gangliosidosis, where T1W is better than T1W/IR. Enhancement is better appreciated on T1W than T1W IR. T1W is recommended in children less than 12 months & T2W for the 12–18 month-age group for better delineation of myelin. Modular IR better delineates small lesions in the brainstem and deep gray matter nuclei. FLAIR differentiates cystic lesions from T2 hyperintensities of white matter (WM). T2W images are more sensitive than FLAIR for brainstem lesions. Longer TE and TR times should be used in T2W imaging to compensate for longer T2 relaxation due to higher water and lower myelin/lipid content in newborns and infants. FLAIR imaging is not very useful except in delineating cystic lesions as in Van der Knaap disease. The conventional spin echo technique is more sensitive than the fast spin echo technique but may not be practical at times due to longer scan times.

4.2 Structures to be assessed

Certain structures are more vulnerable at certain ages due to their specific energy and nutrient requirements [25]. Cerebral WM is vulnerable before 32nd week of gestation, while BG is vulnerable during the last three gestational months and first 3 years of life due to high metabolic rate. Myelinating and myelinated WM is involved in neonatal maple syrup urine disease (**Figure 1**). Homocystine accumulating in

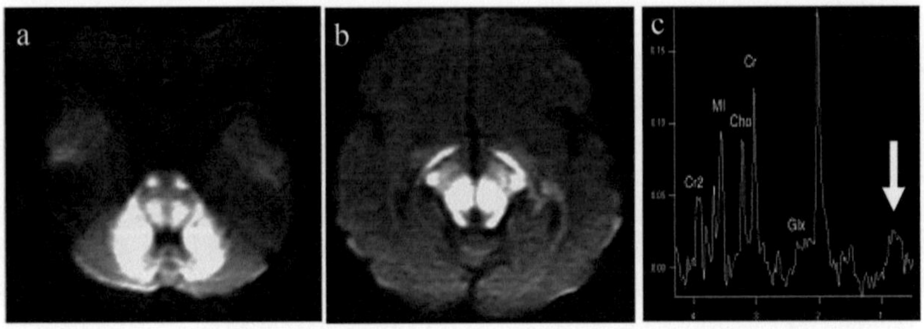

Figure 1.
A five day neonate with poor feeding, vomiting and seizures. a and b: DW images showing diffusion restriction in myelinated WM. c: Proton spectroscopy showing branched chain amino and keto acids at 0.9 ppm (arrow). Maple syrup urine disease.

DOI: http://dx.doi.org/10.5772/intechopen.1002290

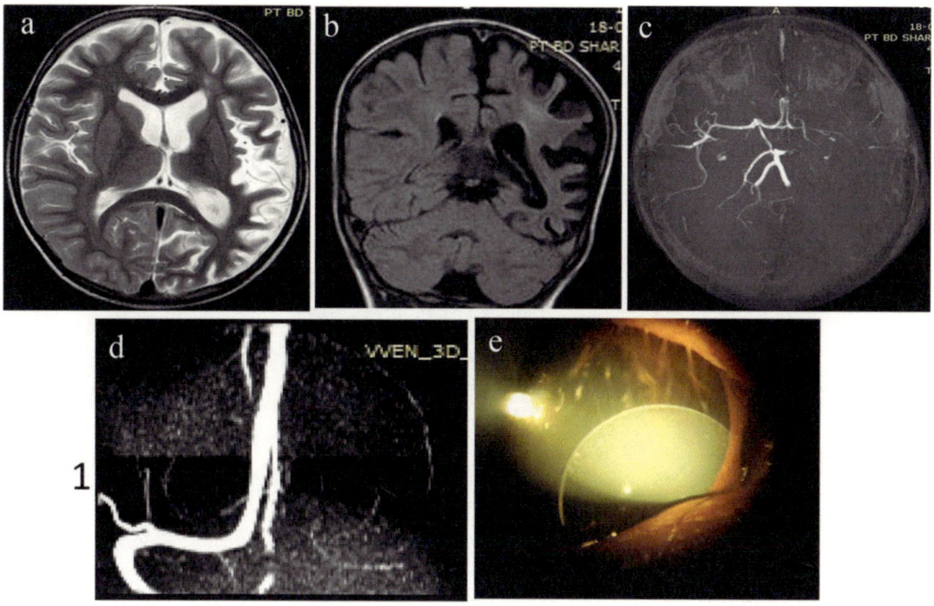

Figure 2.
A one year child with right sided hemiparesis, loose skin. a and b: Axial T2W and coronal T2W/FLAIR images showing encephalomalacia suggestive of old infarct in left temporoparietal area. c: Time of flight MR angiography showing blocked left middle cerebral artery, left posterior cerebral artery and left posterior communicating artery. d: MR venography showing blocked left transverse sinuse: Fundoscopy image showing inferomedial dislocation of lens. Homocystinuria.

homocystinuria is destructive to fibrillin (resulting in lens subluxation) and toxic to vascular endothelium (predisposing to thrombus formation) (**Figure 2**). Hence, some brain structures need special attention while reading MRI of a patient suspected of having neurometabolic disorder. WM structures to be assessed are cerebral white matter, subcortical 'U' fibers, extreme capsule, external capsule, internal capsule, medullary laminae, corpus callosum, anterior commissure, mamillary bodies, central tegmental brainstem tract, and cerebellar white matter. GM structures to be assessed are cerebral cortex, claustrum, caudate nucleus, putamen, globus pallidus, thalamus, subthalamic nucleus, red nucleus, substantia nigra, dentate nucleus, and cerebellar cortex.

4.3 Approach to read MRI

A structured systematic approach that takes into account clinical information as detailed above usually helps define at least a broad group of disorders if not the disorder itself and gives further direction for work-up.

4.3.1 Rule out mimics of neurometabolic disorders

There is considerable overlap of MRI findings in neurometabolic brain disorders with other conditions like hypoxic ischemic encephalopathy (HIE), TORCH, viral infections, post viral demyelination, and so on (**Figure 3**). Newborns with HIE mostly stabilize 1–2 weeks after birth, while those with IEM mostly show progressive deterioration. WM changes of inborn errors of metabolism (IEM) need to be

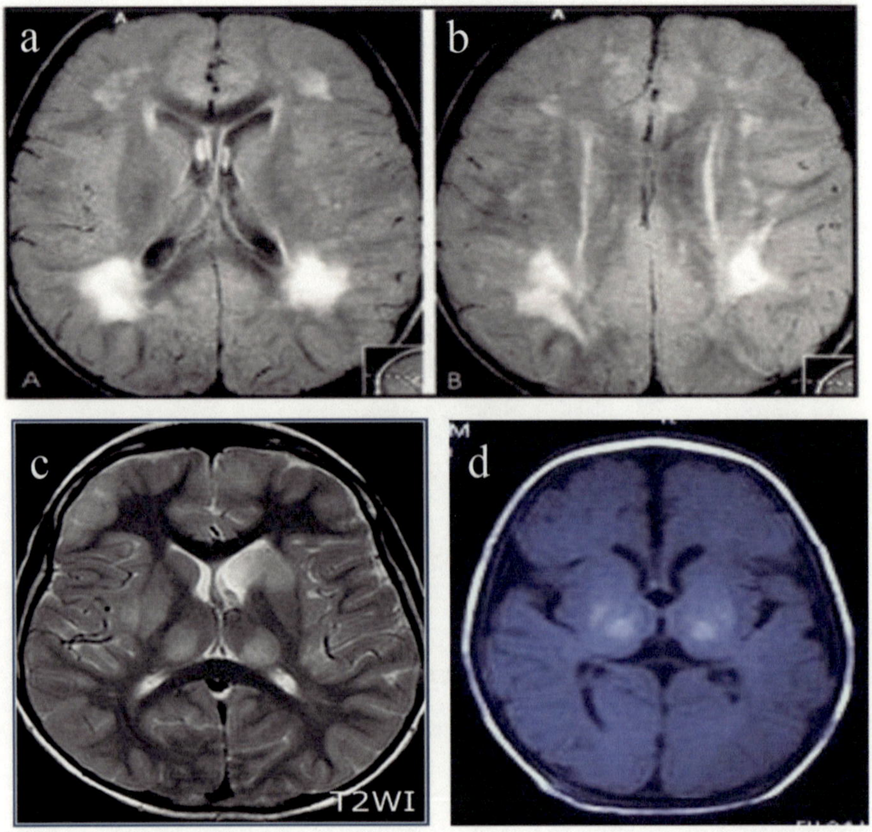

Figure 3.
a and b: Axial T2W images showing periventricular T2 hyperintensities representing demyelination in a child with congenital rubella. c: Axial T2W image showing asymmetric T2 hyperintensities in left caudate nucleus, left lentiform nucleus (anteriorly), right lentiform nucleus (posteriorly), B/L thalami, left superior and right middle frontal gyri & right external capsule in a child with acute disseminated encephalomyelitis. d: Axial T1W image showing hyperintensities in B/L posterior lentiform nuclei and B/L thalami in a patient with HIE.

differentiated from periventricular leukomalacia, vasculitis, progressive multifocal leukoencephalitis, demyelinating diseases, HIV encephalitis, brucellosis, and toxic and postirradiation encephalopathy. Basal ganglia involvement should be distinguished from extrapontine myelinolysis, sequelae of prolonged hypoxemia, or anoxia [26]. Involvement of BG (globi pallidi, caudate nuclei and putamina) without thalamic involvement suggests metabolic diseases, while the thalamic and posterior parts of putamina are mostly affected in perinatal hypoxic-ischemic brain damage. Moreover, altered utilization of ATP may increase creatine in milder forms of HIE [27]. Wernicke encephalopathy may show hyperintensity in putamina, thalami, periaqueductal gray matter, and tectal plate, which may resemble Leigh disease, but hypothalamus and/or mamillary bodies are preferentially involved in Wernicke encephalopathy [28]. Superficial layers of cortex are typically involved in hypoglycemia, while deeper layers are involved in HIE [29]. Demyelination of the dorsal and lateral columns of the spinal cord in hyperhomocysteinemia may be confused with subacute combined degeneration [30].

4.3.2 Myelination pattern

The myelination pattern assessment is of the utmost importance, whether myelination is normal or abnormal for the age. T1W images are better in assessing myelination before 12 months of age, while T2W images are better for children above 12 months. Myelinated structures appear slightly hyperintense on T1W and hypointense on T2W images. Normal myelination proceeds from central to peripheral, caudal to rostral, and dorsal to ventral. Sensory parts myelinate before motor parts. The brainstem, cerebellum, posterior limb of the internal capsule, optic tract, and perirolandic regions are myelinated in term neonates and seen on both T1W as well as T2W images. After that, T2W images lag behind T1W images in identifying myelination. Myelination of the anterior limb of the internal capsule is seen at 2–3 months on T1W images and 7–11 months on T2W images; that of the splenium of the corpus callosum is seen at 3–4 months on T1W images and 4–6 months on T2W images; and that of the genu of the corpus callosum at 4–6 months on T1W and 5–8 months on T2W images.

Abnormal myelination may include delayed myelination, demyelination, or dysmyelination. In addition to referring to the normal age of myelination, some illnesses in the first 18 months of age should also be taken into account before labeling delayed myelination. This is because myelination needs energy and nutrition, and any systemic (respiratory or cardiac) or neurologic disease such as meningoencephalitis during the initial 18–24 months of age can delay myelination, and the child can later catch up with myelination. Hence, it is important to repeat MRI at a gap of 6–12 months and look for the progress of myelination before labeling myelination delay as pathological. Demyelination refers to the loss of normal myelin, while dysmyelination refers to abnormal myelin. Such myelin is unstable and can lead to secondary demyelination. Demyelination appears hypointense on T1W images and hyperintense on T2W images, while hypomyelination is an unchanged pattern of deficient myelination on two successive MRI scans at least 6 months apart. Dysmyelination shows increased radial but normal axial diffusivities [31]. Metabolic disorders having a postnatal onset have normal myelin produced before the onset of metabolic derangement, while myelin produced after birth is defective and fragile. They show a myelination pattern like neonates or early infants with the oldest myelinated structures like the brainstem, cerebellum, and central corticospinal tracts being normal, while younger white matter structures show demyelination. L-hydroxyglutaric aciduria and homocystinuria show such a pattern.

4.3.3 Pattern recognition

Identifying the pattern of abnormal signal goes a long way in disease recognition [32]. It is important to recognize terminal zones of myelination that are classically located in the posterior periventricular region as well as frontotemporal subcortical regions and are normally seen up to the age of two years (**Figure 4**).

4.3.3.1 WM signal abnormalities' pattern

WM abnormalities provide significant insight into the pathology. Anteroposterior gradient means signal abnormality starts anteriorly and is more prominent anteriorly

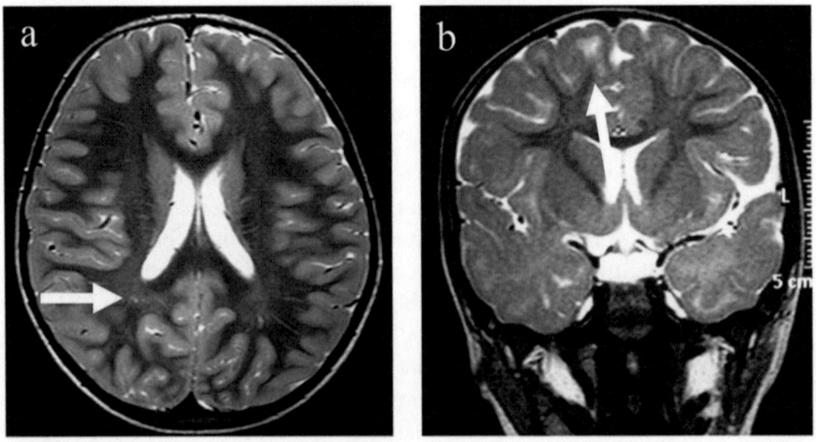

Figure 4.
a and b: Axial and coronal T2W images showing normal terminal zones of transition (arrows). These are abnormal above two years of age.

(**Figure 5a**). This pattern is seen in Van der Knaap, Canavan, and Alexander diseases and L2-hydroxyglutaric aciduria, while posteroanterior gradient (disease starts posteriorly and is more prominent posteriorly) (**Figure 5b**) is seen in Krabbe disease and ALD. The centripetal gradient (signals abnormality progressing from the subcortical to the periventricular area) (**Figure 5a**) is seen in Canavan disease, Alexander disease, L2-hydroxyglutaric aciduria, and Van der Knaap disease, while the centrifugal gradient (signals abnormality progressing from the periventricular to the subcortical area) (**Figure 5b**) is seen in MLD, Krabbe disease, and ALD. External and extreme capsules are involved in L-2-hydroxyglutaric aciduria and fucosidosis (**Figure 5a**). Corpus callosum should be evaluated for signal and volume. It reflects the magnitude and possible progression gradient of involvement of the hemispheric WM. The inferior aspect of the body of corpus callosum shows prominent signal changes in Van der Knaap disease. The involvement of central tegmental structures of pons is nonspecific but sensitive for metabolic and neurodegenerative processes. Corticospinal tracts should be analyzed from precentral gyrus, posterior limbs of the internal capsules, and cerebral peduncles up to decussation at the level of medulla (**Figure 5c**). The tigroid pattern of demyelination due to the sparing of perivenular white matter is seen in MLD and Palaezius Merzbacher disease (**Figure 5d**). Cerebellar hemispheric WM may be involved in Canavan disease, Krabbe disease, Van der Knaap disease, MLD, and ALD.

4.3.3.2 GM signal abnormalities' pattern

Just like WM, GM signal abnormalities also help in suggesting diagnosis. Cortex is thin in GM2 gangliosidosis, Van der Knaap disease, and Canavan disease. Zellweger disease and fumaric aciduria may be associated with cortical dysplasias. The important thing to note is that diseases that are associated with structural malformations of the brain start prenatally and hence affect the normal development of the brain. Hypointensities suggestive of calcification or premature iron deposition suggest Wilson disease. The involvement or sparing of some structures helps in narrowing down the differentials. Claustra are spared in L-2-hydroxyglutaric aciduria but involved in Wilson

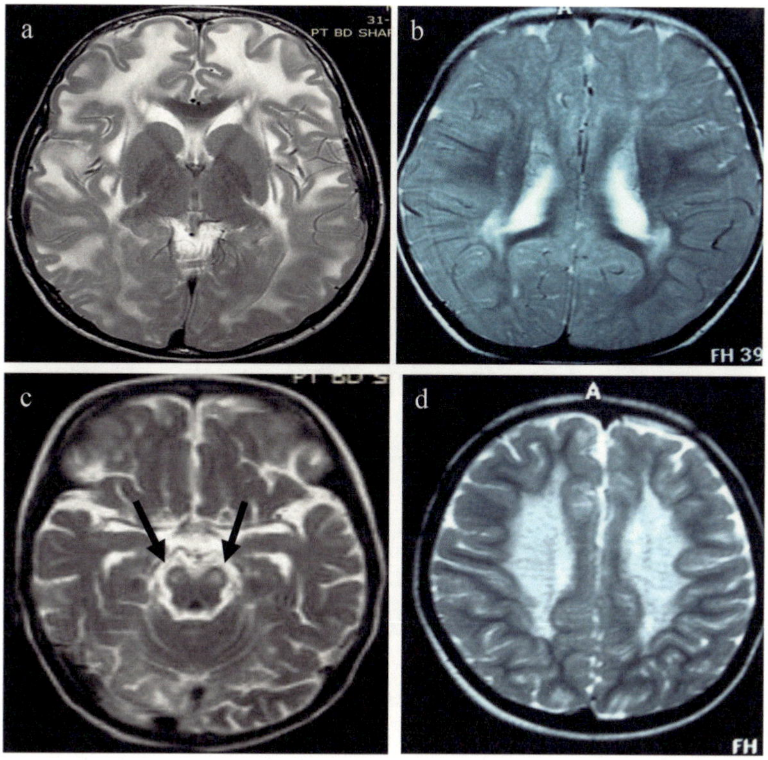

Figure 5.
a: Axial T2W image showing more WM signal abnormalities in anterior aspect than posterior (anteroposterior gradient) and subcortically than in periventricular aspect (centripetal gradient). b: Axial T2W image showing more WM signal abnormalities in posterior aspect than anterior (posteroanterior gradient) and periventricularly than in subcortical aspect (centrifugal gradient). c: Axial T2W image showing hyperintensity in corticospinal tracts in cerebral peduncles (arrows). d: Axial T2W image showing T2 hyperintensity in B/L centrum semiovale sparing perivenular area giving tigroidappearance.

disease (**Figure 6a** and **b**). Subthalamic nuclei are involved in kernicterus and leigh disease. Giant panda face is seen in Wilson disease and glutaric aciduria type I (**Figure 6c**). This happens due to the sparing of red nucleus, which stands out as hypointense in the background of hyperintense substantia nigra and periaqueductal WM on T2W images. Dentate nucleus is involved in organic acidopathies and cerebrotendinous xanthomatosis (**Figure 6d**). BG show signal changes in acute metabolic crises, kernicterus, and Wilson disease (**Figure 7a**) and are swollen in GM1 & GM2 gangliosidoses (**Figure 7b**). Cerebellar atrophy is seen in neuronal ceroid lipofuscinosis, 3-methylglutaconic aciduria, carbohydrate deficient glycoprotein syndrome, many lysosomal storage diseases, Menke's disease, and mitochondrial diseases. Concomitant brainstem and cerebellar atrophy are suggestive of a neurodegenerative disease.

4.3.3.3 Spinal cord involvement

Involvement of the spinal cord also gives some clue to the disease. Cauda equina shows contrast enhancement in Krabbe disease [33]. Brainstem shows hyperintensity on T2W images in leukodystrophy with brainstem and spinal cord involvement and high lactate [34].

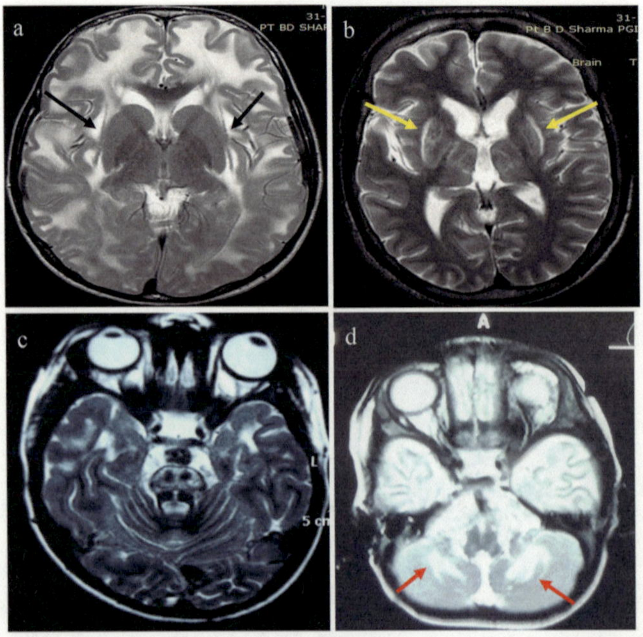

Figure 6.
a: Axial T2W image showing normal claustra in L2-hydroxyglutaric aciduria (white arrows). b: Axial T2W image showing T2 hyperintensity in claustra in Wilson disease (yellow arrows). c: Axial T2W image showing T2 hyperintensity in substantia nigra and periaqueductal WM with sparing of red nucleus giving 'giant panda face appearance'. d: Axial T2W image showing T2 hyperintensity seen in B/L dentate nuclei (red arrows).

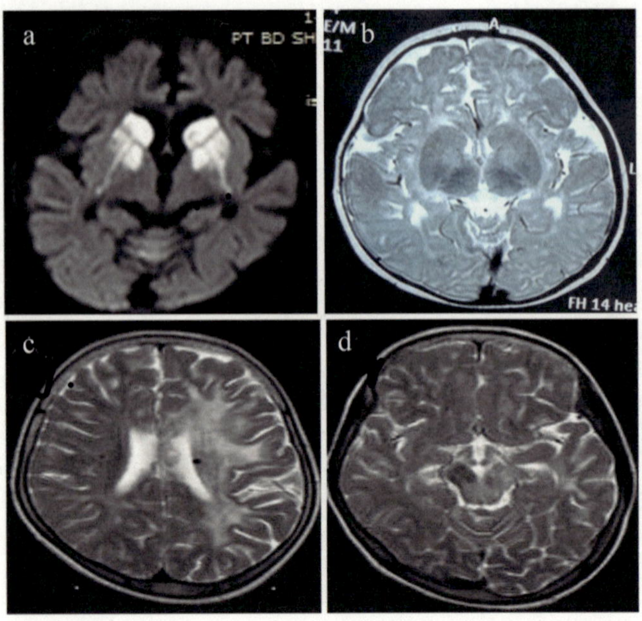

Figure 7.
a: Axial DW image showing diffusion restriction in basal ganglia in acute metabolic crisis. b: Axial T2W image showing swollen basal ganglia in GM2 gangliosidosis. c and d: Axial T2W images showing hyperintensity in left centrum semiovalein a patient with MLD (asymmetric involvement). Though both crus cerebri show signal abnormality, but left crus cerebri is more prominently involved.

4.3.4 Evolving lesions

Lesions evolve over time. In MLD, the subcortical 'U' fibers are initially spared but involved later on.

4.3.5 Symmetry

Looking for symmetry is equally important. Most of the neurometabolic disorders have a symmetric pattern of abnormality, but neurodegenerative diseases and toxic and hypoxic-ischemic encephalopathies are also symmetric. There may, however, always be some exceptions to this rule (**Figure 7c** and **d**).

4.3.6 Contrast enhancement

Few of the neurometabolic disorders show contrast enhancement. Most typical, rather diagnostic enhancement is seen in ALD where actively demyelinating inflammatory zone shows enhancement (**Figure 8a**). Alexander disease shows enhancement along the ependymal lining of lateral ventricles sometimes extending to more remote areas of frontal lobes and within deep GM structures. Krabbe disease shows patchy enhancement in periventricular white matter and cauda equina nerve roots [33] (**Figure 8b**).

4.3.7 Associated findings

4.3.7.1 Subdural hematoma (SDH)

SDH may be seen in many disorders when atrophy sets in like glutaric aciduria type I (**Figure 8c**) [35], 3-methyl-crotonyl-glycinuria, and Menkes disease. This may be mistaken for child abuse.

4.3.7.2 Malformations

Some malformations are associated with particular neurometabolic disorders. Dysmorphic facies are seen in lysosomal storage disorders, peroxisomal disorders [36], and golgi complex disorders. Bilateral perisylvian polymicrogyria and germinolytic cysts are found in Zellweger disease [37], diffuse polymicrogyria and open operculae in fumaric aciduria [38], and pachygyria in glutaric aciduria type 2 and

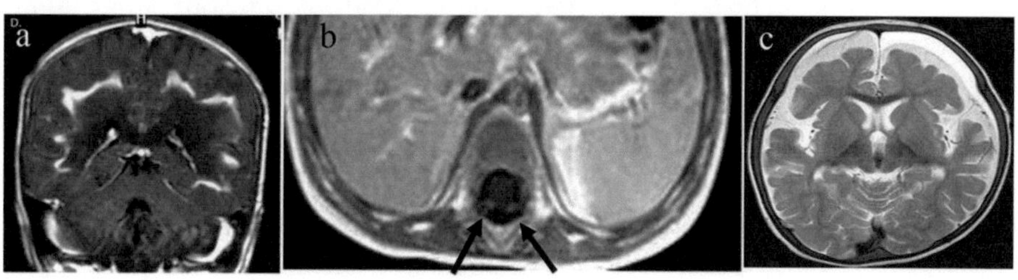

Figure 8.
a: T1W contrast enhanced coronal image shows enhancement of actively demyelinating zone in ALD. b: T1W contrast enhanced image shows enhancing cauda equina nerve roots in Krabbedisease (arrows). c: T2W axial image shows SDH in B/L frontal areas in a child with glutaric aciduria type I.

non-ketotic hyperglycinemia [39]. Callosal abnormalities are seen in nonketotic hyperglycenemia, glutaric aciduria type 2, pseudoneonatal adrenoleukodystrophy, salla disease, and mucolipidosis type IV [40–42]. Operculization is disturbed in glutaric aciduria type 1 [43]. Ethylmalonic aciduria shows Chiari I malformation and tethered cord [44].

4.3.8 Role of diffusion weighted imaging

DW imaging is based on the Brownian motion of particles. Neuropathologically, four types of edema are identified. Cytotoxic and myelin edema show restricted diffusion, while vasogenic and interstitial edema show increased diffusion, which is isotropic. These can be differentiated on DW imaging and not on T1W and T2W images. Hence, DW images enhance specificity. Vasogenic edema of non-myelinated WM is common in UCDs and sulfite oxidase deficiency. Scalloped ribbon pattern of diffusion restriction in the sulcal depth points toward UCDs where T1W and T2W images are non-specific [29]. In the context of neurometabolic disorders, cytotoxic edema is seen in acute gray matter diseases. Myelin edema is seen in active demyelination. In fact, we diagnosed a case of neonatal maple syrup disease on the basis of restricted diffusion (**Figure 1**). Diffusion restriction was seen in BG in patients of glutaric aciduria type I in a metabolic crisis (**Figure 7a**) and another patient with mitochondrial disease. Vasogenic edema may be seen in metabolic crises. DWI also helps in monitoring disease progression and differentiating between the active and burnt-out phase of diseases in both polio and leukodystrophies.

DTI detected differences in corticospinal tracts of neonates with Krabbe disease having an early onset of the disease. This is significant as DTI has the potential to be used as a marker of disease progression in neonates suspected to have Krabbe through screening programs, especially because enzyme activity and genetic mutation both cannot fully predict phenotype [45].

4.3.9 Proton spectroscopy

Proton spectroscopy provides molecular signatures of the tissue by identifying different biomolecules in the substrate. Short TE spectroscopy allows the detection of more metabolites and has a greater signal-to-noise ratio than longer TE; however, it is better to add long TE, too [46]. Being conversant with the normal spectrum at different ages helps. Generally, the N-acetyl aspartate (NAA) peak is small while choline is the most prominent in neonates. By 4 months of age, NAA becomes the most prominent peak; by 6 months of age, the spectrum assumes an "adult" appearance [47]. Lactate may be seen in the brain of premature infants and the first couple of weeks in term infants.

Lactate peak is seen in mitochondrial disorders, systemic lactic acidosis, metabolic crises of IEMs, hypoperfusion, and inflammation. We were able to diagnose a case of mitochondrial disorder correctly based on the very prominent lactate peak on spectroscopy, while the pediatrician suspected vanishing white matter disease. A genetic study revealed NDUFV1 mutation, suggesting mitochondrial disorder [48]. Estimating the lactate peak is better than CSF or plasma lactate in monitoring therapy in leigh disease. Moreover, demonstrating the lactate peak in a normal-appearing brain tissue better suggests IEM than lactate peak associated with focal lesion [27]. Glutamine and glutamate suggest UCDs, propionic acidemia, hepatic encephalopathy, and hypoxic-ischemic brain damage [49]. Phenylalanine (at 7.37 ppm) is the hallmark of phenylketonuria [50], and branched chain amino acids and ketoacids (at 0.9 ppm) of maple syrup urine disease, while glycine (at 3.55 ppm) is seen in nonketotic hyperglycinemia. Increased NAA is seen in Canavan disease [51]. The absence of creatine peak suggests guanidoacetate methyl-transferase deficiency. Spectroscopy may even prognosticate IEMs. The Myoinositol peak shows an inverse relation with the severity of UCD [46].

4.3.10 Pathognomic MRI patterns

Based on the above detailed approach to reading MRI, some neurometabolic disorders have pathognomonic MRI patterns. These include L-2-hydroxyglutaric aciduria (**Figure 9**), glutaric aciduria type 1 (**Figure 10**), neonatal maple syrup urine

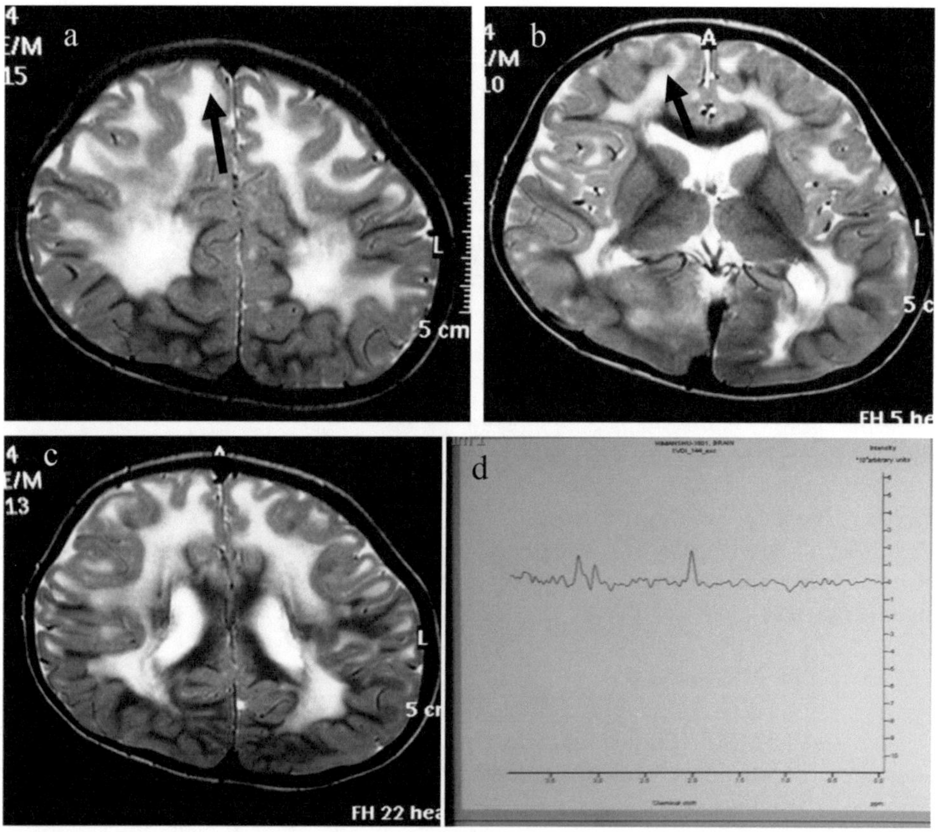

Figure 9.
Two year female had delayed milestones and learning disabilities. a–c: Axial T2W images at different levels showing T2 hyperintensities in WM with clear anteroposterior and centripetal gradients. Subcortical 'U' fibresare destroyed at many places (arrows). d: MR spectroscopy in involved areas shows reduced NAA and choline peaks. L2-hydroxyglutaric aciduria.

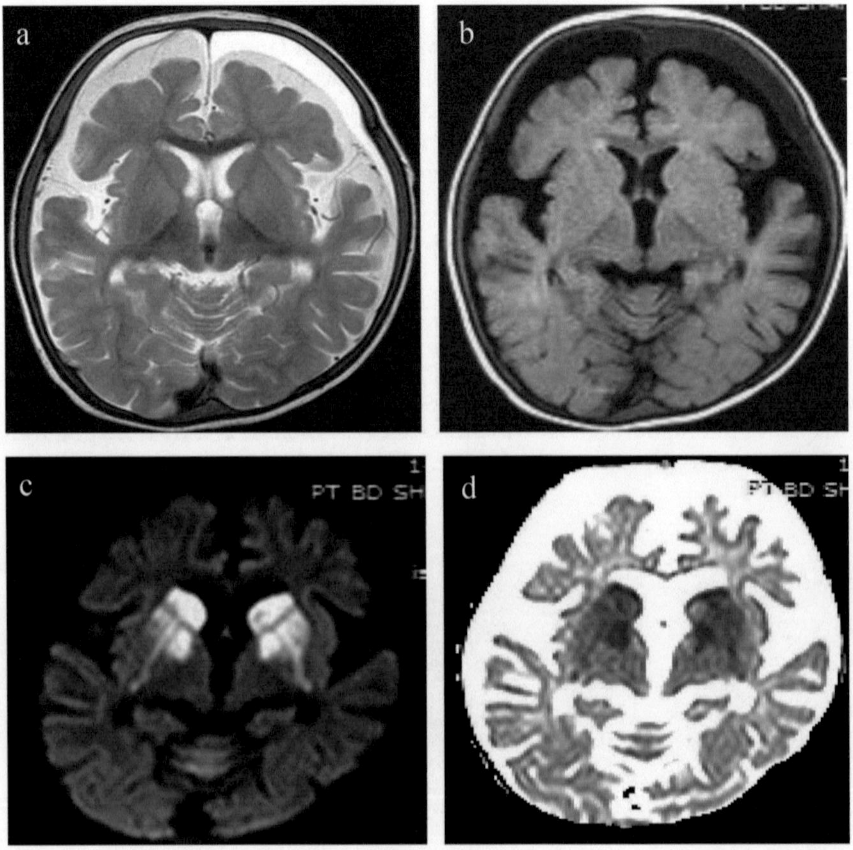

Figure 10.
A 1.5 year old boy had seizures, vomiting and altered sensorium after fever. a and b: Axial T2W and T2W/FLAIR axial images showing atrophy in B/L frontal and temporal areas with improper operculization seen as open operculae. SDH of different ages is seen in B/L frontal areas, subacute on left side and chronic on right side. c and d: DW and ADC maps show diffusion restriction in B/L corpora striata suggestive of acute metabolic crisis consistent with clinical presentation. Glutaric aciduria type I with acute metabolic decompensation.

disease (**Figure 1**), Zellweger disease, X-linked ALD (**Figure 11**), Canavan disease, Alexander disease (**Figure 12**), Van der Knaap disease (**Figure 13**), leukodystrophy with brainstem and spinal cord involvement and high lactate, and mucopolysaccharidoses (**Figure 14**).

4.3.11 Suggestive MRI patterns

Diseases like MMA (**Figure 15**), 3-methyl glutaconic aciduria, beta-ketothiolase deficiency, the late onset form of maple syrup urine disease, homocystinuria (**Figure 2**), Krabbe disease (**Figure 16**), MLD (**Figure 17**), GM2 gangliosidosis (**Figure 18**), vanishing white matter disease (**Figure 19**), leigh disease (**Figure 20**), Menke disease (**Figure 21**), Wilson disease (**Figure 22**), and mitochondrial disorders (**Figure 23**) have suggestive MRI patterns. Though not having exactly suggestive patterns, but we were able to diagnose UCD (**Figure 24**) based on the age of presentation, hyperammonemia, spectroscopy, and other clinical features.

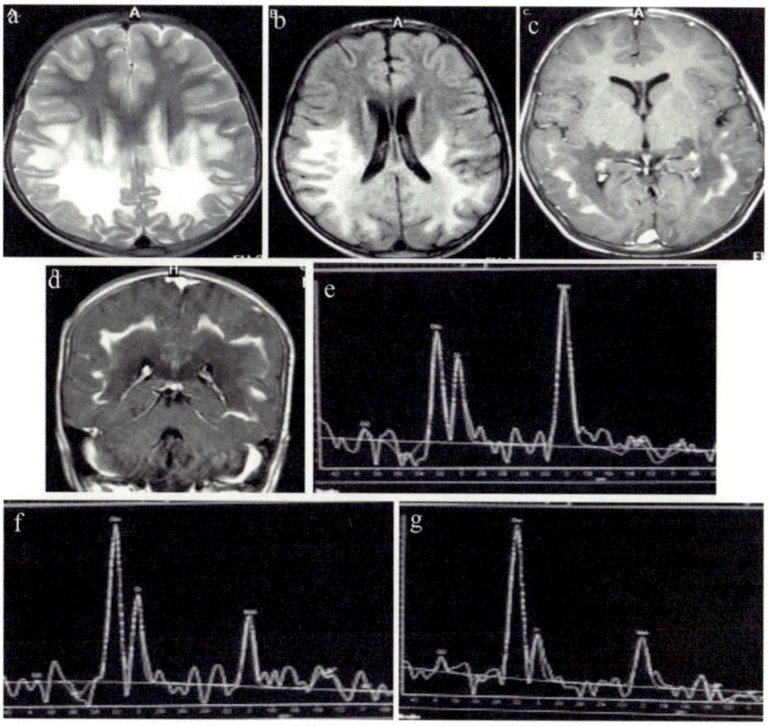

Figure 11.
An 8 year male with declining academic performance, loss of speech, and spasticity. a: Axial T2W image shows T2 hyperintensity in WM mainly in periventricular area in B/L parietal lobes and splenium of corpus callosum. b: Axial T2W/FLAIR images showing some suppression of signal centrally, not peripherally suggesting central necrosis and peripheral edema. c and d: Axial and coronal T1W contrast images showing enhancement of actively demyelinating intermediate zone. e: MR spectroscopy in outer edematous zone showing normal peaks. f: MR spectroscopy in intermediate zone showing increased choline and reduced NAA peak suggestive of active demyelination. g: MR spectroscopy in inner zone showing prominent choline peak. While NAA and creatine peaks are even smaller than intermediate zone suggestive of necrotic inner zone (burnt out area). X-linked adrenoleukodyatrophy.

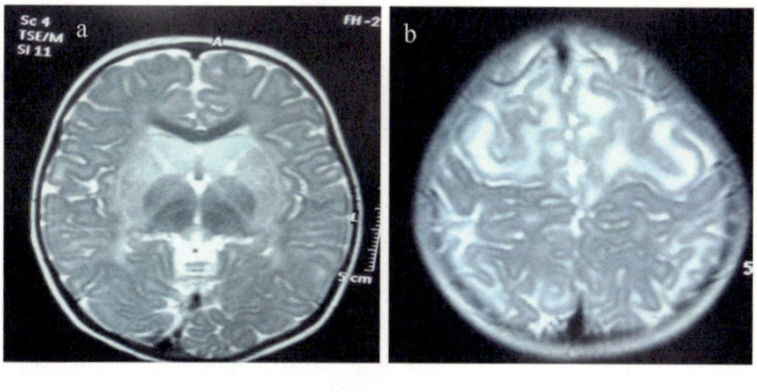

Figure 12.
A one year old macrocephalic female child had delayed milestones, failure to thrive and difficulty in swallowing. a: Axial T2W image showing hyperintense signal in B/L caudate and lentiform nuclei which are also slightly swollen. There is sparing of thalami. b: Axial T2W image at a slightly higher level shows hyperintensity in WM of B/L frontal area with involvement of subcortical 'U' fibers. Alexander's disease.

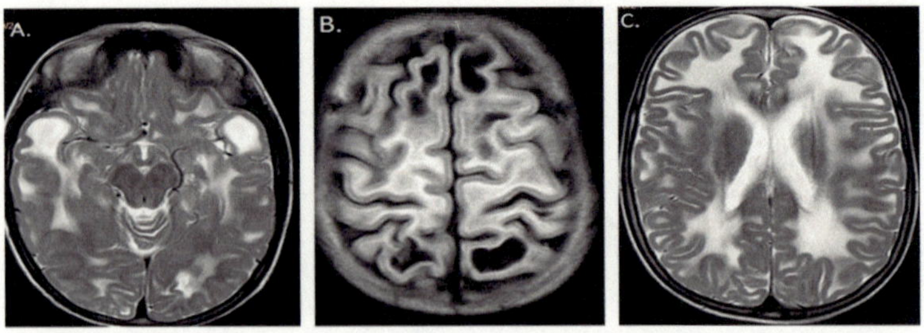

Figure 13.
A seven year Aggarwal boy had delayed milestones and learning disability. a & b: Axial T2W and T2W/FLAIR images showing subcortical cysts in B/L temporal, frontal and parietal areas. c: Axial T2W image at a higher level showing hyperintensity in WM of B/L frontal and parietal areas, more prominent in frontal areas along with destruction of 'U' fibers in frontal areas, showing anteroposterior and centripetal gradient of signal change. Van der knap disease.

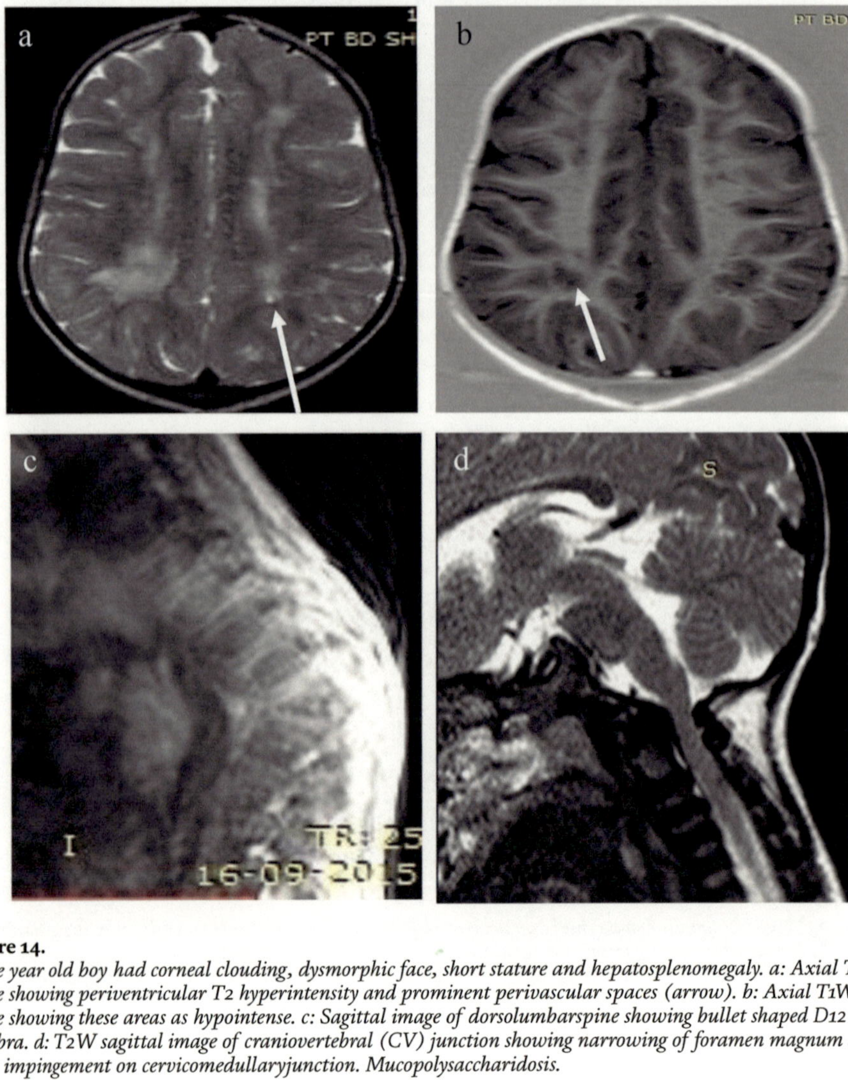

Figure 14.
A five year old boy had corneal clouding, dysmorphic face, short stature and hepatosplenomegaly. a: Axial T2W image showing periventricular T2 hyperintensity and prominent perivascular spaces (arrow). b: Axial T1W image showing these areas as hypointense. c: Sagittal image of dorsolumbarspine showing bullet shaped D12 vertebra. d: T2W sagittal image of craniovertebral (CV) junction showing narrowing of foramen magnum and slight impingement on cervicomedullaryjunction. Mucopolysaccharidosis.

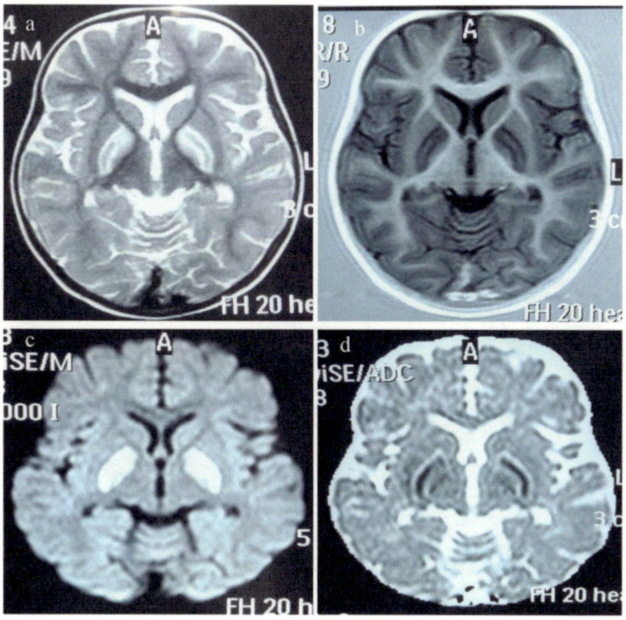

Figure 15.
A 2.5 month female had seizures, failure to thrive and poor feeding. a: Axial T2W image showing hyperintensity in B/L globipallidi and intermedullary laminae. b: Axial T1W image shows the involved areas as hypointense. c and d: DW and ADC map show diffusion restriction in B/L globipallidi methylmalonic acidemia.

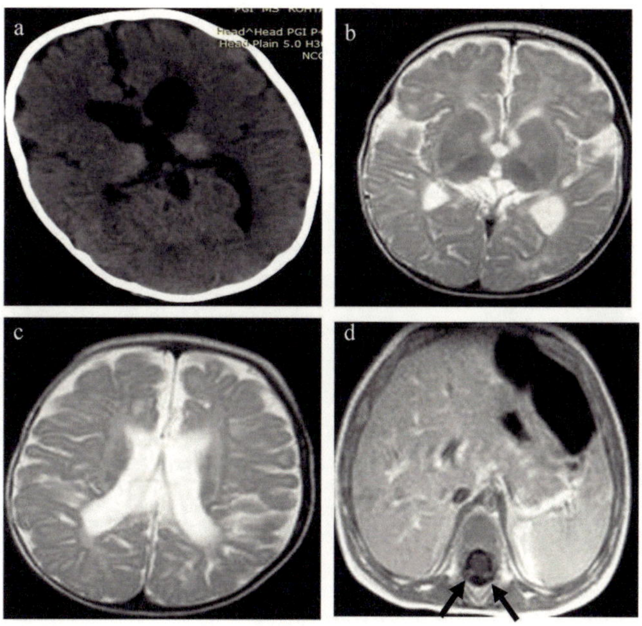

Figure 16.
A six month male presented with irritability and refusal to feed along with episodes of tonic spasms. a: CT scan showing hyperdense thalami b: Axial T2W image showing subtle hyperintensity in posterior limbs of internal capsules (posteroanterior gradient) c: Axial T2W image at a higher level showing periventricular hyperintensity more prominent posteriorly. d: Axial T1W contrast enhanced image showing enhancement of cauda equina nerve roots (arrows).

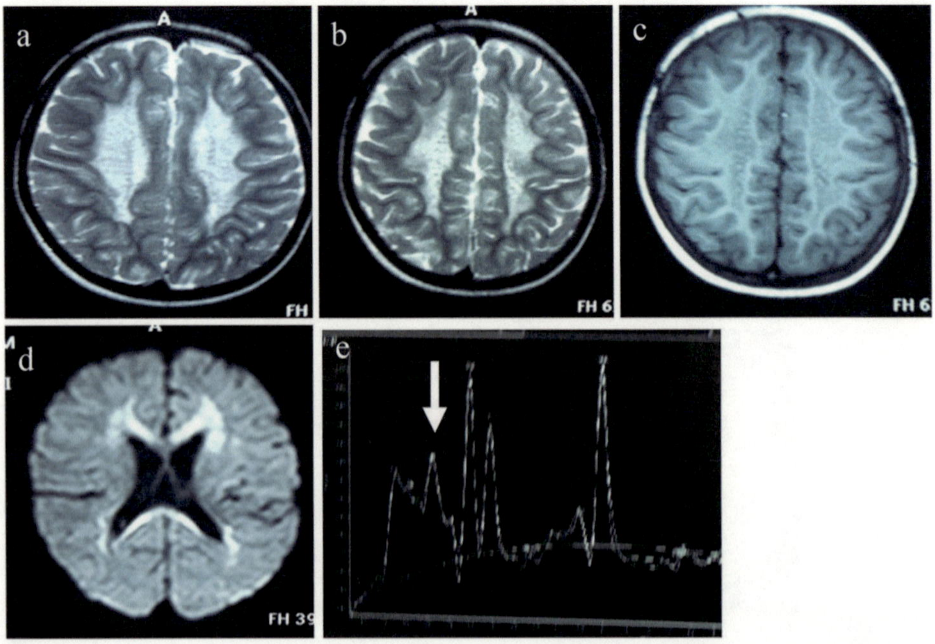

Figure 17.
A five year old boy presented with ataxia and regression of milestones. a & b: Axial T2W images at slightly different levels show hyperintensity in B/L centrum semiovalehaving typical tigroidpattern due to sparing of perivenular area. Though the signal abnormality is quite widespread, there is sparing of subcortical 'U' fibers. c: Axial T1W image shows hypointensityin same area. d: DW image shows hyperintensity in both genu and splenium of corpus callosum. Note that splenium is thin as compared to genu suggesting that atrophy has set in splenium, while involvement of genu is comparatively recent. This indirectly reinforces posteroanterior gradient. e: MR spectroscopy shows an mI peak at 3.56 ppm (arrow). Patient had elevated urinary sulfatides thus confirming metachromatic leukodystrophy.

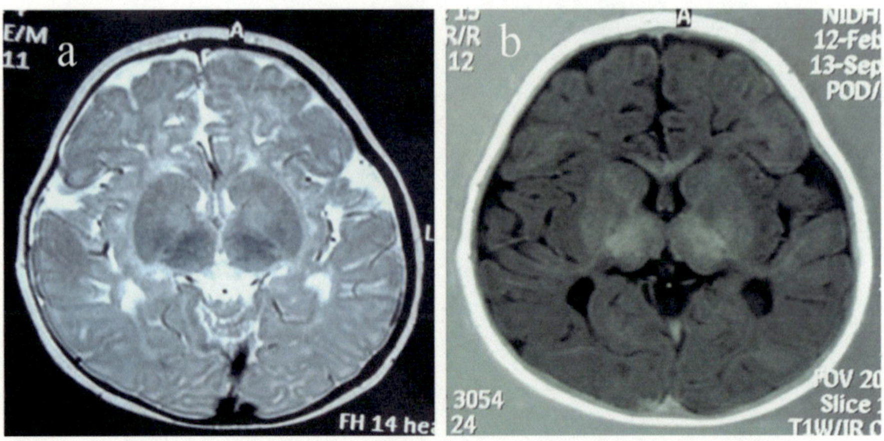

Figure 18.
A seven month old female had failure to thrive and generalized tonic clonicseizures. Her head circumference was also increased. a: Axial T2W image showing comparatively swollen corpora striata, slight hyperintensity in B/L external and extreme capsules and hypointensityin B/L thalami. b: Axial T2W/FLAIR image shows swollen corpora striata and hyperintense thalami. Fundus examination of the child showed cherry red spots suggesting GM2 gangliosidosis.

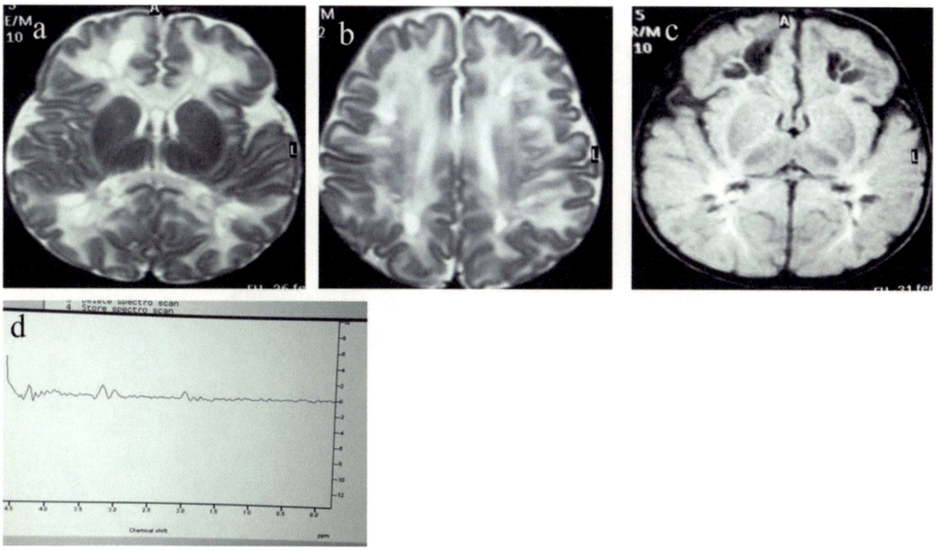

Figure 19.
A three year female showed gait disturbance and mild learning disability a and b: Axial T2W images show wide gyri, destruction of subcortical 'U' fibers at places, rarefaction with cyst formation in B/L periventricular areas, more prominently seen radiating along frontal and occipital horns of B/L lateral ventricles. c: Axial T2W/FLAIR image shows fluid signal in cystic areas WM. d: MR spectroscopy shows significantly reduced NAA, choline and creatinine peaks. Vanishing white matter disease.

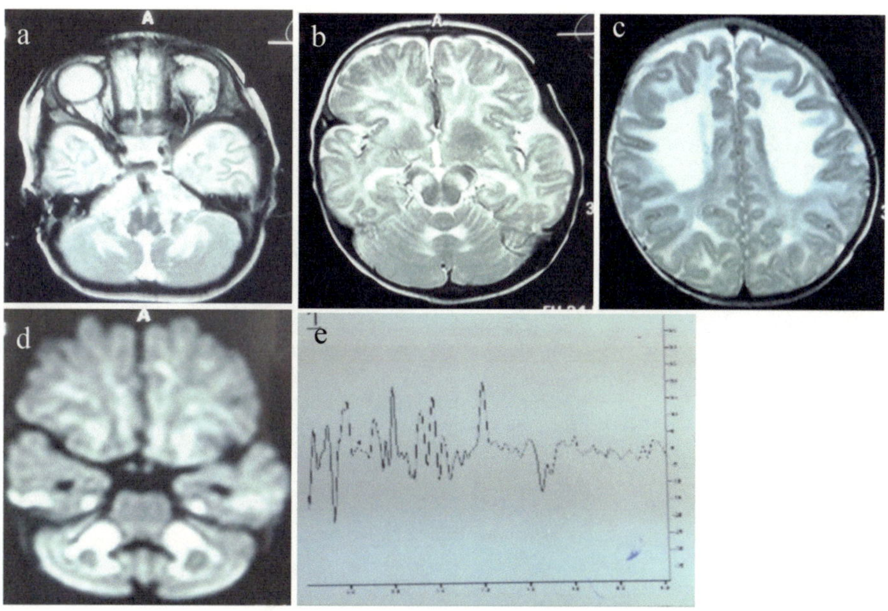

Figure 20.
A six month old male had delayed milestones, nystagmus and seizures. a–c: Axial T2W images at different levels show hyperintensity in B/L dentate nuclei, WM of B/L frontotemporal areas, B/L external capsules and corticospinal tracts in crus cerebri. d: DW image showing diffusion restriction in B/L frontal areas and B/L dentate nuclei. e: MR spectroscopy in normal appearing WM shows lactate peak. Leigh disease.

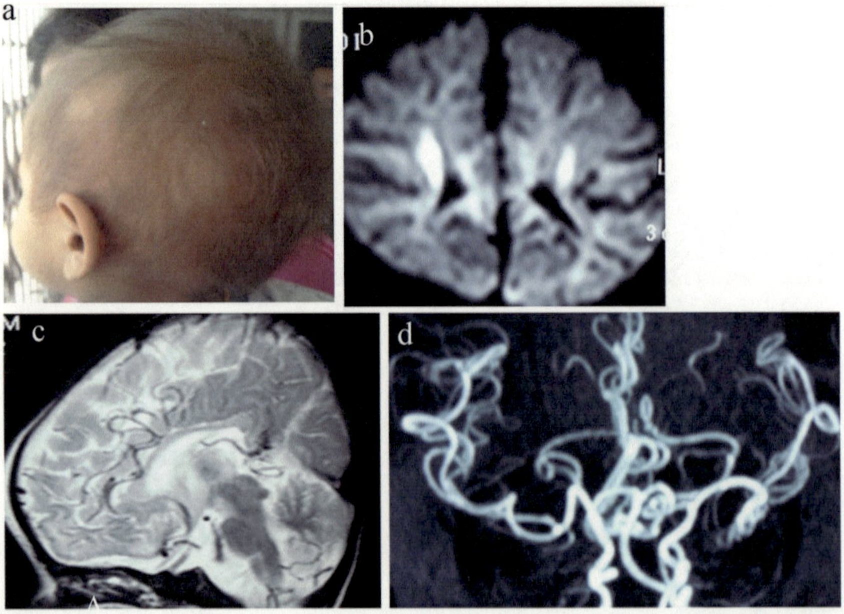

Figure 21.

A six month male child presented with seizure and lethargy. a: Photograph of head showing coarse, dry, lusterless, fragile hair (pili torti). b: DW axial image showing diffusion restriction in B/L periventricular area. c: Sagittal T2W image showing tortuous anterior cerebral arteries. d: Time of flight MR angiogram showing all intracranial arteries and circle of willisto be tortuous. Menkes disease.

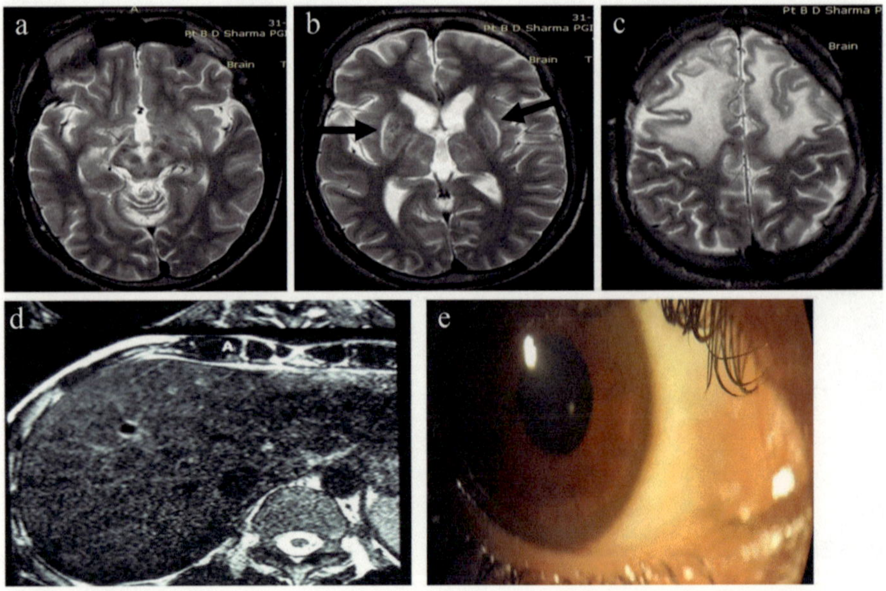

Figure 22.

A five year old boy had dystonia and swallowing difficulties. a: Axial T2W image at the level of midbrain shows 'giant panda face'. b: Axial T2W image at the level of basal ganglia shows necrosis of claustra (arrows) and subtle hyperintensity in B/L basal ganglia and thalmi c: Axial T2W image at higher level shows hyperintensity in WM of B/L frontal areas. d: Axial T2W image of liver shows mixed density of liver suggestive of cirrhosis. e: Slit lamp examination of eyes shows the pathognomonic Kaiser Fleischer ring at the periphery of cornea. Wilson disease.

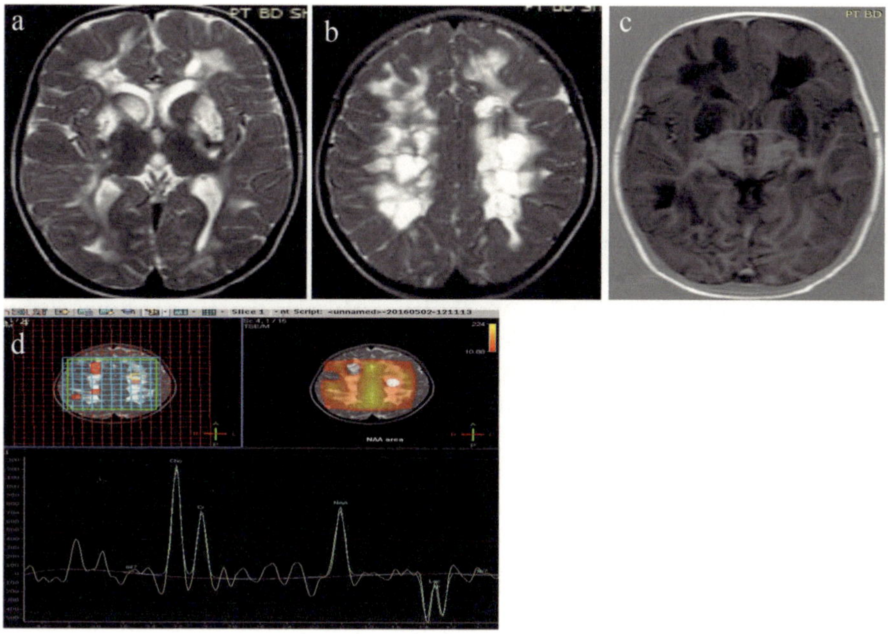

Figure 23.
A 2.5 year old male child had developmental delay, learning disability and myopathy. a and b: Axial T2W images at different levels show hyperintensity along with cyst formation in B/L corpora striata, periventricular area and deep WM. c: Axial T1W image shows the involved areas/cysts to be hypointense. d: MR spectroscopy shows a prominent lactate peak and reduced NAA peak. Mitochondrial leukodystrophy.

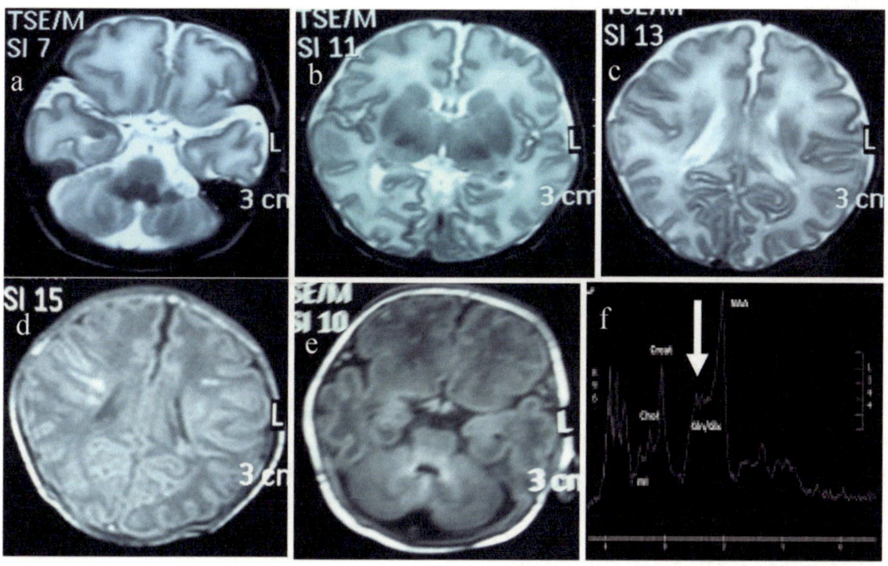

Figure 24.
A 20 days ole neonate presented with lethargy, vomiting, hypotonia, hypothermia, and hyperventilation. a-c: Axial T2W images at different levels show brain swelling and vasogenic edema in B/L frontal and peri-insular areas. d and e: Axial T1W images show hypointensityin same areas. f: MR spectroscopy shows prominent glutamine-glutamate peaks at 2.2–2.4 ppm (arrow). The child had respiratory alkalosis. Blood ammonia level was elevated. A diagnosis of urea cycle disorders was made.

5. Associations

Some inborn errors may coexist, making the picture even more complex. Aminoacidurias may be associated with organic acidemias (e.g., association of homocystinuria with MMA).

6. Biochemical investigations

Analysis of body fluids (blood, urine, CSF), blood pH, glucose, ammonia, lactic acid, urine ketone bodies, and hepatic profile can help a lot in arriving at a diagnosis. Thrombocytopenia may be seen in organic acidemias like methylmalonic, propionic, and isovaleric acidemias [4]. Ammonia is normal or borderline elevated in maple syrup urine disease, UCDs, and organic acidemias. However, blood pH shows respiratory alkalosis in UCDs and metabolic acidosis in organic acidemias. Lactic acidosis with hypoglycemia is seen in HMG CoA lyase deficiency [52], some subtypes of 3-methylglutaconic acidemia, glutaric aciduria type 2, and medium and long chain fatty acid oxidation disorders. Oxidative phosphorylation diseases like primary lactic acidosis show lactic acidosis and normal glucose levels. Different forms of lactic acidosis like pyruvate dehydrogenase deficiency, pyruvate carboxylase deficiency, and cytochrome c oxidase deficiency may be identified with the help of the pyruvate-lactate ratio. Severe metabolic acidosis without lactic acidosis and ketosis is seen in 5-oxoprolinuria. Hypoglycemia is always present in fatty acid oxidation disorders, holocarboxylase synthetase deficiency, and neonatal onset 3-methylglutaconic aciduria and frequent in HMG coenzyme A lyase deficiency and can be seen in pyruvate carboxylase deficiency, propionic, methylmalonic ethylmalonic, and isovaleric acidemias. Fatty acid oxidation defect and HMG coenzyme A lyase deficiency show nonketotic hypoglycemia. Persistent hyperinsulinemic hypoglycemia in newborns of diabetic mothers and patients on insulin treatment may present as nonketotic hypoglycemia. Ketotic hypoglycemia can be seen in defects of gluconeogenesis, glycogenolysis, organic acidemias (isovaleric, propionic, and methylmalonic acidemia), galactossemia, and fructosemia. It may also be found in sepsis, adrenal insufficiency, dehydration, and acute GIT problems (vomiting, diarrhea). Hypoglycemia is never seen in beta-ketothiolase deficiency, 4-hydroxybutyric aciduria, late onset 3-methylglutaconic aciduria, biotinidase deficiency, glutaric aciduria type 1, and the late onset form of maple syrup urine disease. Diabetic ketoacidosis may be associated with hyperglycemia. Liver disease is seen in fatty acid oxidation and oxidative phosphorylation disorders. High plasma levels of phytanic, pipecolic, and very long chain fatty acids (VLCFA), and bile acid intermediates are common in peroxisomal disorders. CSF examination may be helpful in glutaric aciduria type I, L-2-hydroxyglutaric aciduria, propionic acidemia, methylmalonic acidemia, and certain mitochondrial diseases as the levels of abnormal metabolites in CSF may exceed those in plasma [53].

7. Advanced laboratory methods

Gas chromatography and mass spectroscopy of urine, high pressure liquid chromatography, tandem mass spectroscopy of blood, specific enzyme activity studies of fibroblasts, peripheral blood cell culture, and biopsy specimen are some other methods that can be helpful. PET may be more sensitive than MRI in the early detection of hypometabolism. Phosphorus MRS is particularly helpful in mitochondrial diseases. ^{31}P MRS is very helpful in imaging organic acidurias (especially during metabolic decompensations and monitoring response to therapy) as it can measure in vivo pH. ^{13}C isotope has low abundance in nature. To measure it, carbon MRS requires a high magnetic field strength. A technique referred to as proton observed carbon edited spectroscopy may be implemented on commercially available 1.5 T systems. Various metabolic pathways and their functions may be studied by administering ^{13}C labeled metabolites.

8. Histological diagnosis

Some diseases are amenable to histopathologic diagnosis like peripheral nerve biopsy in MLD and Krabbe disease, muscle biopsy in mitochondrial disorders, and skin, mucosa, or liver biopsy in storage diseases and Wilson disease.

9. Diagnostic pitfalls

It is important to be mindful that one enzyme deficiency may affect other metabolic pathways also, thus complicating the diagnosis. Propionyl coenzyme A inhibits pyruvate dehydrogenase (energy production and gluconeogenesis), N-acetyl-glutamate synthetase (urea cycle), and glycine cleavage system. Hence, propionic acidemia presents with acidosis (metabolic and lactic), hypoglycemia, hyperammonemia, ketosis, and increased glycine level (as also seen in methylmalonic acidemia). Hyperammonemia may erroneously suggest UCD. Because the cofactor of the enzyme is biotin, other enzyme defects related to biotin deficiency (impairment of holocarboxylase synthetase or biotinidase) may cause differential diagnostic problems. Likewise, fatty acid synthesis, gluconeogenesis, and amino acid catabolism are impaired in 3-methyl-crotonyl-glycinuria, leading to diverse presentations [3].

10. Proteomics-based diagnosis

The proteomics approach allows the studying, identification, and quantification of total protein contents of a cell, some of which may act as markers for the disease. Mass Spectroscopy (MS), 2D Electrophoresis, LC-MS-MS, and MALDI-TOF/TOF are major proteomics methods in use. Mass spectroscopy is a promising analytical technique that allows semiquantitative and qualitative assessments of proteins by measuring the mass-to-charge ratio, thus allowing protein sequencing and identification with high sensitivity and accuracy [54]. Mass spectroscopy may allow the analysis and quantification of thousands of proteins in a single go. However, despite substantial advances in sample throughput, sensitivity, specificity, and reproducibility, concerns about the presence of false positive, time, speed, and cost remain. Automation in mass spectrometry made it possible to use this technology for newborn screening. Tandem mass spectrometry (TMS) is a sophisticated proteomic technique whereby two mass spectrometers are made to operate in tandem to analyze, quantify, and determine the structure of proteins. With just a drop of blood, more than 30 disorders may be quickly screened in newborns with no or minimal false positives.

11. Molecular genomic aspects

Whereas the conventional biochemical tests are time consuming, the metabolomics-based tests and procedures compounded with the Systems Medicine approach are more precise to comprehensively address IEMs, many of which are greatly influenced by complex gene-environment interactions [55, 56]. Any genetic disease can be studied at the level of genes/genome/DNA (genomics), RNA (transcriptomics), or proteins (proteomics). Gene sequencing enables to decode base by base information of the genome. The conventional Sanger Sequencing was difficult and cumbersome to perform. Its automation provided a robust, speedy, and cost-effective sequencing solution. Next Generation Sequencing (NGS) is a preferred genome-wide tool for diagnosing genomic imbalances for which there are multiple identifiable molecular targets. It is a massively parallel sequencing technology allowing ultra-high throughput, scalability, and speed.

Whole genome sequencing (WGS), Whole exome sequencing (WES), targeted exome sequencing (TES), and clinical exome sequencing (CES) can be used for comprehensively analyzing entire genomes. WGS provides a high resolution one-to-one viewing of the whole of the bases on the genome, capturing both large and small variants. Tremendous amount of data is generated in a short time, which enables the assembling of novel genomes. Gene expression array, chromosomal microarray analysis (CMA), and the array comparative genome hybridization (array CGH) are whole-genome high resolution diagnostic procedures that enable the detection of genome-wide gene expression profile, deletion and/or duplication of one or more sections of DNA, or detection of large deletions/duplications in the genome. In recent years, all these methods have been used with an attempt to capture the metabolic signatures in several neurometabolic diseases and IEMs [57–59]. Using WGS, single nucleotide variations may be studied to pin point functional variants to find the association of polymorphic genes to diseases, thus allowing predicting disease susceptibility. There may be situations where looking for genetic variations across the entire length of genome might be of potential benefit as the decision to go for a specific customized and personalized treatment would not be possible otherwise in the absence of the desired diagnosis. Because WGS may also cover variants involving InDels, chromosomal rearrangements, copy number variations, as well as the tri-nucleotide expansions, it is considered to be more sensitive.

In situations where the gene product might be of pathological interest, whole exome sequencing (WES) or clinical exome sequencing (CES) may be the preference. WES involves sequencing the protein-coding regions of the genome, which constitutes less than 2% of the genome but contains ~85% of known disease-related variants [60]. It detects variations in the coding regions. WES allows to focus on genes most likely to affect the phenotype. However, DNA variations outside the exons can also affect gene activity and hence phenotype. These variations may be missed by WES but may possibly be detected by combining the DNA and RNA-Seq analyses of specific genes [61]. WES is a cost-effective alternative to WGS where more manageable and analyzable data are produced compared to WGS. CES is used for the detection of exomic variants with known clinical association with a disease and has been gradually recognized as an affordable option as specifically the clinical exome is sequenced and only the variants of plausible clinical relevance are reported.

Alternatively, only the specific region of the genome that is of clinical relevance is sequenced instead of the whole genome. This approach is called targeted sequencing and is better in terms of cost and speed as WGS and WES are prohibitively expensive.

Targeted sequencing enables multiple genes to be assessed across many samples in parallel and generates a focused and manageable amount of data, with a higher coverage allowing accurate identification of rare variants with high sensitivity and specificity. It is ideal for the detection of causative mutations and variants like Single Nucleotide Polymorphisms (SNPs) and InDels across multiple genomic regions with a short turnaround time and high depth. It can also detect copy number variations (CNVs) and the structural variants (SVs). Targeted sequencing allows the identification of variants at low allele frequencies and identifies causative novel or inherited mutations in a single assay. When a set of genes is known to cause a disease, targeted gene panel sequencing (TGPS) is performed. Gene panels are basically collections of genes grouped for the purpose of simultaneous testing of all the genes known to cause a particular disease, syndrome, or phenotype and enable deep sequencing. Although data are only generated for genes on the panel, virtual panels can also be added to WES or WGS-generated data to analyze sequencing information only relevant to the genes in the virtual panel(s). When there are multiple genomic areas of interest, gene panel sequencing is preferred. Focused panels have been devised, which contain a select set of genes or gene regions that are either known to cause a disease or have known or suspected associations with the disease or phenotype under investigation. Since a limited number of genes are included in the gene panel, it limits the number of variants requiring interpretation as well as results in fewer variants of uncertain significance (VUS). Compared to WGS and WES, TGPS allows greater depth and coverage. In the event of using a virtual panel, reanalysis of data in future is possible particularly for the patients in whom no variants were initially found. This is how additional genes associated with a disease can be analyzed for variants over time. Targeted gene panel sequencing has been successfully used for investigating complex neurometabolic phenotypes [62–64]. It, however, is unable to identify novel causative genes as it is limited to only those genes already known to cause the disease. Also, once a gene panel has been devised, it is challenging to add new genes to it. Besides gene panel sequencing is incapable of detecting structural rearrangements or copy number variants.

12. Collaborative multi'omics' approach

Neurometabolic imaging coupled with modern genomics, proteomics, and system medicine tools have revolutionized both the accuracy and precision of diagnosis of IEMs. Molecular imaging further adds to diagnostic accuracy and efficiency. Whereas CT and conventional MR imaging provide mere structural and anatomical details, molecular imaging allows the assessment of fine details of the molecular and cellular interplay of physiological events. Molecular imaging allows the metabolic activity of the affected cells to be directly visualized in vivo [27, 65, 66] and hence may be very useful in planning personalized therapy.

Although INMDs are now being diagnosed at a greater rate and precision owing to advances in next-generation sequencing technology, the pace of their diagnoses still remains slow particularly due to a lack of data on immediate functional significance of an identified variant in terms of uncertainty of its pathogenic effect, the challenges associated with prioritization of variants of unknown significance, or the candidate disease genes for potential differential diagnosis. The 'Phenome' signifies the sum of all the traits and characteristics expressed by a cell. 'Phenomics' is the study of the summation of qualitative and quantitative traits including clinical, biochemical, and imaging characteristics and may be treated as the metabolic fingerprint of a cell. It is about the changes that occur in response to genetic mutation and environmental influences. Combined use of genomics, proteomics and metabolomics may be of immense utility in understanding the metabolic diseases where the causation and connection between the genetic makeup and disease predisposition pose challenges for diagnosis [67]. With improvement in knowledge and technology, the term deep clinical phenotyping is increasingly gaining significance. Phenotyping enables comprehensive characterization of the discrete components of a patient's clinical and biochemical phenotype. The "multiomics" approaches combined with phenomic annotation are increasingly gaining importance for the development of a stronger knowledge base, improvement in diagnostic procedures, and expansion of genomics, epigenomics, and metabolomics data interpretation tools. A cohesive and integrated effort involving state-of-the-art NGS, metabolomics technologies, and in depth clinico-radiological-cellular & molecular phenotyping should definitely prove valuable for developing newer diagnostic modalities for the diseases that otherwise remain difficult to diagnose at present due to their inherent complexity [68, 69].

13. Relevance

The phenotypical complexities often lead to delay or underdiagnosis of INMDs. Even after diagnosis, the prognosis is mostly guarded. This has led to a comparative lack of interest in such patients and hence slow progress in this field. This is also evident from the fact that most of the literature that we can refer to is quite old. In view of guarded prognosis, genetic counseling, early diagnosis, and preventive strategies are as important as ever in management. With more precise and early diagnosis, prognosis and quality of life in some of the diseases has improved. Early diagnosis can take the form of antenatal or postnatal screening/diagnosis. Deficient enzyme activity can be demonstrated in cultured amniocytes and chorionic villous samples as in propionic acidemia, UCDs, or Menke disease. Prenatal US and MRI may suggest diseases such as Zellweger disease, glutaric aciduria type 1, and nonketotic hyperglycinemia. Tandem mass spectroscopy (TMS) in neonatal urine and blood samples can screen for glutaric aciduria type I, classical phenylketonuria, homocystinuria, tyrosinemia, and histidinemia [70]. This preclinical screening can help in early intervention, leading to possible prevention or minimizing of the effects of the disease. Single gene testing may be done in cases where MRI is almost diagnostic. Suggestive MRI patterns may point to a disease category where a particular gene panel can be analyzed.

Some INMDs are incompatible with life, and even early diagnosis does not help in such cases. Few examples being neonatal peroxisomal disorders, severe forms of propionic acidemia, and maple syrup urine disease. Dietary control and/or supplementation may help others. Biotin supplementation may prevent irreversible brain damage in 3-methyl-crotonyl-glycinuria. High protein intake may aggravate UCDs. Bone marrow transplantation may be helpful in MLD, Krabbe disease, and some mucopolysaccharidoses [71]. It works well in MLD in early stages (preferably before symptoms appear) but can work even late in Krabbe disease, even reversing some symptoms. The transplantation of umbilical cord blood stem cells from unrelated donors before the onset of symptoms in Krabbe disease may help improve the outcome [72]. There can be various approaches for removing enzyme-related defects—restoration of a minimal enzymatic activity/enzyme substitution for achieving the optimal metabolic function, limiting or lessening of the accumulation of toxic substrates, or substitution of the deficient product. The mutated genes may be repaired or replaced with the normal copy of genes to allow the cell to resynthesize the normal protein. Intervention may be done at a metabolite level in order to regulate the metabolic flux [73]. Given the accessibility to the newer genomics, proteomics, and metabolomics tools and the issues of affordability, efficacy, and safety with the new therapeutic options, gene- and cell-based therapies [74–76] and fetal neuronal transplants [77] may prove successful in treating INMDs. Transplantation of kidney, liver or both is an option to manage late systemic complications of some diseases like Wilson disease or MMA.

This is just a glimpse of now available management options of INMDs to emphasize the role and relevance of early and proper diagnosis. Detailed description of treatment options is outside the scope of the present chapter.

14. Conclusion

Though properly diagnosing IEM is a challenge, an integrated structured approach taking into account the age and type of presentation, clinical features, odor, skin stigmata, imaging (both conventional and molecular imaging), biochemistry, histology, metabolomics (including genomics, transcriptomics and proteomics), and phenomics should pave the way for early diagnosis and new therapeutic regimens to effectively treat inborn neurometabolic disorders [78].

Author details

Seema Rohilla[1*], Vikas[1], Yamini Wadhwa[1], Deepak Singla[1] and Dhara B. Dhaulakhandi[2]

1 Department of Radiodiagnosis, Pt. B. D. Sharma Postgraduate Institute of Medical Sciences, Rohtak, Haryana, India

2 Department of Biotechnology and Molecular Medicine, Pt. B. D. Sharma Postgraduate Institute of Medical Sciences, Rohtak, Haryana, India

*Address all correspondence to: seemarohilla@yahoo.co.in

References

[1] Ortigoza-Escobar JD. A proposed diagnostic algorithm for inborn errors of metabolism presenting with movements disorders. Frontiers in Neurology. 2020;**11**:582160. DOI: 10.3389/fneur.2020.582160

[2] Navarrete R, Leal F, Vega AI, Morais-López A, Garcia-Silva MT, MartínHernández E, et al. Value of genetic analysis for confirming inborn errors of metabolism detected through the spanish neonatal screening program. European Journal of Human Genetics. 2019;**27**(4):556-562. DOI: 10.1038/s41431-018-0330-0

[3] Yoon HJ, Kim JH, Jeon TY, Yoo SY, Eo H. Devastating metabolic brain disorders of newborns and young infants. Radiographics. 2014;**34**(5):1257-1272. DOI: 10.1148/rg.345130095

[4] Fischer AQ, Challa VR, Burton BK, McLean WT. Cerebellar hemorrhage complicating isovaleric acidemia: A case report. Neurology. 1981;**31**(6):746-748. DOI: 10.1212/wnl.31.6.746

[5] Shigematsu Y, Mori I, Nakai A, Kikawa Y, Kuriyama M, Konishi Y, et al. Acute infantile hemiplegia in a patient with propionic acidemia. European Journal of Pediatrics. 1990;**149**(9):659-660. DOI: 10.1007/BF02034758

[6] Ruano MM, Castillo M, Thompson JE. MR imaging in a patient with homocystinuria. American Journal of Roentgenology. 1998;**171**:1147-1149

[7] Mamourian AC, du Plessis A. Urea cycle defect: A case with MR and CT findings resembling infarct. Pediatric Radiology. 1991;**21**(8):594-595. DOI: 10.1007/BF02012608

[8] Thompson JE, Smith M, Castillo M, Barrow M, Mukherji SK. MR in children with L-carnitine deficiency. American Journal of Neuroradiology. 1996;**17**(8):1585-1588

[9] Sperl W, Felber S, Skladal D, Wermuth B. Metabolic stroke in carbamyl phosphate synthetase deficiency. Neuropediatrics. 1997;**28**(4):229-234. DOI: 10.1055/s-2007-973705

[10] Steen C, Baungartner ER, Duran M, Lehnert W, Suormala T, Fingerhut SR, et al. A metabolic stroke in isolated 3-methylcrotonyl-CoA carboxylase deficiency. European Journal of Pediatrics. 1999;**158**(9):730-733. DOI: 10.1007/s004310051189

[11] Mize C, Johnson JL, Rajagopalan KV. Defective molybdopterin biosynthesis: Clinical heterogeneity associated with molybdenum cofactor deficiency. Journal of Inherited Metabolic Disease. 1995;**18**(3):283-290. DOI: 10.1007/BF00710416

[12] Van Geet C, Jaeken J. A unique pattern of coagulation abnormalities in carbohydrate- deficient glycoprotein syndrome. Pediatric Research. 1993;**33**(5):540-541. DOI: 10.1203/00006450-199305000-00024

[13] Hoon AH, Reinhardt EM, Kelley RI, Breiter SN, Morton H, Naidu S, et al. Brain magnetic resonance imaging in suspected extrapyramidal cerebral palsy: Observations in distinguishing genetic-metabolic from acquired causes. The Journal of Pediatrics. 1997;**131**(2):240-245. DOI: 10.1016/s0022-3476(97)70160-4

[14] Garcia-Cazorla A, Ortez C, Pérez-Dueñas B, Serrano M, Pineda M,

Campistol J, et al. Hypokinetic-rigid syndrome in children and inborn errors of metabolism. European Journal of Paediatric Neurology. 2011;**15**(4):295-302. DOI: 10.1016/j.ejpn.2011.04.013

[15] Kurian M, McNeill A, Lin JP, Maher ER. Childhood disorders of neurodegeneration with brain iron accumulation (NBIA). Developmental Medicine and Child Neurology. 2011;**53**:394-404. DOI: 10.1111/j.1469-8749.2011.03955.x

[16] Pierson TM, Adams D, Bonn F, Martinelli P, Cherukuri PF, Teer JK, et al. Whole-exome sequencing identifies homozygous aFG3L2 mutations in a spastic ataxia-neuropathy syndrome linked to mitochondrial m-AAA proteases. PLoS Genetics. 2011;**7**(10):e1002325. DOI: 10.1371/journal.pgen.1002325

[17] Poggi-Travert F, Fournier B, Poll-The BT, Saudubray JM. Clinical approach to inherited peroxisomal disorders. Journal of Inherited Metabolic Disease. 1995;**18**(Suppl 1):1-18. DOI: 10.1007/BF00711425

[18] Estrov Y, Scaglia F, Bodamer OA. Psychiatric symptoms of inherited metabolic disease. Journal of Inherited Metabolic Disease. 2000;**23**(1):2-6. DOI: 10.1023/a:1005685010766

[19] Al Essa M, Rahbeeni Z, Jumaah S, Joshi S, Al Jishi E, Rashed MS, et al. Infectious complications of propionic acidemia in Saudi Arabia. Clinical Genetics. 1998;**54**(1):90-94. DOI: 10.1111/j.1399-0004.1998.tb03702.x

[20] Ozand PT, Rashed M, Millington DS, Sakati N, Hazzaa S, Rahbeeni Z, et al. Ethylmalonic aciduria: An organic acidemia with CNS involvement and vasculopathy. Brain & Development. 1994;**16**(Suppl):12-22

[21] Kahler SG, Sherwood WG, Woolf D, Lawless ST, Zaritsky A, Bonham J, et al. Pancreatitis in patients with organic acidemias (comment). The Journal of Pediatrics. 1994;**124**(2):239-243. DOI: 10.1016/s0022-3476(94)70311-6

[22] Simon P, Weiss FU, Zimmer KP, Koch HG, Lerch MM. Acute and chronic pancreatitis in patients with inborn errors of metabolism. Pancreatology. 2001;**1**(5):448-456. DOI: 10.1159/000055846

[23] Brusilow S, Horwich A. Urea cycle enzymes. In: Scriver CR, Beaudet AL, Sly WS, Valle D, Childs B, Kinzler KW, et al., editors. The Metabolic and Molecular Bases of Inherited Disease. 8th ed. New York: McGraw-Hill; 2001. pp. 1909-1963. Chapter 85

[24] Edwards MC, Johnson JL, Marriage B, Graf TN, Coyne KE, Rajagopalan KV, et al. Isolated sulfite oxidase deficiency: Review of two cases in one family. Ophthalmology. 1999;**106**(10):1957-1961. DOI: 10.1016/S0161-6420(99)90408-6

[25] Johnston MV, Hoon AH Jr. Possible mechanisms in infants for selective basal ganglia damage from asphyxia, kernicterus, or mitochondrial encephalopathies. Journal of Child Neurology. 2000;**15**(9):588-591. DOI: 10.1177/088307380001500904

[26] Ho VB, Fitz CR, Chuang SH, Geyer CA. Bilateral basal ganglia lesions: Pediatric differential considerations. Radiographics. 1993;**13**(2):269-292. DOI: 10.1148/radiographics.13.2.8460220

[27] Lai LM, Gropman AL, Whitehead MT. MR Neuroimaging in pediatric inborn errors of metabolism. Diagnostics. 2022;**12**(4). DOI: 861, 10.3390/diagnostics12040861

[28] de Oliveira AM, Paulino MV, Vieira APF, McKinney AM, da Rocha AJ, dos Santos GT, et al. Imaging patterns of toxic and metabolic brain disorders. Radiographics. 2019;**39**(6):1672-1695. DOI: 10.1148/rg.2019190016

[29] Poretti A, Blaser SI, Lequin MH, Fatemi A, Meoded A, Northington FJ, et al. Neonatal neuroimaging findings in inborn errors of metabolism. Journal of Magnetic Resonance Imaging. 2013;**37**(2):294-312. DOI: 10.1002/jmri.23693

[30] Hao M, Zhang Y, Hou S, Chen Y, Shi M, Zhao G, et al. Spinal cord demyelination combined with hyperhomocysteinemia: A case report. Neuropsychiatric Disease and Treatment. 2014;**10**:2057-2059. DOI: 10.2147/NDT.S70963

[31] Song SK, Sun SW, Ramsbottom MJ, Chang C, Russell J, Cross AH. Dysmyleination revealed through MRI as increased radial (but unchanged axial) diffusion of water. NeuroImage. 2002;**17**(3):1429-1436. DOI: 10.1006/nimg.2002.1267

[32] van der Knaap MS, Valk J, de Neeling N, Nauta JJ. Pattern recognition in magnetic resonance imaging of white matter disorders in children and young adults. Neuroradiology. 1991;**33**(6):478-493. DOI: 10.1007/BF00588038

[33] Vasconcellos E, Smith M. MRI nerve root enhancement in Krabbe disease. Pediatric Neurology. 1998;**19**(2):151-152. DOI: 10.1016/s0887-8994(98)00033-2

[34] van de Knap MS, van der Voorn P, Barkhof F, van Coster R, Krageloh-Mann I, Feigenbaum A, et al. A new leukoencephalopathy with brainstem and spinal cord involvement with high lactate. Annals of Neurology. 2003;**53**(2):252-258. DOI: 10.1002/ana.10456

[35] Osaka H, Kimura S, Nezu A, Yamazaki S, Saitoh K, Yamaguchi S. Chronic subdural hematoma, an initial manifestation of glutaric aciduria type-1. Brain & Development. 1993;**15**(2):125-127. DOI: 10.1016/0387-7604(93)90049-e

[36] Clayton PT, Thompson E. Dysmorphic syndromes with demonstrable biochemical abnormalities. Journal of Medical Genetics. 1988;**25**(7):463-472. DOI: 10.1136/jmg.25.7.463

[37] Russel IM, van Sonderen L, van Straaten HLM, Barth PG. Subependymal germinolytic cysts in Zellweger syndrome. Pediatric Radiology. 1995;**25**(4):254-255. DOI: 10.1007/BF02011090

[38] Kerrigan JF, Aleck KA, Tarby TJ, Bird CR, Heidenreich RA. Fumaric aciduia: Clinical and imaging features. Annals of Neurology. 2000;**47**(5):583-588

[39] Fletcher JM, Bye AME, Nayanar V, Wilcken B. Nonketotic hyperglycinemia presenting as pachygyria. Journal of Inherited Metabolic Disease. 1995;**18**(6):665-668. DOI: 10.1007/BF02436754

[40] Frei KP, Patronas NJ, Crutchfield KE, Altarescu G, Schiffmann R. Mucolipidosis type IV: Characteristic MRI findings. Neurology. 1998;**51**(2):565-569. DOI: 10.1212/wnl.51.2.565

[41] Sonninen P, Autti T, Varho T, Hamalainen M, Raininko R. Brain involvement in Salla disease. American JournalofNeuroradiology.1999;**20**(3):433-443

[42] Kyllerman M, Blomstrand S, Mansson JE, Conradi NG, Hindmarsh T.

Central nervous system malformations and white matter changes in pseudo-neonatal adrenoleukodystrophy. Neuropediatrics. 1990;**21**(4):199-201. DOI: 10.1055/s-2008-1071495

[43] Forstner R, Hoffmann GF, Gassner I, Heideman P, De Klerk JB, Lawrenz-Wolf B, et al. Glutaric aciduria type I: Ultrasonographic demonstration of early signs. Pediatric Radiology. 1999;**29**:138-143

[44] Nowaczyk MJ, Blaser SI, Clarke JT. Central nervous system malformations in ethylmalonic encephalopathy. American Journal of Medical Genetics. 1998;**75**(3):292-296

[45] Escolar ML, Poe MD, Smith JK, Gilmore JH, Kurtzberg J, Lin W, et al. Diffusion tensor imaging detects abnormalities in the corticospinal tracts of neonates with infantile Krabbe disease. American Journal of Neuroradiology. 2009;**30**(5):1017-1021. DOI: 10.3174/ajnr.A1476

[46] Enokizono M, Aida N, Yagishita A, Nakata Y, Ideguchi R, Kurokawa R, et al. Neuroimaging findings of inborn errors of metabolism: Urea cycle disorders, aminoacidopathies, and organic acidopathies. Japanese Journal of Radiology. 2023. DOI: 10.1007/s11604-023-01396-0

[47] van der Knap MS, van der Grond J, van Rijen PC, Faber JA, Valk J, Willemse K. Age-dependent changes in localized proton and phosphorous MR spectroscopy of the brain. Radiology. 1990;**176**(2):509-515. DOI: 10.1148/radiology.176.2.2164237

[48] Wadhwa Y, Rohilla S, Kaushik JS. Cystic leukoencephalopathy in NDUFV1 mutation. Indian Journal of Pediatrics. 2018;**85**(12):1128-1131. DOI: 10.1007/s12098-018-2721-1

[49] Bergman AJ, van der Knap MS, Smeitink JA, Duran M, Dorland L, Valk J, et al. Magnetic resonance imaging and spectroscopy of the brain in propionic acidemia: Clinical and biochemical considerations. Pediatric Research. 1996;**40**(3):404-409. DOI: 10.1203/00006450-199609000-00007

[50] Biswas A, Malhotra M, Mankad K, Carney O, D'Arco F, Muthusamy K, et al. Clinico-radiological phenotyping and diagnostic pathways in childhood neurometabolic disorders—a practical introductory guide. Translational Pediatrics. 2021;**10**(4):1201-1230. DOI: 10.21037/tp-20-335

[51] Reddy N, Calloni SF, Vernon HJ, Boltshauser E, Huisman TAGM, Soares BP. Neuroimaging findings of organic Acidemias and Aminoacidopathies. Radiographics. 2018;**38**(3):912-931. DOI: 10.1148/rg.2018170042

[52] Gibson KM, Breuer J, Kaiser K, Nyhan WL, McCoy EE, Ferreira P, et al. 3-hydroxy-3-methylglutaryl-coenzyme A lyase deficiency: Report of five new patients. Journal of Inherited Metabolic Disease. 1988;**11**:76-87

[53] Hoffmann GF, Meier-Augenstein W, Stockler S, Surtees R, Rating D, Nyhan WL. Physiology and pathophysiology of organic acids in cerebrospinal fluid. Journal of Inherited Metabolic Disease. 1993;**16**(4):648-669. DOI: 10.1007/BF00711898

[54] Clayton PT. Applications of mass spectrometry in the study of inborn errors of metabolism. Journal of Inherited Metabolic Disease. 2001;**24**(2):139-150. DOI: 10.1023/a:1010358715835

[55] JJM J, Broeks MH, Verhoeven-Duif NM. Metabolomics in diagnostics

of inborn metabolic disorders. Current Opinion in Systems Biology. 2022;**29**:100409. DOI: 10.1016/j.coisb.2021.100409

[56] Costanzo M, Zacchia M, Bruno G, Crisci D, Caterino M, Ruoppolo M. Integration of proteomics and metabolomics in exploring genetic and rare metabolic diseases. Kidney Diseases. 2017;**3**(2):66-77. DOI: 10.1159/000477493

[57] Hernandez MA, Schulz R, Chaplin T, Young BD, Perrett D, Champion MP, et al. The diagnosis of inherited metabolic diseases by microarray gene expression profiling. Orphanet Journal of Rare Diseases. 2010;**5**:34. DOI: 10.1186/1750-1172-5-34

[58] Wang J, Zhan H, Li FY, Pursley AN, Schmitt ES, Wong LJ. Targeted array CGH as a valuable molecular diagnostic approach: Experience in the diagnosis of mitochondrial and metabolic disorders. Molecular Genetics and Metabolism. 2012;**106**(2):221-230. DOI: 10.1016/j.ymgme.2012.03.005

[59] Pinheiro MI, Silva C, Lourenço L, Gonçalves D, Dória S, Guardiano M, et al. Array-CGH: Importance in the study of developmental delays in pediatrics. Revue Neurologique. 2020;**71**(5):171-176. DOI: 10.33588/rn.7105.2020211

[60] Gilissen C, Hoischen A, Brunner HG, Veltman JA. Disease gene identification strategies for exome sequencing. European Journal of Human Genetics. 2012;**20**(5):490-497. DOI: 10.1038/ejhg.2011.258

[61] Soriano-Sexto A, Gallego D, Leal F, Castejón-Fernández N, Navarrete R, Alcaide P, et al. Identification of clinical variants beyond the exome in inborn errors of metabolism. International Journal of Molecular Sciences. 2022;**23**(21):12850. DOI: 10.3390/ijms232112850

[62] Reid ES, Papandreou A, Drury S, Boustred C, Yue WW, Wedatilake Y, et al. Advantages and pitfalls of an extended gene panel for investigating complex neurometabolic phenotypes. Brain. 2016;**139**(11):2844-2854. DOI: 10.1093/brain/aww221

[63] Yubero D, Brandi N, Ormazabal A, Garcia-Cazorla À, Pérez-Dueñas B, Campistol J, et al. Targeted next generation sequencing in patients with inborn errors of metabolism. PLoS One. 2016;**11**(5):e0156359 doi.org/10.1371/journal.pone.0156359

[64] Barbosa-Gouveia S, Vázquez-Mosquera ME, González-Vioque E, Álvarez JV, Chans R, Laranjeira F, et al. Utility of gene panels for the diagnosis of inborn errors of metabolism in a metabolic reference Center. Genes (Basel). 2021;**12**(8):1262. DOI: 10.3390/genes12081262

[65] Sharma V, Luker GD, Piwnica-Worms D. Molecular imaging of gene expression and protein function in vivo with PET and SPECT. Journal of Magnetic Resonance Imaging. 2002;**16**(4):336-351. DOI: 10.1002/jmri.10182

[66] Gropman AL, Anderson A. Novel imaging technologies for genetic diagnoses in the inborn errors of metabolism. Journal of Translational Genetics and Genomics. 2020;**4**:429-445. DOI: 10.20517/jtgg.2020.09

[67] Rahman J, Rahman S. The utility of phenomics in diagnosis of inherited metabolic disorders. Clinical Medicine (London, England). 2019;**19**(1):30-36. DOI: 10.7861/clinmedicine.19-1-30

[68] Biswas A, Malhotra M, Mankad K, Carney O, D'rco F, Muthusamy K, et al.

Clinico-radiological phenotyping and diagnostic pathways in childhood neurometabolic disorders—A practical introductory guide. Transl Pediatr. 2021;**10**(4):1201-1230. DOI: 10.21037/tp-20-335

[69] Guéant JL, Feillet F. Inherited metabolic disorders beyond the new generation sequencing era: The need for in-depth cellular and molecular phenotyping. Human Genetics. 2022;**141**(7):1235-1237. DOI: 10.1007/s00439-022-02467-4

[70] Rashed MS, Bucknall MP, Little D, Awad A, Jacob M, Al-Amoudi M, et al. Screening blood spots for inborn errors of metabolism by electrospray tandem mass spectroscopy with a microplate batch process and a computer algorithm for automated flagging of abnormal profiles. Clinical Chemistry. 1997;**43**(7):1129-1141

[71] Peters C, Steward CG. National Marrow Donor Program, international bone marrow transplant registry, working party on inborn errors, European bone marrow transplant group. Hematopoietic cell transplantation for inherited metabolic diseases: An overview of outcomes and practice guidelines. Bone Marrow Transplantation. 2003;**31**(4):229-239. DOI: 10.1038/sj.bmt.1703839

[72] Escolar ML, Poe MD, Provenzale JM, Richards KC, Allison J, Wood S, et al. Transplantation of umbilical-cord blood in babies with infantile Krabbe's disease. The New England Journal of Medicine. 2005;**352**(20):2069-2081. DOI: 10.1056/NEJMoa042604

[73] Fernández-Eulate G, Carreau C, Benoist JF, Lamari F, Rucheton B, Shor N, et al. Diagnostic approach in adult-onset neurometabolic diseases. Journal of Neurology, Neurosurgery, and Psychiatry. 2022;**93**(4):413-421. DOI: 10.1136/jnnp-2021-328045

[74] Willemsen MA, Harting I, Wevers RA. Neurometabolic disorders: Five new things. Neurology: Clinical Practice. 2016;**6**(4):348-357. DOI: 10.1212/CPJ.0000000000000266

[75] Yilmaz BS, Gurung S, Perocheau D, Counsell J, Baruteau J. Gene therapy for inherited metabolic diseases. Journal of Mother and Child. 2020;**24**(2):53-64. DOI: 10.34763/jmotherandchild.20202402si.2004.000009

[76] Ahrens-Nicklas RC. Heal thyself: The promise of autologous hematopoietic stem cell gene therapy in neurometabolic disorders. Molecular Therapy. 2022;**30**(4):1353-1354. DOI: 10.1016/j.ymthe.2022.03.006

[77] Ozand PT, Gascon CG. Treatment of inherited neurometabolic diseases: The future. Journal of Child Neurology. 1992;**7**(Suppl):S132-S140. DOI: 10.1177/08830738920070011711

[78] Ginocchio VM, Brunetti-Pierri N. Progress toward improved therapies for inborn errors of metabolism. Human Molecular Genetics. 2016;**25**(R1):R27-R35. DOI: 10.1093/hmg/ddv418

Section 2

Novel Monitoring Technologies with Neuropediatric Patients

Chapter 3

The Role of Monitoring the Electrical Activity of the Diaphragm in a Comprehensive Assessment of the Effectiveness of Intensive Treatment in Premature Infants with Extremely Low Birth Weight

Aleksei Anurev, Vladimir Gorbachev, Tatiana Pavlova and Alexander Pavlov

Abstract

Premature newborns are patients who need detailed monitoring of vital processes such as respiration, blood circulation, central and peripheral perfusion, and brain activity. From this point of view, the use of modern methods of visualization of respiratory activity, which can be implemented in the NAVA mode, is a very promising solution to this problem. Our study shows that adequate respiratory support not only contributes to the prevention of ventilator-induced diseases but also reduces the duration of ventilation and the length of stay of patients in the intensive care unit. In addition, this study presents a comparative description of some indicators of ventilation parameters such as peak pressure and tidal volume. We also analyzed the values of gas composition of the venous blood during the first three days. The incidence of bronchopulmonary dysplasia, intraventricular hemorrhages and retinopathy depending on the mode, parameters and duration of ventilation in premature newborns with extremely low birth weight was estimated.

Keywords: electrical activity of the diaphragm, premature newborns, extremely low birth weight, bronchopulmonary dysplasia, intraventricular hemorrhages, retinopathy

1. Introduction

Adequate monitoring of vital functions in preterm infants in the intensive care unit (ICU) is an urgent and quite complicated problem. To get a more complete picture of the severity of child's condition, the dynamics of the disease and possible outcomes doctors often have to analyze large amounts of information. This implies the study of the maternal history with clarification of somatic or obstetric pathology, interpretation of the results of laboratory and instrumental studies, probing of prescription sheets, which, together with "paper" work, leaves practically no time for direct "communication" with the patient. A substantial problem in the neonatal ICU is lack of objective methods of monitoring the vital functions. Routine measurement of venous blood saturation, heart rate and blood pressure does not adequately assess the severity of the child's condition and the effectiveness of newly prescribed cardiotonic therapy or the correction of mechanical ventilation (MV) parameters, especially in patients with extremely low body weight (ELBW). Therefore, the doctor has to rely on his own knowledge and experience. In this regard, key points in the progression of the disease may be missed, so it becomes much more difficult to provide quality care to the child. Currently, there is no specialized equipment adapted for this category of patients, which would allow for a combined assessment of the child's condition, taking into account his neurological deficit, the state of systemic hemodynamics, and the severity of respiratory failure. That is why the issue of using neuromonitoring of the electrical activity of the diaphragm (Edi) of the patient treated in the ICU and requiring MV is extremely promising and interesting.

1.1 Development of the nervous system in a newborn

For a more complete understanding of the principles of action of various aspects of intensive care, whether it is respiratory or cardiotonic support, it is necessary to understand in detail the anatomy and physiology of the respiratory and cardiovascular systems of the premature newborn. The development of the central nervous system (CNS) begins early in utero and continues into the postnatal period. The human brain undergoes slow development from embryonic conception to early adulthood, this being preceded by many events occurring in a strictly limited sequence [1]. The brain develops from the neuroectoderm in the neural plate on the dorsal side of the embryo. Brain stem cells temporarily proliferate with the formation of neurons and glial cells [2]. During pregnancy, the brain undergoes gradual development of various sections, while the central part is formed first and then the peripheral one: proliferative zones (ventricular and subventricular zones), intermediate zone, future white matter (WM), sublamina, cortical plate (future cortex) and marginal zone [3]. Proliferation and migration of neurons predominate in the first trimester of pregnancy, while growth of axons and dendrites occurs mainly in the second and third trimesters. Subsequently, the phenomena of advanced maturation with the mechanisms of synaptogenesis and myelination, neurochemical maturation are observed. At the macroscopic level, intensive brain growth is observed in the last trimester of pregnancy and in the first two years of postnatal period with a significant increase in gray matter volumes and WM [4]. Cortical volume increases from ~10 to ~150 cm^3 between 18 and 39 weeks of gestational age and from 200 to 600 cm^3 between 1 and 24 months of postnatal age [5]. It is mainly based on an exponential increase in the surface area of the cortex: from ~150 cm^2 at 27 weeks and ~2000 cm^2 at 1 and 24 months after birth, respectively [6]. This is accompanied by the complication of brain morphology and the formation of convolutions, primary, secondary, and tertiary sulci from 20, 32, and 40 weeks of gestational age [7]. These intense macroscopic changes in volume, surface area and folding are probably visible markers of changes in the microstructure of the cortical plate (the future cortex), which develops by different mechanisms in the preterm and postterm periods. Following the migration of neurons the number of interneuronal connections increases, synaptogenesis actively develops, and the structure of the dendritic tree grows and becomes more complex. In parallel, myelination of intracortical fibers begins, mainly in the early postpartum period. These mechanisms of connection growth, synapse development, and myelination occur at different time periods depending on cortical areas [8]. If we talk about the timing of myelination of specific nerves it should be noted that more primitive, unmyelinated nerve fibers mature first. It is mainly the vagus nerve, which is the first autonomic branch and does not have significant functions before the birth period. [9]. It is followed by the development of the sympathetic department of the nervous system, which develops steadily throughout the prenatal period. [10]. Fetus in utero and preterm infants have natural variability in sympathetic tone, in contrast to parasympathetic tone, which plays an important role in the control of heart rate and blood pressure. On the other hand, the parasympathetic division of the CNS represented by the vagus nerve develops later. The parasympathetic division has little effect until 25–30 weeks of gestation. And at 37–38 weeks there is a sharp increase in the tone of the vagus nerve [11]. Under conditions of intrauterine stress and hypoxia, primitive unmyelinated vagus nerve systems contribute to bradycardia due to imperfect autoregulation [12]. The sucking reflex appears at the 16th week of fetal development, the sucking/swallowing coordination occurs at the 32–34th week of pregnancy, and the interaction of sucking/swallowing with the act of breathing appears only by the end of the 37th week of pregnancy and later. These processes require the involvement of many neuronal signals, including afferent and efferent fibers of the cranial nerves (IV, V, VII, IX, X, XII), nuclei of the inferior medulla oblongata, and motor cortical circuits [13]. Violations in these areas lead to the inability to suck, swallow and breathe. Nervous system symptoms include impaired growth and development of the brain, which are prominent in a variety of emotional, cognitive, motor and social skills. Early assessment and diagnosis of typical signs of developmental anomalies is critical for effective intervention aimed at speedy treatment and minimization of neurological and functional deficits [14]. Otherwise, the disease may progress and result in disability and in some cases death of the child.

In the structure of early neonatal mortality, cerebral injuries occupy a leading place, and, as a rule, they are the result of preterm birth. Brain damage occurs both in the early neonatal and late postnatal periods. Research on neurological diseases in premature babies began in the 1970s. Both experimentally and clinically, a correlation has been found between visualization of cerebral injury and functional outcomes. Since then, much more information has been obtained on the pathophysiology of early brain injury [15]. The most significant acquired brain diseases in preterm infants are periventricular hemorrhages (PVH) and diffuse white matter injury (WMI). The diagnosis of PVH is confirmed by ultrasound examination of the head at the patient's bedside. For a more complete picture of the nature of brain damage, classifications have been proposed that identify the severity of ischemia and hemorrhage. The most commonly used classifications are Volpe, Papile, Levene, Sarnat, and others. PVH occurs when the fragile vascular network of the germinal matrix (GM) is damaged, at the site where neurons and glial cells are formed. In humans, GM begins to involute around the 28th week of pregnancy and almost completely disappears by the time of birth. The predisposing factors of PVH include the immaturity of the vascular wall of the GM, the dependence of cerebral blood flow on the systemic one, and hemodynamic disorders in premature infants, especially in children with ELBW [16].

In more than 90% of cases, PVH occurs within the first 3 days after birth, when hemodynamic restructuring occurs, and the immature cardiovascular system is maladjusted [17]. Another form of brain damage in preterm infants is white matter damage, with periventricular leukomalacia (PVL) being the main and best known finding. PVL is a focal periventricular necrosis associated with diffuse reactive gliosis and microglial activation in the surrounding white matter [18]. Banker and Larroche were the first to describe cerebral injury in detail and associated it with cardiorespiratory changes and cerebral ischemia [19]. More recently, the neuropathology of WMI was developed by Volpe et al. and received the name "encephalopathy of prematurity", consisting of a primary destructive disease (acute cell death) and secondary disorders of maturation and trophism, causing insufficiency of differentiation and hypomyelination [20]. It is generally accepted that the main initiating pathogenetic mechanisms of PVL are ischemia and inflammation, and further WMI occur as a result of myelination deficiency and disruption of communication with the CNS pathways. Inflammation leads to microglial activation, free radical attack, and excitotoxicity [21]. Evidence for an association of brain injury caused by hemorrhagic infarction and WMI with poor neurodevelopmental outcomes has been confirmed by neuroimaging and in cohorts around the world. As a rule, cerebral deficiency is manifested by movement disorders, changes in cognition and behavior, deafness and blindness. These manifestations may persist in adult survivors [22].

1.2 Pain and phrenic nerve in premature newborns

Before 1980, there was a long-standing misconception that newborns did not experience pain. However, recent studies have shown that newborns not only experience pain but they are hypersensitive to painful stimuli due to their immature nervous system. The lack of treatment of pain in the neonatal period can lead to negative long-term consequences [23]. Knowledge about pain in newborns has increased dramatically over the past three decades. It is well known that neonates can detect, process and respond to noxious stimuli [24]. Extremely preterm infants are even more hypersensitive to pain due to immature pain suppression mechanisms at birth [25]. Excessive and prolonged painful phenomena in newborns have an adverse effect on all organs and systems, and therefore can be potentially life-threatening [26]. Another problem is determined by inadequate and inconsistent treatment of pain syndrome in newborns. In particular, this applies to the implementation of invasive procedures and care. Despite the fact that neonatology is a progressive science, research on pain in preterm infants is extremely lacking. In 2015, an Oxford research team found evidence that children experience pain in the same way as adults do. MRI scans of ten infants and adults were compared in the presence of a painful stimulus. The results showed that 18 of the 20 brain regions active in adults experiencing pain are also active in newborns. The brain of infants showed the same level of response as in adults, when exposed to a stimulus four times weaker [27]. These results directly contradict the common belief that newborns are unable to perceive pain [28]. At the same time, there were hypotheses confirming this statement. Newborns were thought to be unable to interpret pain due to their inability to create memories. Combined with fears of the side effects of anesthesia, neonatologists performed surgeries such as circumcision without anesthesia until the 1990s [29].

The question of whether term and preterm infants have the necessary anatomy and physiology to sense and respond to pain has been of concern to many researchers. The ability to feel pain occurs at key stages in the development of the nervous system. At the beginning, nociceptors, which perceive a painful stimulus, are involved in the formation of pain reaction. Then they transmit information to the cells surrounding the nociceptors, chemicals are released, which, in turn, act on pain stimuli. In the presence of pain stimuli, the nociceptor transforms the pain signal into an impulse that propagates along the cluster of neurons to the dorsal horns, where sensory information arrives [30]. At this point, the impulse splits: one returns to the original site of pain to trigger a reflex response, the other reaches the thalamus. The thalamus localizes pain and the brain forms information about the nature of pain and how it can be prevented [31]. Each stage of the nociceptive pain pathway corresponds to a specific phase of embryonic development. By the seventh week of pregnancy, nociceptive nerve endings begin to develop around the mouth. And by the 20th week, nociceptive development is completed around the mucous membranes of the body and extremities [32]. However, without any connection to the spine, nociceptor signals are not active and have limited utility. The interaction between nociceptive nerve endings and the posterior horn begins at the 13th week and becomes functional by the 30th week. During this period, the fetus is able to respond to painful stimuli. Cortical pain perception develops after the 24th week of gestation, when the thalamic pathway completes its connection to the dorsal horns. In short, the neonate will be able to localize pain and make reflex movements to try to avoid it after 24 weeks, thus completing the nociceptive pain pathway [33]. Another important component of the pain pathway is the myelin sheath and its role in pain modulation. The myelin sheath acts as an electrical insulator, increasing the speed of signal travel from the peripheral to the central nervous system. Myelination develops after 25 weeks of pregnancy and is completed by the 37th week [34]. Pain modulation is also critical in pain management. Descending signaling pathways exit to the posterior horn, where pain transmission is halted by release of endogenous opioids or activation of inhibitory pathways. However, both of these mechanisms are much more common in adults than in neonates [35]. Thus, in premature infants, the pain threshold is 30–50% lower than in adults, so they have a lower pain tolerance. Subsequent, fatal and recurring painful phenomena have a negative impact on the structures of the brain and the body as a whole. Moreover, they can be life-threatening and have long-term cumulative effects, including altered neurobehavioral development [36].

Another nerve that is of great importance in the intranatal and early postnatal period in newborns is the phrenic nerve. It is the largest nerve of the cervical plexus and is a mixed motor and sensory nerve that originates from the C3–C5 spinal nerves in the neck. The nerve plays a key role in the act of breathing because it provides exclusive motor control of the diaphragm. Any damage at the C4 level or higher can lead to disruption of the connection between the respiratory centers of the brain and the diaphragm. From this point of view, the impact on the phrenic nerve is considered promising in the treatment of cervical injuries and high spinal blocks. Dysfunction of the phrenic nerve plays an important role in the development of respiratory failure in newborns. Because preterm infants, especially those with ELBW, have an underactive peripheral nervous system, they are extremely susceptible to poor phrenic nerve-diaphragm interaction. A similar problem is faced by newborns who have been on MV for a long time. In this case, the main cause is atrophy and secondary weakness of the muscles involved in breathing (including the diaphragm). And, finally, the third category of patients is children with severe neurological deficits, usually of central origin. Thus, all patients are united by one problem—a violation of adequate interaction between the central, peripheral nervous system and the diaphragm. What has been suggested to solve this problem? The first reports of effects on the phrenic nerve appeared in 1976 in patients with tetraplegia [37]. By applying an electrical current to the phrenic nerve, it was possible to cause the diaphragm to contract and thus initiate inspiration. Theoretically, this technique has been known for a long time but the technology that allows stimulation of the phrenic nerve as an alternative to mechanical positive pressure ventilation has existed for only four decades [38]. Establishing phrenic nerve stimulation consists of several steps. The patient's phrenic nerve and diaphragm must first be assessed to ensure they are interacting and contracting sufficiently to provide adequate airflow. This is done by applying an external current to a transcutaneous nerve in the neck to measure diaphragmatic contraction, and is confirmed by X-ray or ultrasound. If sufficient contraction is demonstrated radioelectrodes are surgically implanted bilaterally and placed directly on the phrenic nerve, and the radio receiver is placed subcutaneously on the chest or abdomen [39, 40]. After that, the technique of endoscopic access to the phrenic nerve appeared. However, both the first and second technologies are accompanied by the invasiveness of the intervention, significant pain syndrome, the need for anesthesia, and the risk of infectious complications. Therefore, these methods are not used in infants. Attempts to treat the phrenic nerve percutaneously in neonates have proved painful and potentially dangerous [41]. From this point of view, the use of NAVA ventilation is not only a painless option for maintaining breathing, but also quite effective in terms of restoring connections between the peripheral nervous system and the diaphragm in extremely immature children. Another key reason for the need for MV in preterm infants is significant lung damage. With the development of neonatal medicine and intensive care, the concepts and methods of treating respiratory diseases in newborns are constantly changing. However, the goal is the same—to minimize lung damage and reduce the incidence of respiratory support related illnesses.

1.3 The negative impact of MV and the development of ventilator-induced diseases in infants

Respiratory distress syndrome (RDS) is a major cause of respiratory failure in preterm infants due to immature lung tissue and surfactant deficiency. This problem does not lose its relevance since the strategies for protecting the lung tissue are not fully understood, although it has been determined that exogenous surfactant therapy, the use of non-invasive ventilation and various ventilation modes to prevent intubation significantly reduce the risks of ventilation-induced lung damage (VILD) and associated diseases [42]. When ventilating the lungs, it is necessary to control the duration of respiratory support, oxygenation targets and peak pressure values. These principles must be followed from the first hours after birth until the moment of extubation. Among conventional ventilation modes, there is strong evidence that volume-triggered ventilation is superior to pressure-limited ventilation. This ventilation reduces the risk of bronchopulmonary dysplasia (BPD), death, and improves long-term outcomes [43]. In addition to BPD, premature infants may suffer from chronic respiratory diseases that prevent them from enduring heavy loads even in adolescence and adulthood [44]. Other complications of ventilation include intracerebral hemorrhages, which often end in cerebral palsy, and retinopathy of prematurity (RP), which ends in blindness [45]. The development of these diseases directly depends on the oxygen concentration in the inhaled mixture, since hyperoxia leads to the development of reactive oxygen species and triggers the process of aseptic inflammation in the corresponding organs [46]. On the other hand, hypoxia increases morbidity and mortality [47]. Thus, saturation level is decisive in clinical practice for correcting the oxygen concentration in the inhaled mixture. This is the ventilation parameter that doctors most often have to change when performing lung ventilation. It should be noted that ventilation is an important aspect of patient care in the intensive care unit especially when it comes to preterm infants. While in past years the main concept of ventilation in newborns was the absence of spontaneous breathing, now it is considered necessary to use modes that promote the preservation of spontaneous breathing and reduce VILD [48]. These include: synchronized intermittent mandatory ventilation (SIMV), assisted controlled ventilation (A/C), and pressure support ventilation (PSV) [49]. In these modes, the start of inspiration is determined by the child's inspiratory effort, while in A/C mode, all inspiratory attempts that exceed the critical trigger level are supported. In SIMV mode, the ventilator maintains a certain number of breaths set by the doctor, and in the pauses between "hardware" breaths, the patient can breathe on his own. Inspiration occurs when the child's respiratory activity exceeds the trigger value of flow or pressure, i.e. the patient must create a sufficient change in pressure or flow to induce ventilator support [50]. PSV is a widely used ventilator assist mode, especially during weaning. Although it has proven its value in some clinical conditions, not all of its parameters change depending on the needs of the patient [51]. Using these modes, the doctor arbitrarily sets the values of the peak pressure (PIP) that is supplied to the child, regardless of his needs. Not infrequently, this leads to excess tidal volume, damage to the alveoli and the occurrence of complications. It became possible to reduce the risks of ventilatory complications due to the use of the guaranteed volume (VG) function, which allows you to control the tidal volume [52]. The significance of the effect of tidal volume on the development of complications during MV was proved in the course of a randomized controlled trial, in which two ventilation strategies were evaluated: the first—MV with a high tidal volume (12 ml/kg), the second—with a low tidal volume (6 ml/kg) in adult patients with acute lung injury. The study was terminated prematurely when an interim analysis revealed a significant reduction in mortality and ventilation duration in the low tidal volume group [53]. The use of adequate tidal volume improves stability and reduces lung damage. In addition, limiting rapid changes in arterial carbon dioxide partial pressure by maintaining stable minute ventilation can stabilize cerebral perfusion and reduce brain damage [54]. Despite the constant efforts of doctors to improve the quality of respiratory support using modern ventilation regimens, 40% of children under 28 weeks of age develop BPD [55]. Respiratory therapy strategies for BPD aim to prevent alveolar overexpansion and damage and include avoiding endotracheal intubation when possible, use of non-invasive positive end-expiratory pressure (PEEP) ventilation, and timely administration of surfactant [56]. When a newborn requires endotracheal intubation and MV, it is advisable to use minimal parameters, adhere to permissive hypercapnia, and think about extubation as early as possible [57]. The problem of finding the optimal ventilation mode in children with ELBW and very low birth weight (VLBW) contributed to the introduction of NAVA ventilation into practice. NAVA is a MV mode that initiates inspiration at the same time as the infant attempts to inhale and delivers it in proportion to the Edi, allowing infants to control their own PIP and tidal volume based on the number of inhalations and exhalations. Neural breathing patterns in preterm infants are highly variable, and constant adjustment of NAVA according to inspiratory time and respiratory rate may better adapt to extrauterine life [58]. It is important to remember that whichever ventilation mode or setting you choose, the most important thing is to ensure that the child is adequately ventilated and to minimize lung damage, since the diseases such as BPD, PVH, RP directly depend on the appropriateness and duration of MV. It is these factors that prompted us to use NAVA ventilation as a starting method of respiratory therapy in premature infants, as well as to implement the effectiveness of the proposed therapy by continuously monitoring the Edi.

2. Experience with the use of NAVA ventilation in premature infants in the intensive care unit

2.1 Methods

The study was conducted on the basis of the Irkutsk Regional Perinatal Center. The clinical trial protocol was approved by the ethical committee of this center (decision of the ethical committee No. 10 dated December 27, 2021). The provision of primary resuscitation care to these patients began immediately after birth. A set of measures was carried out in the delivery room, which included the prevention of hypothermia, methods of respiratory stabilization, and surfactant therapy. Respiratory support in the delivery room was performed using the CPAP method with a pressure of 5–6 cm H_2O within 10 s followed by an assessment of the heart rate. If spontaneous breathing was not restored within 5 min, ventilation was started with a mask with the following parameters: PIP—20-22 cm H_2O, PEEP—5 cm H_2O, respiratory rate—60 per minute, fraction of inspired oxygen (FiO_2)—21%. In the absence of effective spontaneous breathing, bradycardia of 60–100 beats per minute, as well as in the presence of signs of severe respiratory failure assessed by the Silverman scale tracheal intubation was performed and MV was started through the endotracheal tube. The main indicator of the effectiveness of the proposed respiratory therapy was the increase in heart rate >100 beats/min. Surfactant was administered at a dose of 200 mg/kg in the first 20 min to infants less than 30 weeks gestational age who required tracheal intubation in the delivery room, and to neonates over 30 weeks gestational age who required tracheal intubation in the delivery room with continued FiO_2 dependence of more than 40%. Surfactant was administered by the traditional method. Prenatal prevention of RDS was carried out in full in 19 mothers of children of the first group and in 17 mothers of children of the second group. Transportation of patients from the delivery room to the ICU was carried out in a plastic film, in a transport incubator under the control of pulse oximetry by at least two medical workers. In the ICU, all children underwent general clinical, laboratory methods of research, as well as ultrasound examination with Doppler cerebral vessels, echocardiography. Therapeutic measures, which included: infusion and cardiotonic therapy, parenteral nutrition, care features, were performed in accordance with generally accepted clinical protocols.

The work was performed in the design of a cohort, prospective, single-center study. Clinical, instrumental (including monitoring of the Edi), laboratory and statistical research methods were used. The object of the study were premature newborns with ELBW and VLBW at birth with a gestational age of less than 32 weeks.

The aim of the study was to evaluate the role of monitoring the Edi in the complex treatment of premature infants with severe respiratory failure on the background of RDS. Two groups of patients were formed who had common signs: VLBW and ELBW at birth, gestational age 25–32 weeks, need for MV, stable cardiohemodynamics, absence of cerebral lesions according to neurosonography performed on the first day of life, normal gas and electrolyte blood composition before the study, the absence of a generalized infectious process and congenital malformations. Patients of both groups underwent the same complex of diagnostic and treatment measures. In the control group, during respiratory support the SIMV + PS mode with pressure control and flow triggering was used, in the main group the NAVA mode was used, since it is this mode that allows you to continuously monitor the work of the diaphragm. The SIMV + PS mode was used on Avea fans made in the USA and MAQUET Servo-n,

Sweden. NAVA ventilation was carried out on MAQUET Servo-n fans with special software, Edi module with cable. The effectiveness of respiratory support was carried out taking into account the assessment of the patient's respiratory comfort, the presence or absence of asynchrony, the need for sedation, constant monitoring of blood saturation and radiological picture.

To assess gas composition and acid-base composition (ABC) of blood, 0.2 ml of venous blood was taken from the umbilical cord at birth, as well as from the central vein during the first three days. Then pH, partial pressure of carbon dioxide ($hvCO_2$), partial pressure of oxygen (pvO_2), base deficiency (BE) and lactate concentration were analyzed during the first three days. In addition, the duration of MV and the duration of treatment in the ICU were analyzed in all patients. The incidence of ventilation associated diseases was also determined.

Statistical data processing was performed using the STATISTICA 10.0 program for Windows. Quantitative data are presented as medians and quartiles (25–75% of the interquartile range). The analysis of the significance of statistical differences in quantitative traits for two independent groups was performed using the Mann-Whitney test, to compare the significance of differences in several traits over time, the Kruskal-Wallis test was used. The analysis of the reliability of statistical differences in qualitative characteristics was carried out using the Pearson x-square test. The value of $p < 0.05$ was taken as the level of statistical significance.

2.2 Results

2.2.1 Changes in PIP and tidal volume depending on MV

In order to assess the effectiveness and safety of the ventilation modes used in preterm infants, the actual ventilation parameters were studied during the first three days. The tactics of respiratory support in both groups was the same and consisted in using the most sparing parameters to maintain adequate oxygenation and respiratory comfort of the patient. During MV in patients of the first group, we managed to maintain spontaneous breathing, eliminate episodes of asynchrony, and maintain a saturation level of ≥92%. However, to achieve these goals, we were forced to apply a PIP of 16 [15; 17] cm H_2O. At the same time, the tidal volume exceeded the physiological norm by several times and amounted to 15.6 [14.6; 16.7] ml. Attempts to reduce PIP in order to restore tidal volume led to the decreased saturation. In order to adequately assess PIP and tidal volume, the same values of PEEP and the FiO_2 were used in patients of both groups. PEEP corresponded to 4–5 cm H_2O, FiO_2 did not exceed 40%. Given that in NAVA mode there is no possibility to arbitrarily set the PIP and its function is performed by the NAVA level which converts the electrical impulse generated by the diaphragm into pressure, our task was to choose the right NAVA level. It allowed us to control the PIP, which changed its value with each breath of the patient. Due to high sensitivity of the trigger, even the smallest attempt to inhale was supported by the ventilator, in proportion to the child's needs. Thus, the PIP was completely dependent on the patient and amounted to 9 [8; 10] cm H_2O ($p < 0.01$). Despite clear differences with the PIP values obtained during MV in the SIMV+PS mode, in patients with NAVA ventilation we did not observe either a decrease in saturation or changes in the blood gas composition, or a violation of respiratory discomfort. On the contrary, it gave us the opportunity to stabilize the tidal volume and maintain it at the level of 1.5 [1.4; 1.7] ml ($p < 0.01$). Indicators of PIP and tidal volume in various ventilation modes are shown in **Figures 1** and **2**.

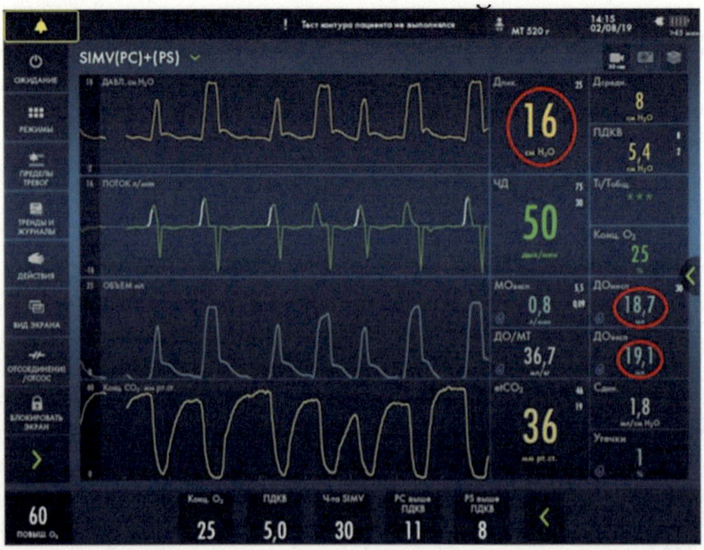

Figure 1.
Indicators of PIP and tidal volume in a premature baby (body weight 520 g) with respiratory support in the SIMV + PS mode.

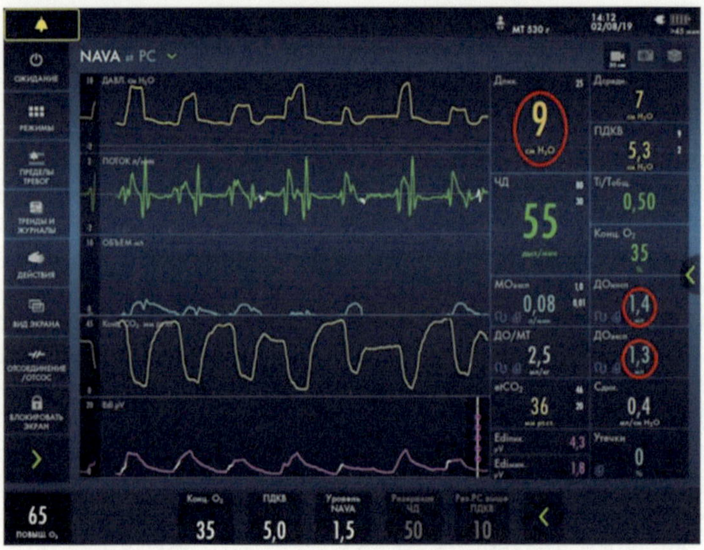

Figure 2.
Indicators of PIP and tidal volume in a premature baby (body weight 530 g) with respiratory support in NAVA mode.

Statistically significant differences in PIP and tidal volume values were obtained. The dynamics of PIP and tidal volume in premature newborns during the first three days depending on the ventilation mode is presented in **Table 1**.

So, high PIP and excess tidal volume in patients with respiratory support in SIMV + PS mode are the result of ineffective triggering. In this case, the ventilator does not recognize the child's breathing attempts, and breaths are delivered automatically.

Values	Day					
	1		2		3	
	SIMV + PS	NAVA	SIMV + PS	NAVA	SIMV + PS	NAVA
PIP (cm H_2O)	16 [15; 17]	9 [8; 10]	17 [16; 18]	11 [9; 13]	15 [14; 16]	10 [9; 11]
	$p < 0.01$					
Volume tidal (ml)	15.6 [14.6; 16.7]	1.5 [1.4; 1.7]	16.0 [15.2; 17.0]	1.8 [1.5; 2.0]	15.0 [14.0; 16.0]	1.7 [1.4; 1.8]
	$p < 0.01$					

Note: p—the significance of differences between groups according to the Mann-Whitney test.

Table 1.
Dynamics of PIP and tidal volume in premature newborns during the first 3 days depending on the mode of MV.

2.2.2 Dynamics of indicators of gas composition and ABC of blood

The analysis of blood gas composition in patients of the first group revealed hypocapnia. Low levels of $pvCO_2$ in these patients were recorded during the first three days. Despite a significant decrease in $pvCO_2$ in children of the first group, respiratory alkalosis was not observed, which can be explained by compensatory mechanisms. The dynamics of base deficit indicators reflects the compensation of hyperventilation in these patients. The $pvCO_2$ values at birth did not differ significantly and corresponded to normal values. On the first day, children of the control group had hypocapnia. $pvCO_2$ was 32.0 [24.9; 37.8] mm Hg, while in children of the main group $pvCO_2$ values were close to the reference and amounted to 36.0 [32.5; 42.2] mm Hg ($p < 0.01$). Similar results were obtained on the second and third days. The $pvCO_2$ level in newborns of the control group on the second day was 32.0 [26.7; 38.1] mm Hg, in children of the main group—35.9 [34.2; 40.3] mm Hg ($p < 0.01$). On the third day $pvCO_2$ values in children receiving MV in the SIMV + PS mode were 33.0 [28.0; 38.3] mm Hg, in children ventilated in the NAVA mode—39.9 [33.7; 43.4] mm Hg ($p < 0.02$). The dynamics of $pvCO_2$ indicators is shown in **Figure 3**.

The pvO_2 values of venous blood at birth in children of the first group were reduced to 22.4 [14.8; 39.4] mm Hg, in children of the second group—to 19.7 [17.8; 25.0] mm Hg, which corresponded to the norm, since the fetus is in a state of physiological hypoxia in utero. Subsequently, there were no significant differences in pvO_2 between the groups. On the first day in patients with MV in the SIMV + PS mode, pvO_2 values were 37.7 [33.3; 46.8] mm Hg, in patients with NAVA ventilation—43.6 [39.3; 46.9] mm Hg ($p = 0.1$). On the second and third days, pvO_2 was 36.3 [32.9; 42.2] mm Hg and 34.1 [31.0; 40.6] in patients of the control group and 42.4 [37.5; 47.0] mm Hg, 41.2 [36.4; 44.8] mm Hg in patients of the main group ($p = 0.2$). The daily dynamics of pvO_2 indicators is shown in **Figure 4**.

The BE indices at birth in children of both groups corresponded to the norm, however, in dynamics in children of the control group, the base deficiency was more pronounced and reached a maximum on the 3rd day. On the first day in children of the control group, the BE values were 5.0 [−7.1; −2.8] mmol/l, in the main group −3.0 [−4.0; −2.0] mmol/l ($p < 0.01$). On the second day, the level of BE in children of the control group corresponded to −5.7 [−6.8; −4.4] mmol/l, in children of the main

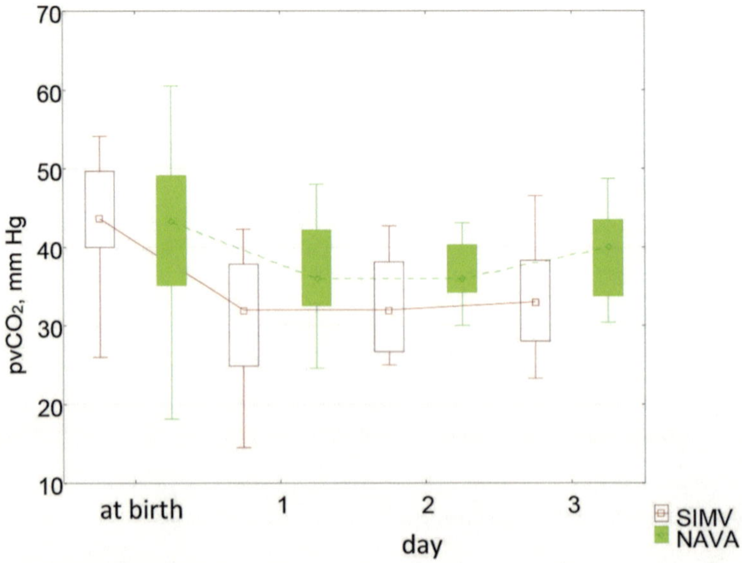

Figure 3.
Dynamics of $pvCO_2$ indicators by day.

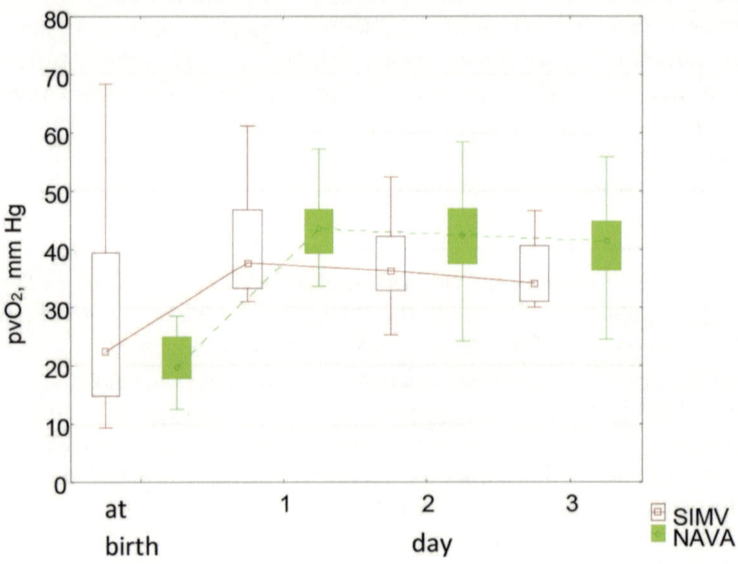

Figure 4.
Dynamics of pvO_2 indicators by day.

group - to-4.0 [−5.2; −2.7] mmol/l ($p < 0.01$). On the third day it comprised −6.3 [−6.8; −5.2] mmol/l in children of the control group and – 4.7 [−6.0; −3.1] mmol/l in children of the main group ($p < 0.02$). Changes in the indicators of BE in patients of both groups are shown in **Figure 5**.

The level of lactate at birth and during the first three days in children of both groups corresponded to normal values. At birth, its concentration was 2.1 [1.5; 2.6] mmol/l in children of the control group and 2.6 [1.7; 3.7] mmol/l in children of the

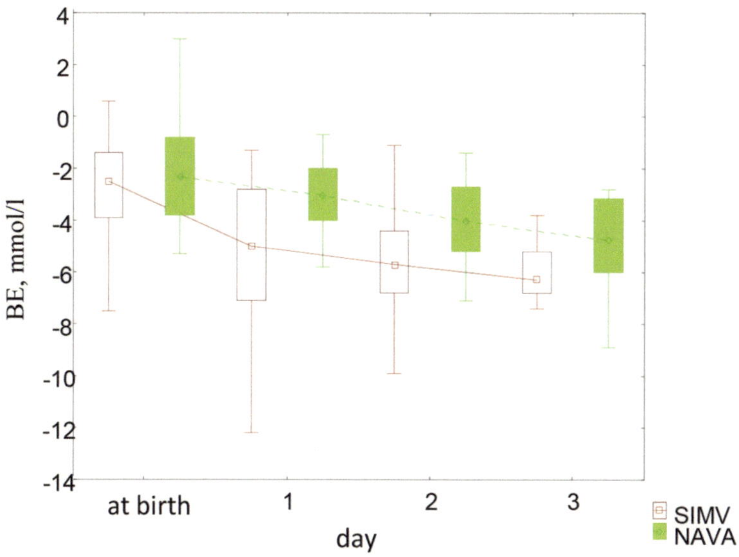

Figure 5.
Dynamics of BE indicators by day.

main group. On the first day in children of the control group, the lactate level was 2.8 [2.5; 4.0] mmol/l compared with 2.5 [2.0; 2.7] mmol/l in children with NAVA ventilation ($p = 0.2$). On the second day, lactate values in children receiving respiratory support in the SIMV + PS mode corresponded to 2.5 [1.9; 3.5] mmol/l, in children of the main group – to 2.2 [2.1; 2.5] mmol/l ($p = 0.26$). On the third day, lactate values were 2.6 [2.2; 2.7] mmol/l and 2.1 [1.7; 2.5] mmol/l in children of the first and second groups, respectively ($p = 0.11$). Thus, the ventilation mode does not affect the level of lactate in the blood. The daily dynamics of lactate concentration is shown in **Figure 6**.

Ph indicators at birth and in dynamics in children of both groups corresponded to the norm and had no statistically significant differences.

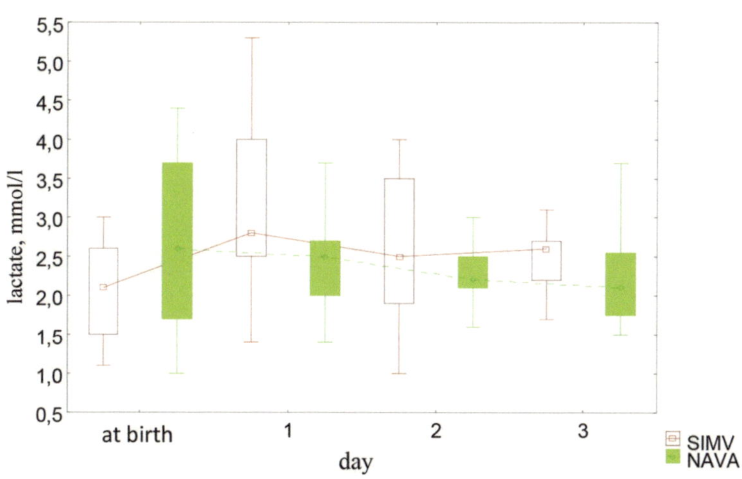

Figure 6.
Dynamics of lactate by day.

2.2.3 Analysis of the incidence of MV associated diseases, the duration of ventilation and the duration of treatment at the intensive care unit

Diseases associated with the damaging effect of MV include PVH of varying severity, BPD and RP. PVH was diagnosed using neurosonography performed on the first, third and seventh days of life. They were verified as thrombi located subependymally (PVH 1st degree), in the lumen of the ventricle without its expansion (PVH 2nd degree), in the lumen of the ventricle with its expansion (PVH 3rd degree), and hemorrhages with a breakthrough into the brain parenchyma (PVH 4th degree). In addition to the direct diagnosis of PVH, some indicators of cerebral hemodynamics were analyzed: blood flow velocity in the anterior, middle and basilar arteries, as well as their resistance indices. PVH was found in 8 patients who underwent MV in the SIMV + PS mode, among them grade 1 hemorrhages were revealed in 5 patients, grade 3 PVH—in 3 patients, grade 2 hemorrhages were not observed. In patients with NAVA ventilation, PVH was diagnosed in 3 cases, with 2 children having grade 1 PVH and 1—grade 2 PVH ($p = 0.24$). The distribution of patients with PVH depending on the ventilation mode is shown in **Figure 7**.

The results obtained during the processing of cerebral hemodynamic parameters on the first and third days did not reveal a statistically significant difference either in speed indicators or in the resistance index.

BPD developed in 7 patients of the control group, and there was a clear relationship between the incidence of BPD and the duration of MV. Invasive lung ventilation in these patients was 5 [2; 10] days, and it was noted that the longer the patients underwent MV, the more difficult it was for them to ensure effective spontaneous breathing. In this regard, the duration of treatment in the ICU increased significantly. By the time of transfer to the pathology department for further observation and nursing, the patients developed oxygen dependence. In this regard, they underwent oxygen therapy with the use of binasal cannulas, face masks, or in the form of a

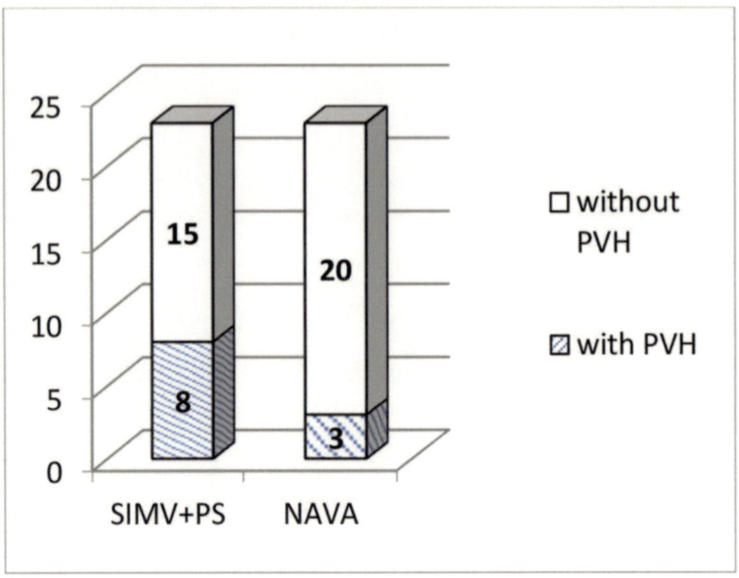

Figure 7.
Distribution of patients with PVH depending on the ventilation mode.

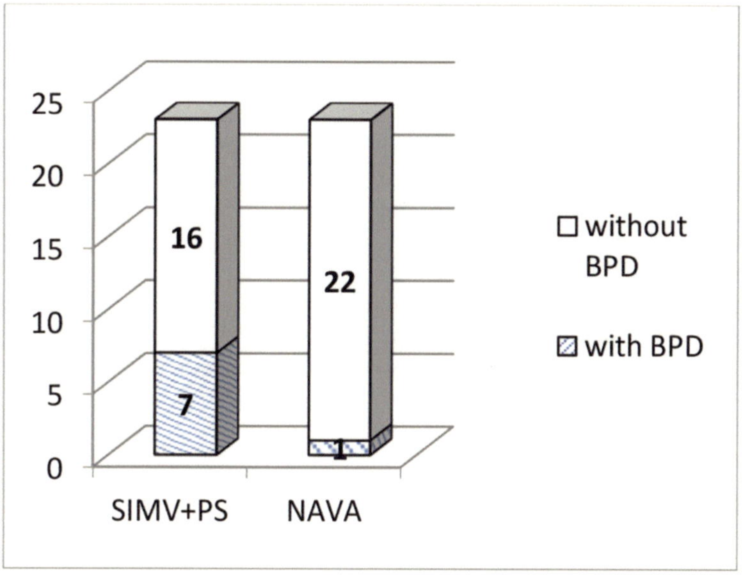

Figure 8.
Incidence of BPD in preterm infants.

background subsidy in the incubator. In the NAVA ventilation group, BPD developed in 1 patient ($p < 0.04$). The incidence of BPD is shown in **Figure 8**.

All patients included in the study were at risk for developing RP. Primary ophthalmological examination of premature babies born with a gestational age of 25–26 weeks was carried out at 30–31 weeks of postconceptual age; at 27–31 weeks - from 4 weeks of life; at 32 weeks—from 3 weeks of life. The results of the

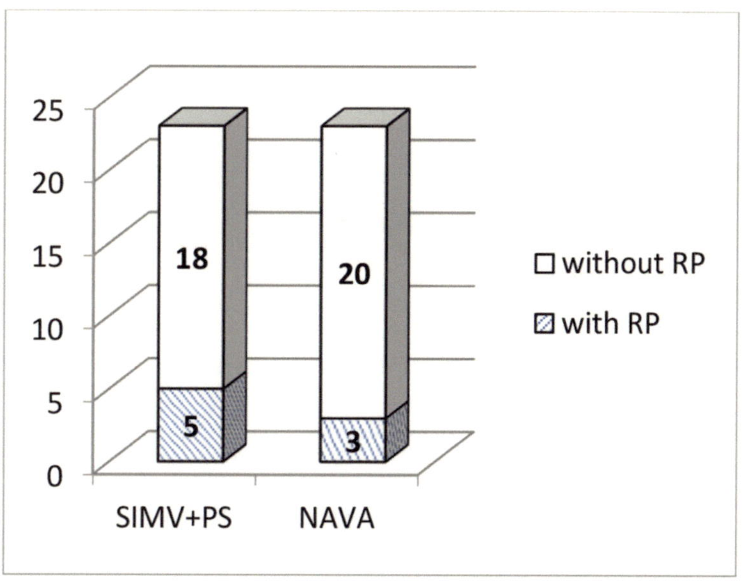

Figure 9.
The incidence of RP in premature newborns.

initial examination showed that 5 patients of the control group had RP of various stages, so 3 children had stage 2 RP when the retina in the area of the demarcation line thickened and protruded into the vitreous body. 2 children were diagnosed with stage 3 RP. In the group of children who underwent NAVA ventilation, 3 patients were diagnosed with stage 2 RP ($p = 0.35$). The outcome of the disease in these patients was as follows: in all patients with stage 2 and in 1 patient with stage 3 RP, the disease regressed, and they did not require surgical treatment. One child had progression of the disease, for which he underwent transpupillary laser coagulation of the retina. The incidence of RP is shown in **Figure 9**.

The duration of respiratory support in patients of the control group was 5 [2; 10] days, in patients of the main group—4 [3; 8] days ($p = 0.66$), and the duration of stay in the ICU in children of the control group—14 [11; 33] days, in children of the main group—7.0 [6; 15] days ($p < 0.01$).

3. Conclusion

The performed clinical study showed that continuous monitoring of the Edi not only gives us an idea of the severity of the patient's condition but also describes in detail his respiratory status and allows you to select ventilation parameters in proportion to the needs of the child, while maintaining a normal blood gas composition. The control of the diaphragm function and the timely adjustment of the ventilator settings allow to maintain spontaneous breathing, ensure good interaction between the child and the ventilator, and reduce the risks of VILD. As a result, the duration of ventilation and the length of stay in the ICU are reduced.

Conflict of interest

The authors declare no conflict of interest.

Author details

Aleksei Anurev[1*], Vladimir Gorbachev[2], Tatiana Pavlova[1] and Alexander Pavlov[1]

1 Irkutsk Regional Perinatal Center, Irkutsk, Russia

2 Irkutsk Academy of Postgraduate Education, Irkutsk, Russia

*Address all correspondence to: anurev.lesha@mail.ru

References

[1] Dubois J, Alison M. Editors. MRI of the neonatal brain: A review of methodological challenges and neuroscientific advances. Journal of Magnetic Resonance Imaging. 2021;**53**(50):1318-1343. DOI: 10.1002/jmri.27192

[2] Lendahl U. Transgenic analysis of central nervous system development and regeneration. Acta Anaesthesiologica Scandinavica Supplementum. 1997;**110**:116-118. DOI: 10.1111/j.1399-6576.1997.tb05524.x

[3] Gao W, Grewen K, Knickmeyer RC. A review on neuroimaging studies of genetic and environmental influences on early brain development. NeuroImage. 2019;**185**:802-812. DOI: 10.1016/j.neuroimage.2018.04.032

[4] Dubois J, Kostovic I, Judas M. Development of structural and functional connectivity. In: Brain Mapping: An Encyclopedic Reference. Vol. 2. Elsevier Cambridge: Academic Press; 2015. pp. 423-437. DOI: 10.1016/B978-0-12-397025-1.00360-2

[5] Knickmeyer RC, Gouttard S, Kang C. A structural MRI study of human brain development from birth to 2 years. The Journal of Neuroscience: The Official Journal of the Society for Neuroscience. 2008;**28**(47):12176-12182. DOI: 10.1523/JNEUROSCI.3479-08.2008

[6] Lyall AE, Shi F, Geng X. Dynamic development of regional cortical thickness and surface area in early childhood. Cerebral Cortex. 2015;**25**(8):2204-2212. DOI: 10.1093/cercor/bhu027

[7] Chi J, Dooling E, Gilles F. Gyral development of the human brain. Annals of Neurology. 1977;**1**(1):86-93. DOI: 101002/ana.410010109

[8] Kostović I, Sedmak G, Judaš M. Neural histology and neurogenesis of the human fetal and infant brain. Neuroimage. 2019;**188**:743-773. DOI: 101016/j.neuroimage.2018.12.043

[9] Porges SW. In: Schore AN, editor. The Polyvagal Theory. 1st ed. New York: W. W. Norton & Company; 2011. 347 p

[10] Longin E, Gerstner T. Maturation of the autonomic nervous system: Differences in heart rate variability in premature vs. term infants. Journal of Perinatal Medicine. 2006;**34**:303-308. DOI: 101515/JPM.2006.058

[11] Faa G, Manchia M. Fetal programming of neuropsychiatric disorders. Birth Defects Research. Part C, Embryo Today: Reviews. 2016;**108**:207-223. DOI: 101002/bdrc.21139

[12] Porges SW, Furman SA. The early development of the autonomic nervous system provides a neural platform for social behavior: A polyvagal perspective. Infant Child Development. 2011;**20**:106-118. DOI: 101002/icd.688

[13] Gewolb I, Vice F. Maturational changes in the rhythms, patterning, and coordination of respiration and swallow during feeding in preterm and term infants. Developmental Medicine and Child Neurology. 2006;**48**(7):589-594. DOI: 101017/S001216220600123X

[14] Friedman H, Soloveichick M. Neuroplasticity in young age: Computer-based early neurodevelopment classifier. In: Neuroplasticity—Insights of Neural Reorganization. Vol. 3. 2017. pp. 47-65. DOI: 105772/intechopen.70894

[15] Salmaso N, Jablonska B, editors. Neurobiology of premature brain injury. Nature Neuroscience. 2014;**17**:341-346. DOI: 10.1038/nn.3604

[16] Perlman JM. The relationship between systemic hemodynamic perturbations and periventricular-intraventricular hemorrhage—A historical perspective. Seminars Pediatric Neurology. 2009;**16**:191-199. DOI: 10.1016/j.spen.2009.09.006

[17] Inder TE, Perlman JM, Volpe JJ. Chapter 24 - preterm intraventricular hemorrhage/posthemorrhagic hydrocephalus. In: Volpe JJ, Inder TE, Darras BT, de Vries LS, du Plessis AJ, Neil JJ, editors. Volpe's Neurology of the Newborn. 6th ed. Elsevier; 2018. pp. 637-698. e21

[18] Volpe JJ. Brain injury in premature infants: A complex amalgam of destructive and developmental disturbances. Lancet Neurology. 2009;**8**:110-124. DOI: 101016/S1474-4422(08)70294-1

[19] Banker BQ, Larroche JC. Periventricular leukomalacia of infancy. A form of neonatal anoxic encephalopathy. Archives of Neurology. 1962;**7**:386-410. DOI: 101001/archneur.1962.04210050022004

[20] Volpe JJ. Confusions in nomenclature: "periventricular leukomalacia" and "white matter injury"-identical, distinct, or overlapping? Pediatric Neurology. 2017;**73**:3-6. DOI: 101016/j.pediatrneurol.2017.05.013

[21] Volpe JJ, Kinney HC. The developing oligodendrocyte: Key cellular target in brain injury in the premature infant. International Journal of Developmental Neuroscience. 2011;**29**:423-440. DOI: 101016/j.ijdevneu.2011.02.012

[22] Linsell L, Malouf R. Prognostic factors for cerebral palsy and motor impairment in children born very preterm or very low birthweight: A systematic review. Developmental Medicine and Child Neurology. 2016;**58**:554-569. DOI: 101111/dmcn.12972

[23] Perry M, Tan Z. Neonatal pain: Perceptions and current practice. Critical Care Nursing Clinics of North America. 2018;**30**(4):549-561. DOI: 101016/j.cnc.2018.07.013

[24] Anand K, Hickey P. Pain and its effects in the human neonate and fetus. The New England Journal of Medicine. 1987;**317**(21):1321-1329. DOI: 101056/NEJM198711193172105

[25] Fitzgerald M, Beggs S. The neurobiology of pain: Developmental aspects. Neuroscientist. 2001;7(3):246-257. DOI: 101177/107385840100700309

[26] Grunau R, Holsti L, Haley D. Neonatal procedural pain exposure predicts lower cortisol and behavioral reactivity in preterm infants in the NICU. Pain. 2005;**113**(3):293-300. DOI: 10.1016/j.pain.2004.10.020

[27] Goksan S, Hartley C. fMRI reveals neural activity overlap between adult and infant pain. Elife. 2015;**4**:1-13. DOI: 107554/eLife.06356

[28] Cong X, Wu J. The impact of cumulative pain/stress on neurobehavioral development of preterm infants in the NICU. Early Human Development. 2017;**108**:9-16. DOI: 101016/j.earlhumdev.2017.03.003

[29] Lippmann M, Nelson R. Ligation of patent ductus arteriosus in premature infants. British Journal of Anaesthesia. 1976;**48**(4):365-369. DOI: 101093/bja/48.4.365

[30] Brown AG. The dorsal horn of the spinal cord. Quarterly Journal of Experimental Physiology. 1982;**67**(2):193-212. DOI: 101113/expphysiol.1982.sp002630

[31] Aziz C, Ahmad A. The role of the thalamus in modulating pain. The Malaysian Journal of Medical Sciences. 2006;**13**(2):11-18

[32] Hatfield L. Neonatal pain: What's age got to do with it? Surgical Neurology International. 2014;**13**(5):479-489. DOI: 104103/2152-7806.144630

[33] Kostovic I, Rakic P. Developmental history of the transient subplate zone in the visual and somatosensory cortex of the macaque monkey and human brain. Journal of Comparative Neurology. 1990;**297**(3):441-470. DOI: 101002/cne.902970309

[34] Hasegawa M, Houdou S. Development of myelination in the human fetal and infant cerebrum: A myelin basic protein immunohistochemical study. Brain Development. 1992;**14**(1):1-6. DOI: 101016/s0387-7604(12)80271-3

[35] Fitzgerald M, Walker S. Infant pain management: A developmental neurobiological approach. Nature Clinical Practice. Neurology. 2009;**5**(1):35-50. DOI: 101038/ncpneuro0984

[36] Slater R, Fabrizi L. Premature infants display increased noxious-evoked neuronal activity in the brain compared to healthy age-matched term-born infants. Neuroimage. 2010;**52**(2):583-589. DOI: 101016/j.neuroimage.2010.04.253

[37] Glenn W, Holcomb W. Central hypoventilation; long-term ventilatory assistance by radiofrequency electrophrenic respiration. Annals of Surgery. 1970;**172**:755-773

[38] Glenn W, Holcomb W. Long-term ventilatory support by diaphragm pacing in quadriplegia. Annals of surgery. 1976;**183**:566-577

[39] Khong P, Lazzaro A, Mobbs R. Phrenic nerve stimulation: The Australian experience. Journal of Clinical Neuroscience: Official Journal of the Neurological Society of Australia. 2010;**17**:205-208. DOI: 101016/j.jocn.2009.06.012

[40] Le Pimpec-Barthes F, Gonzalez-Bermejo J. Intrathoracic phrenic pacing: A 10-year experience in France. Journal of Thoracic and Cardiovascular Surgery. 2011;**142**:378-383. DOI: 101016/j.jtcvs.2011.04.033

[41] Similowski T, Fleury B. Cervical magnetic stimulation: A new painless method for bilateral phrenic nerve stimulation in conscious humans. Journal of Applied Physiology. 1989;**67**:1311-1318. DOI: 10.1152/jappl.1989.67.4.1311

[42] Zifko U, Hartmann M. Diaphragmatic paresis in newborns due to phrenic nerve injury. Neuropediatrics. 1995;**26**(5):281-284. DOI: 101055/s-2007-979774

[43] Schulzke S, Stoecklin B. Update on ventilatory management of extremely preterm infants—A neonatal intensive care unit perspective. Paediatric Anaesthesia. 2022;**32**(2):363-371. DOI: 10.1111/pan.14369

[44] Greenough A. Long-term respiratory consequences of premature birth at less than 32 weeks of gestation. Early Human Development. 2013;**89**:25-27. DOI: 101016/j.earlhumdev.2013.07.004

[45] Chaves-Samaniego M, Garcia CM. Risk calculator for retinopathy of prematurity requiring treatment. Frontiers in Pediatrics. 2020;**8**:529-639. DOI: 103389/fped.2020.529639

[46] Askie L, Henderson-Smart D. Oxygen-saturation targets and outcomes in extremely preterm infants. New England Journal of Medicine. 2003;**349**(10):959-967. DOI: 101056/NEJMoa023080

[47] Saugstad O, Aune D. In search of the optimal oxygen saturation for extremely low birth weight infants: A systematic review and meta-analysis. Neonatology. 2011;**100**(1):1-8. DOI: 101159/000322001

[48] Gorbachev MO. Effect of neonatal respiratory support strategy in the ICU. Anasteziologiia and Reanimatologiia. 2015;**60**(2):39-43

[49] Rocha G. Respiratory care for the ventilated neonate. Canadian Respiratory Journal. 2018;7:29-41. DOI: 10.1155/2018/7472964

[50] Mellot K. Patient-ventilator dyssynchrony: Clinical significance and implications for practice. Critical Care Medicine. 2009;**29**(6):41-55. DOI: 10.4037/ccn2009612

[51] Esteban A. How is mechanical ventilation employed in the intensive care unit? An international utilization review. American Journal Respiratory Critical Care Medicine. 2000;**161**:1450-1458. DOI: 10.1164/ajrccm.161.5.9902018

[52] Gorbachev V, Mitkinov O. The use of VTV ventilation mode in premature newborns. Siberian Medical Journal. 2014;7:72-75

[53] Brower R. Ventilation with lower tidal volumes as compared with traditional tidal volumes for acute lung injury and the acute respiratory distress syndrome. New England Journal of Medicine. 2000;**342**(2):1301-1308. DOI: 10.1056/NEJM200005043421801

[54] Wheeler K. Assist control volume guarantee ventilation during surfactant administration. Archives of Disease in Childhood. Fetal and Neonatal Edition. 2009;**94**(5):336-338. DOI: 10.1136/adc.2008.149583

[55] Stoll B. Trends in care practices, morbidity, and mortality of extremely preterm neonates 1993-2012. Journal of the American Medical Association. 2015;**314**(10):1039-1051. DOI: 10.1001/jama.2015.10244

[56] Jung S. Recent advances in bronchopulmonary dysplasia: Pathophysiology, prevention, and treatment. Lung. 2018;**196**(2):129-138. DOI: 10.1007/s00408-018-0084-z

[57] Fischer H. Avoiding endotracheal ventilation to prevent bronchopulmonary dysplasia: A meta-analysis. Pediatrics. 2013;**132**(5):1351-1360. DOI: 10.1542/peds.2013-1880

[58] Chen I, Chen H. New developments in neonatal respiratory management. Pediatrics and Neonatology. 2022;**63**(4):341-347. DOI: 101016/j.pedneo.2022.02.002

Chapter 4

The Role of Surgical Simulation in the Quality of Health Care for Complex Neurosurgical Patients

Allison Roberto da Silva and Jacqueline Rodrigues da Silva

Abstract

The constant technological evolution allows health professionals possibilities until then only imagined in the pages of science fiction. The three-dimensional reconstruction of real anatomical models, with the help of Virtual Reality, Augmented Reality, and the impression of realistic shadows, provides surgical teams with the possibility of performing complex surgeries without exposing the patient well in advance, allowing us to achieve excellent results, increasing surgeons' precision, and decreasing operating room time and patient exposure to anesthesia. In this way, the results are cost containment and increased the productivity and quality of care. Realistic simulations are an advent that allow not only surgeons but also the entire multidisciplinary team to plan each step of the assistance that will be dedicated to patients throughout the surgical process with greater safety and caution, improving the quality of life and assistance provided to our patients.

Keywords: realistic simulation, surgical nursing, patient safety, pediatric neurosurgery, quality

1. Introduction

1.1 The need for simulations in pediatric neurosurgery

Surgical procedures involving the Central Nervous System are complex by themselves and require specific skills from the neurosurgeon and the entire team involved in the surgical procedure, these skills can take years of practice to be acquired. With technological development; these skills change more quickly when compared to the others, as we can anticipate the learning curve using it as a shortcut. In the case of pediatric surgeries, there are also specific implications with anatomical development, which further limit the acquisition of these skills in the short term. The simulation strategy can be considered as a great facilitator in the acquisition of tactile skills and in the construction of logical reasoning for decision-making and behavior changes, as the experience in simulated situations will be able to provide the surgeon with skill and safety in real situations.

1.2 The use of simulations and their characteristics

The concept of simulation can be defined as the technique where a "simulator" is used in which techniques or behaviors can be replicated in a non-real event so that participants acquire motor skills and/or specific behaviors for each type of event, without exposing them to such situations before they have acquired skills [1, 2].

We can also broaden the concept of "simulator", placing it not only as a real replica of something or someone but also as an event where the interpretation and imitation of a potentially real situation contribute not only to the improvement of motor skills but also to the acquisition of logical and critical reasoning, in addition to more accurate decision-making [1, 2].

These concepts have been widely used in the areas of human knowledge for centuries, in the military field and in the development of technologies, equipment, and products, in addition to medical areas and other segments of human health, such as emergency care or complex surgeries [2–4].

Some areas of human development have among their attributions the use of simulations as a basic requirement in academic training or professional development. From complex equipment simulators such as airplanes and robots to complex neurosurgical procedures.

Graduations in the various areas of human health have been demanding from future professionals a minimum number of hours of simulations or improvement in equipment that can faithfully reproduce the functionalities of specific situations. Thus, they provide the future professional with the experience of contact with materials and equipment or experience with complex situations in a safe place before exposing the professional and the patient to a real situation that exposes them to risks [2, 4, 5].

In this context, Pediatric Neurosurgery becomes one of the medical specialties most benefited from the technological advent of realistic simulations, as we can safely and assertively replicate procedures of different complexities, from a simple trephination to a complex process for separating craniopagus twins, significantly reducing the learning curve of new and experienced surgeons with the acquisition of motor and intellectual skills, preserving the integrity of patients, and minimizing the entire process of caring for children undergoing surgery.

2. Methods

This chapter is a literature review, associated with the experience report of a large Brazilian Hospital in the areas of realistic simulation for specific cases of pediatric neurosurgery.

3. A brief history of simulations

The beginning of the use of simulations dates to the 5th century BC where Greek generals used a board game called Petteia to simulate field battles between two armies and thus define their war strategies, with progression and division of troops across the battlefield. This game was described by Plato in his dialogs with Socrates as the science for logical and strategic reasoning; it was also cited several times by Aristotle and reproduced in Greek art countless times [6–8].

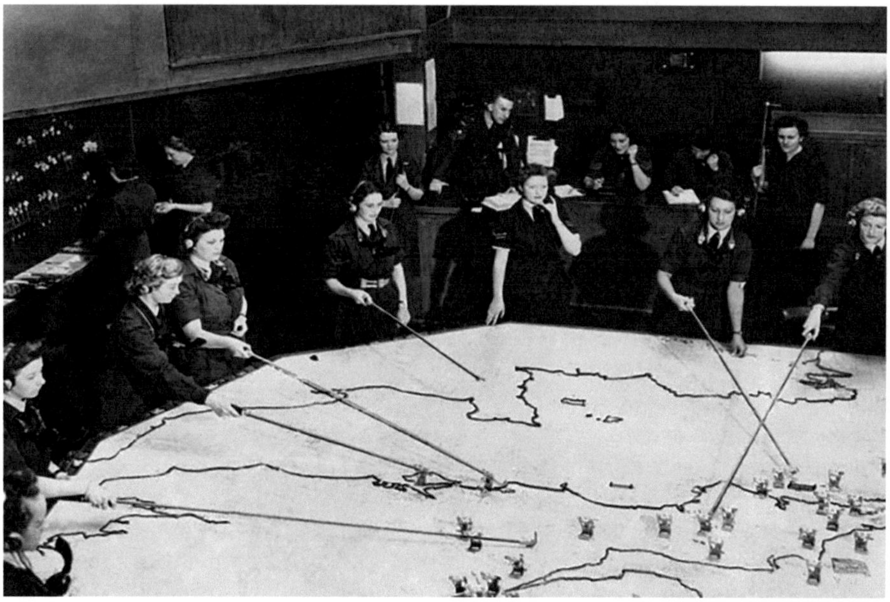

Figure 1.
The operations room at RAF fighter Command's No. 10 Group Headquarters, Rudloe manor (RAF box), Wiltshire, showing WAAF plotters and duty officers at work, 1943. Public domain.

In the Middle Ages, there are reports of generals who played chess and other variations with the same objective. Kings and high-ranking generals used the famous "war tables", on which commanders moved pieces representing military units across the battlefield, simulating maneuvers and decision-making. This strategy was decisive for the Allies in World War II due to territorial proportions and remains active until the twenty-first century (**Figure 1**) [1, 2, 5].

More complex war games were developed and introduced in training as true situational simulators, so the commanders involved can fight battles between two or more armies and develop more advanced strategies, anticipating behaviors and situations on several fronts and managing to project problems and improve decision-making [6].

From the 1940s, with the invention of computers, virtual simulations also gained ground among the military and gave rise to new simulation technologies. During the Cold War, the United States Department of Defense developed networking; this was the world's first multiuser virtual simulator, which simulated real-time strategies with participants from different areas; this program broke major paradigms at the time, as it managed to simulate battles virtually for the first time in history [3, 7, 9].

As seen, the military has benefited from complex simulation strategies throughout history; however, other areas also benefit from simulated situations and simulators, not only for training reasoning but also for acquiring tactile skills. Descriptions of the use of anatomical simulators for education and training are present throughout the development of known civilizations, benefiting patients and health professionals for at least 20,000 years [10–12].

3.1 The importance of anatomical development for simulation

Differently from the military area, the evolution of simulations around human health took place with the use of human and animal cadavers and with the construction and manipulation of anatomical models, which totally or partially replicated human body systems, tissues, or isolated organs [9]. In this context, we cannot talk about simulations without going back to the whole course of anatomical discoveries and how they evolved throughout the history of civilization and influenced the development of these techniques (**Figure 2**) [10–12].

- 24,000 BC: The first human models began with rudimentary sculptures and cave paintings.
- 4000 BC: The first pathological studies began in Eurasia and developed significantly in the Egyptian civilization [11–13].
- 510 BC: Alcménon of Crotona, disciple of the Pythagorean School of Philosophy, dissected a human corpse for the first time with an academic objective and opened up concepts hitherto unknown to men [11, 12].
- 322 BC: Hippocrates dissected several animals and compared his discoveries with similar human characteristics, ended up building the first medical concepts and tracing what would become physiological studies in the future [11, 12].
- 250 BC: Herophilus of Chalcedon carried out relevant anatomical studies and the first public dissections in the ancient world and even wrote the first books on human anatomy [11].
- 200: The works of the Roman physician Claudius Galen provided vital information for human anatomy and for solving complex problems [11, 12].
- 1240: The medical school of Naples introduced the subject of Human Anatomy into the curriculum, a decisive step toward scientific developm4444ent [9–11].

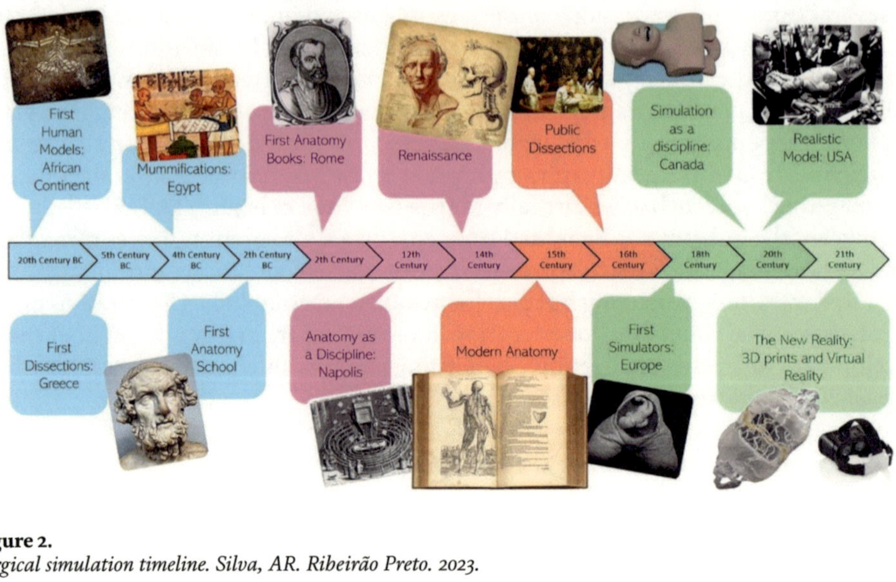

Figure 2.
Surgical simulation timeline. Silva, AR. Ribeirão Preto. 2023.

- 1500: Artists such as Leonardo da Vinci and Michelangelo expanded the human view on the anatomy and concepts of the human body [11–13].

- 1550: The results published by physician Andreas Vesalius in the book "De Humani Corporis Fabrica Libri Septum" were the watershed and transformed rudimentary anatomy into what we know as modern anatomy, with descriptions and drawings of all systems in the most complex form ever seen until then (**Figure 3**) [11–13].

3.2 The development of simulators

The use of cadavers remained standard in European medical schools; however, their use had considerable limitations, such as tissue deterioration and lack of malleability and vascularity, which made the use of these models unfeasible for a long time; in addition, cadavers are difficult to obtain. In view of these limitations, the creation of the first simulators was considered so that educators and professionals would have permanent access to a realistic model of training and teaching [9, 10].

The first models designed for this purpose were described in ancient India, using nasal simulators made with leaves, twigs, and clay, dating from the 6th century BC for the acquisition of specific skills in anatomical manipulations and rudimentary surgical instruments (**Figures 4–6**) [11–13].

The first non-rudimentary models developed specifically for medical procedures date back to the 18th century with anatomical simulators created for training obstetricians and midwives [13].

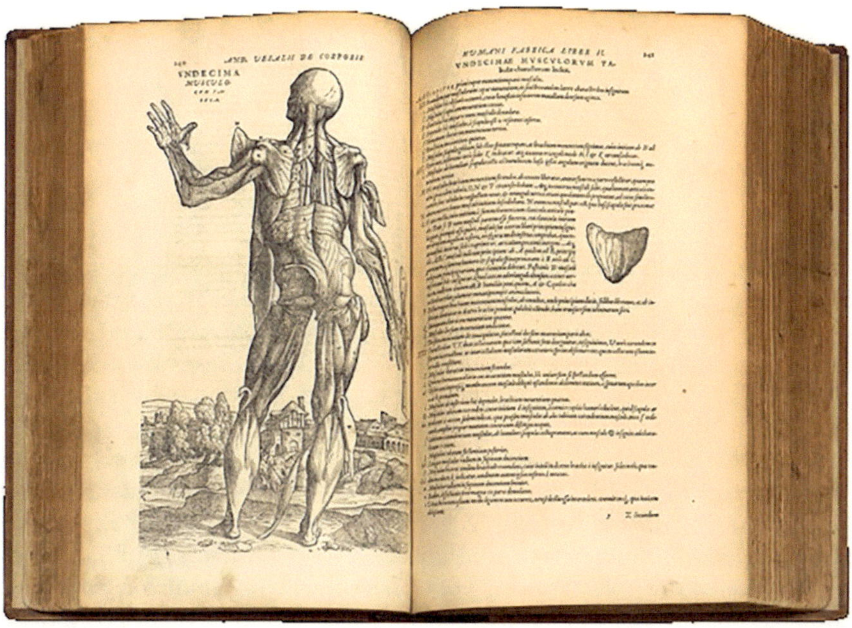

Figure 3.
Book: De Humani Corporis Fabrica Libri septum. Andreas Vesalius. 1555. Museum Für Medizinhistorische Bücher Muri. Available. Muri, Switzerland. 2023.

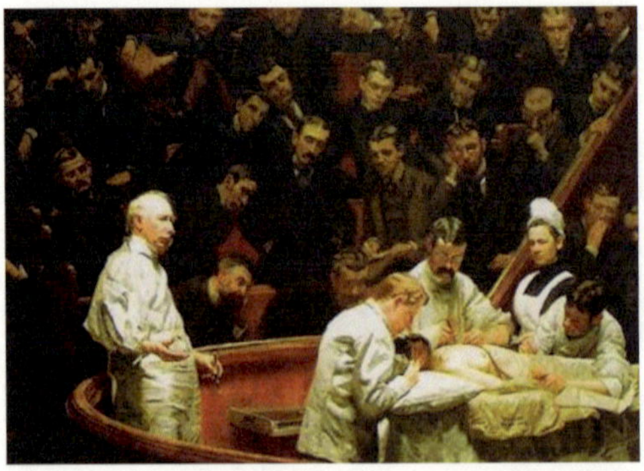

Figure 4.
Anatomy lesson, Dr. van der Meer. Van Mierevelt, 1617. Delft museum. Amsterdam, Nederlands. Starling IG. 2023.

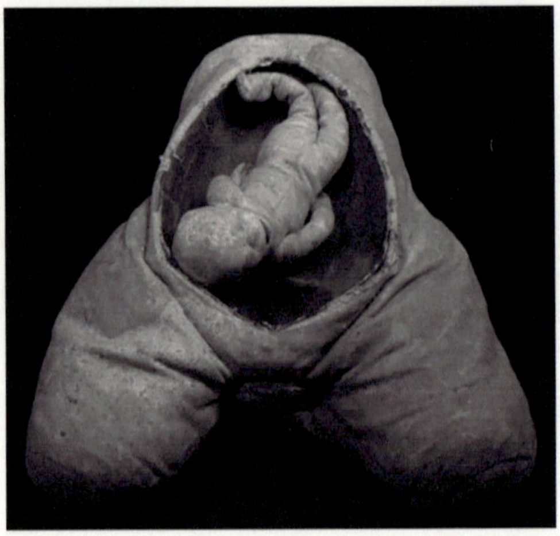

Figure 5.
Obstetric birth simulator dating from the 18th century. Dittrick medical history center, Case Western Reserve University, Cleveland, OH, United States. 2023.

More complex simulators and with more elaborate materials were developed over the years; in this context, we can consider anatomists like Richard Manningham and Marguerite Le Boursier du Coudray as great precursors of surgical simulation and Obstetrics as a pioneering discipline in the development of these technologies [11–13], including the first simulators with simulated venous circulation, which appeared at the same time [14].

The twentieth century, with its technological development, provided the modernization of simulators, mainly from the 1950's, and they gained a new concept among teachers and health professionals [9, 12, 13].

In the late 1960's, Abrahamson and Denson, from the University of Southern California, created the first computer-controlled anesthesia simulator, a device capable of simulating airway definition techniques, changes in vital signs, and physiological responses such as anisocoria, for example (**Figure** 7) [15].

Since then, the concept of "simulators" has also been expanded and real situations have been introduced in a replicated and simulated way in medical schools. Using

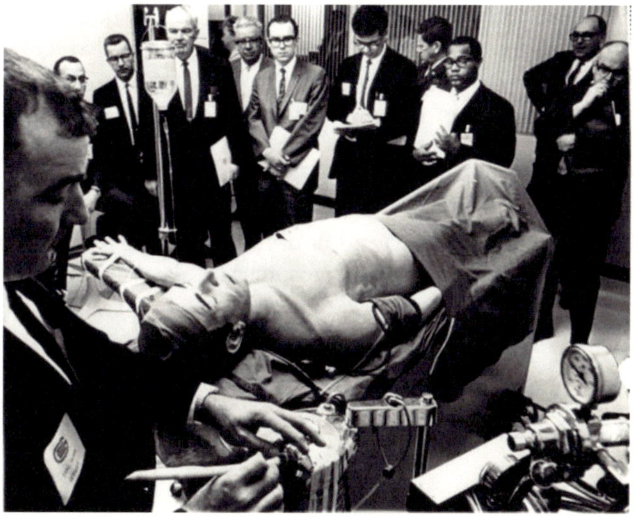

Figure 6.
Dr. Stephen Abrahamson and Dr. Judson Denson with Sim one. Cooper, Taketi. 2004.

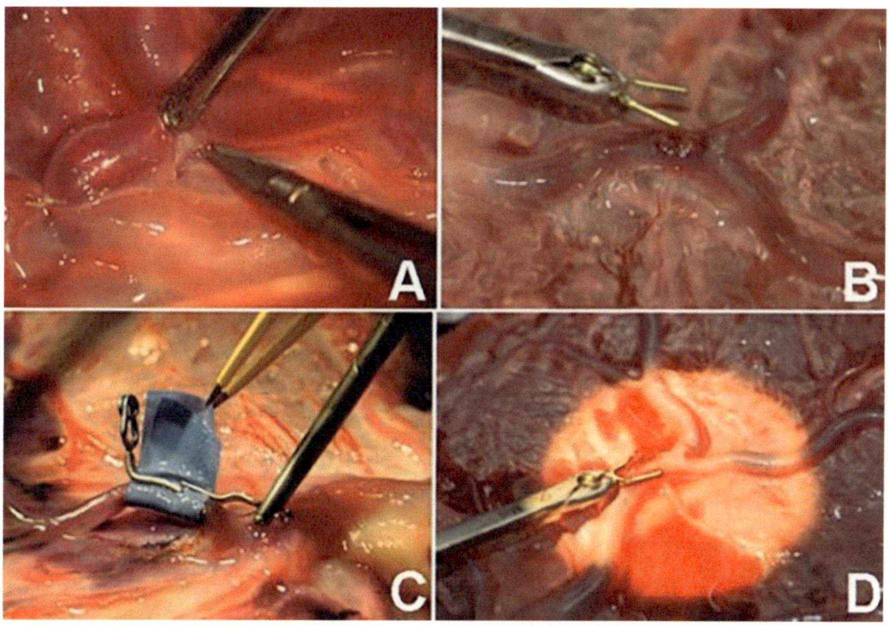

Figure 7.
Brain microsurgery simulation and aneurysm clipping using human placenta. Santos Filho JAM. Belo Horizonte. Brasil. 2015.

interpretation techniques as an ally and hiring actors to perform simulations of meetings with patients for physical examinations and data collection. That is, in this context, the actors, their bodies and their interpretive techniques, are considered simulators [13, 15].

Although the practice presents excellent results, only in 1993 was the first incorporation of this method by the Medical Council of Canada and this practice gained strength and in 2004 became a requirement for medical licensing in the United States [16].

The concept continued to expand in the main academic centers of the world, and currently, the simulation is directly associated with specialized and effective surgical planning, which makes the teams gain time and precision, in addition to reducing the costs generated with the steps of the chain of care [13, 15–18].

3.3 Different techniques for different needs

With technological advancement and nonlinear teaching techniques, we can currently experience two major fronts of surgical simulations: those performed in virtual environments and those performed in physical environments. Therefore, we need to define the simulators and simulation events and know the functionalities of each one.

3.4 Neurosurgical physical simulators

Specifically in Neurosurgery, in most cases, we use biological simulators; these are cadavers or human and animal tissues, where techniques are created and/or trained, with their known and significant limitations, such as difficulties in obtaining fresh cadavers and lack of vascularization and tissue malleability; we will place greater emphasis on non-biological simulators (**Figure 8**) [19].

The technology of printed simulators has been gaining a lot of space among neurosurgery professionals; these can be just for demonstrations of techniques or equipment, such as models for endoscopic third ventriculostomy or aspiration and resection of tumors, where surgeons with experience can test new equipment in practice or even for complex cases; its great advantage is the development of tactile ability (**Figure 9**) [20, 21].

Printed simulators can be divided into three subgroups: low, moderate, and high fidelity. This definition comes from the ability of the equipment to reproduce situations with high fidelity, which may include anatomical and/or physiological reactions, the presence of blood and secretions, and the use of sounds and images:

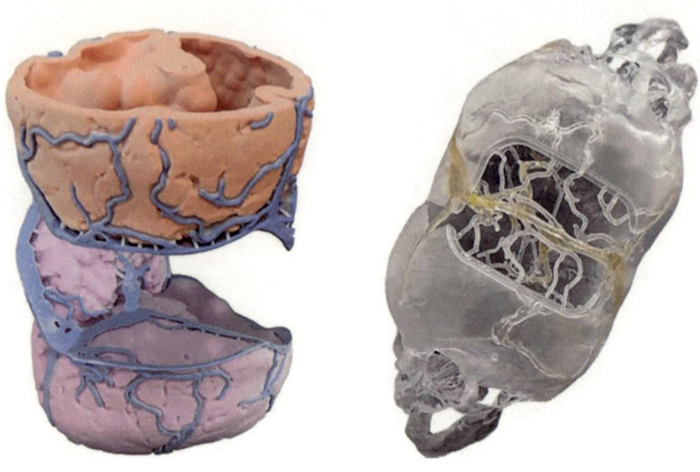

Figure 8.
Specific simulators used for planning the separation of craniopagus twins. HC collection. HCFMRP-USP. Ribeirão Preto. Brazil. 2023.

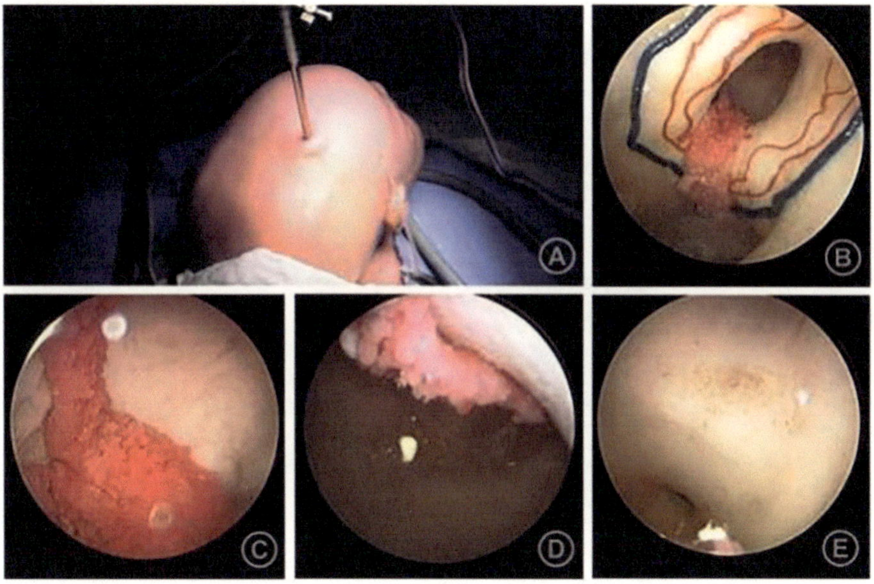

Figure 9.
High fidelity simulator for Neuroendoscopy training for third Ventriculostomy. Caselato GCR. São Paulo, Brazil. 2019.

3.5 Virtual simulators

With the development of high-fidelity neuroimaging reconstruction, virtual simulators began to gain ground in academia and medicine. They are generally used for specific situations and are able to serve teams due to their high level of detail and practical interaction [20, 21].

They also have important limitations, as there is no tactile experience with the patient and the interaction of the instruments with the model; therefore, this type of simulator is not indicated for the development of manual skills. The great advantages of this type of simulator in relation to the physical simulator are the economy with printing and the possibility of restoring the process and restarting it in its initial position; that is, there is no permanent damage to the simulator, which allows its reuse without limits (**Figure 10**) [20, 21].

3.6 Virtual environments for simulation

When we think of a virtual simulation, we need to understand in which environment this simulation takes place; in relation to this technological advent, we can think of three different scenarios: one that takes place entirely in a virtual world, another that takes place in the real world, and one that be able to unify the two realities in real time.

a. Virtual Reality: In this scenario, the entire universe involved in the simulation is reconstructed in a virtual environment; that is, the Operating Room, those involved, the instruments, and the patient are reconstructed and designed completely in a virtual way. This technique allows placing participants in separate locations in the same virtual room, using the concept of shared virtual environment.

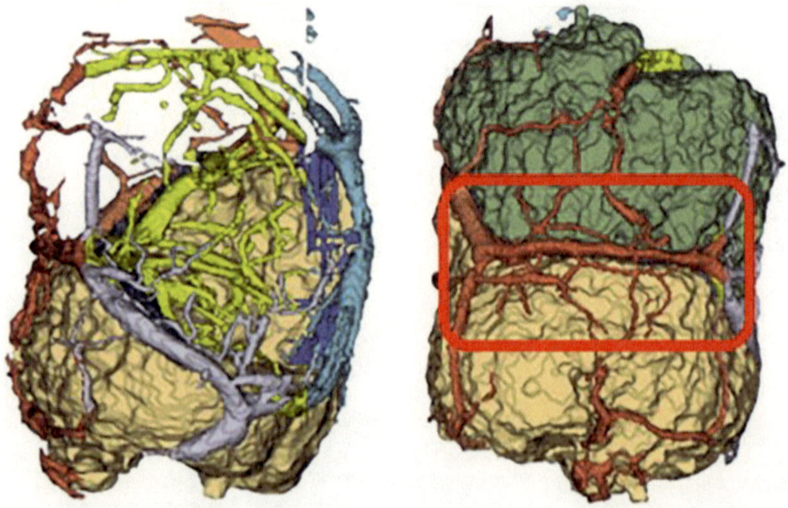

Figure 10.
Virtual simulator for craniopagus separation. HC collection. HCFMRP-USP. Ribeirão Preto. Brazil. 2022.

b. Augmented Reality: This scenario does not reconstruct the universe to be simulated but allows the possibility of applying the virtual simulator as a single object in a non-virtual environment, superimposing the images through glasses or screens and allowing interaction with the object.

c. Mixed Reality: This scenario combines the overlapping of augmented reality elements with the ability of virtual reality to interact and visualize the elements but in a real environment [20, 21].

3.7 Simulations and their subdivisions

Individually, we can use physical or virtual simulators to define and train specific interventions in complex cases and have the first contact with real-size models, allowing the professional to define with greater precision the surgical positioning, instruments, equipment, disposable materials, and techniques necessary for each case, in addition to a considerable decrease in the learning curve of surgical techniques [20–22].

3.8 Situational simulation

Situational simulations are performed for situations or procedures in the same segment, for example, clipping aneurysms or endoscopic surgeries for resection of skull base tumors. They have as their main objective the acquisition of tactile skills; the development of logical and critical reasoning remains as a secondary objective in a situational event, such as the conduct to be taken in a hemorrhage in endoscopic skull base surgeries or the rapid replacement of an engine that malfunctions at the time of craniotomy.

This type of simulation often occurs in pre-congress, extension, or professional training courses. Other segments of the health area use many simulated events for training and skills improvement; and among these, Pediatric Nursing stands out [20–22].

3.9 Realistic simulation of specific patient case

In complex single cases or for the implementation of new techniques in large health services, realistic simulations can be great allies for the quality of surgical intervention.

This type of simulation is used for the surgical planning of complex cases, where each stage of the surgery is simulated, narrated, and discussed among the team, and its main objective is to project a real situation that will happen soon, identify the critical points, and thus plan the intervention before the actual surgery [21, 22].

Neurosurgeons from large centers such as São Paulo, London, Tokyo, or New York, for example, use this technique for extreme cases, thus managing problems even before scheduling surgery, making surgery safer and more economical. As the simulators are built from the child's neuroimaging, it is possible to perform tomography or magnetic resonance imaging of the shadow in the postoperative period and in this way even evaluate the result of the surgical intervention.

3.10 The simulation stages

For the simulations to reach their main objective, it is necessary to be attentive to the three fundamental stages within the process that compose it and to understand the totality of the patient, where the Central Nervous System is just one component of all systems. In this context, these steps are important to define the objectives of the simulation.

a. Briefing: Step that occurs before the simulation event. Dedicated to the case study, clinical evaluation, and discussion among the participating team about the main objectives to be achieved; it is also important to define the place where the simulation will take place, the projection of all the steps and all the necessary instructions in these variables.

b. Action: This step is the simulation event where all pre discussed points will be inserted in a simulated surgical event.

c. Debriefing: Moments after the simulation, where all participants carry out a critical reflection on the simulated event, whether the objectives were fully or partially achieved, where failures occurred, and where intervention is necessary.

It is essential for the simulation leader that all these steps are performed. The critical and constructive vision of this professional must be exposed to the team, and in this way, the disciplines must be reviewed if the objectives are not achieved, and thus, it will be up to the organizer to remind everyone what can be improved and simulated again [21–23].

4. The experience of a University Center in Brazil

The quality in neuroimaging definition already allows 3D reconstructions to be carried out in offices, clinics, and even on home computers that have access to the necessary programs and files. That is, the use of the virtual world in the programming and simulation of large neurosurgical procedures need not be restricted to large health centers. The University Hospital of the Faculty of Medicine of Ribeirão Preto of the University of São Paulo is an example; it already uses this reality and obtains fantastic results (**Figure 11**).

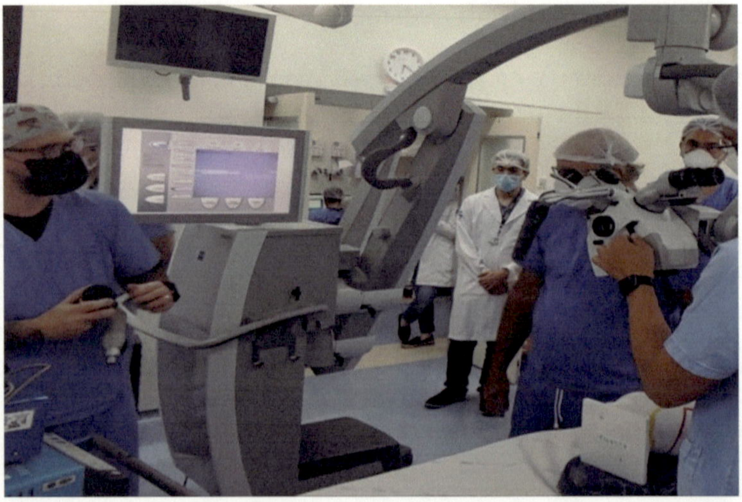

Figure 11.
Realistic simulation for separating craniopagus Siamese. HC collection. HCFMRP. Ribeirão Preto. Brazil. 2023.

In 2018, we carried out the first successful Craniópagus separation in Latin America and the simulation events were decisive for the success of this process; the printing of specific shadows was a watershed for the institution and placed Pediatric Neurosurgery at the forefront of this type of surgical process in the interior of the state of São Paulo.

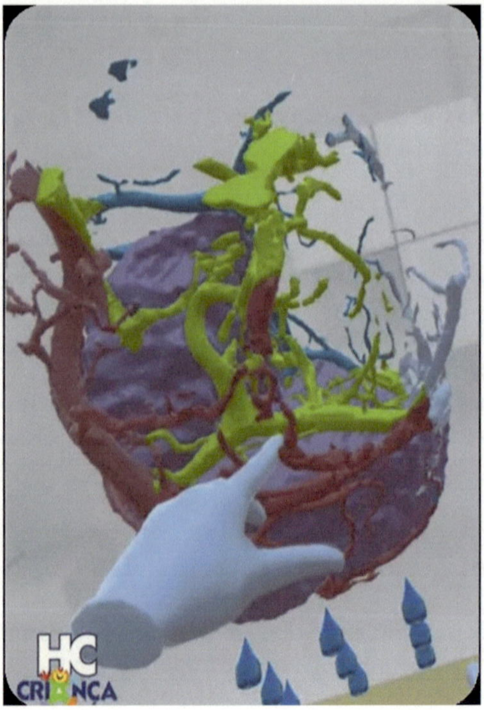

Figure 12.
Virtual simulation for separating craniopagus Siamese. HC collection. HCFMRP. Ribeirão Preto. 2023. HC collection. HCFMRP. Ribeirão Preto. Brazil. 2023.

Until the beginning of the Covid-19 pandemic, 3D printing for specific patients had a unique growth in the institution, with the implementation of new procedures; the anticipation of problems was detected in the first situational simulations and corrected before the realistic simulation, which allowed us to a shorter hospital stay and anesthetic exposure of patients.

After the full resumption of the Surgical Center in the post-pandemic period, we implemented new processes for pediatric neurosurgery with the addition of virtual simulations, even managing to apply augmented reality by integrating a microscope and neuronavigator.

Simulations are used for new procedures and complex surgeries where we need to involve more than one surgical team at the same time, as for fetal surgical corrections of myelomeningocele, for example (**Figure 12**).

In 2022, the institution received a new case of Craniópagus, where the combination of simulations with physical shadows is merging with virtual simulations, bringing fantastic results to children, experienced by the team for the first time.

5. Conclusion

With the popularization of peripherals such as virtual glasses and 3D printers in expansion, we will be able to advance even more in the printing speed of specific simulators for complex simulated events. As the use of realistic simulations is already part of the training curriculum for health professionals in various segments around the world, these are inserted in the daily life of health institutions with much more naturalness for each new generation of professionals.

Would we have imagined mixed reality in the programming of a surgery 15 years ago? Or perform an entire surgery in a virtual environment shared with multidisciplinary teams?

Today, we already use these resources and get fantastic results. Where the future will take us is still a question with many possibilities; the only common answer to these questions is that the objective of providing safer, more assertive, and quality assistance will always guide professionals of this and the next generations.

Author details

Allison Roberto da Silva[1,2*] and Jacqueline Rodrigues da Silva[3,4]

1 Clinical Hospital, Medicine School of Ribeirão Preto, University of São Paulo, São Paulo, Brazil

2 Medicine School of Ribeirão Preto, University of São Paulo, São Paulo, Brazil

3 Children's Clinical Hospital, Medicine School of Ribeirão Preto, University of São Paulo, São Paulo, Brazil

4 Nurse School of Ribeirão Preto, University of São Paulo, São Paulo, Brazil

*Address all correspondence to: alrsilva@hcrp.usp.br

References

[1] Pazin Filho A, Scarpelini S. Simulation: Definition. Medicine Magazine. 2007;**40**(2):162-166. Available from: https://www.revistas.usp.br/rmrp/article/download/312/313/618 [Accessed: June 15, 2023]

[2] Ziv A, Wolpe PR, Small SD, Glick S. Simulation-based medical education: An ethical imperative. Academic Medicine. 2003;**78**(8):783-788. Available from: https://www.researchgate.net/publication/10616959_Simulation-Based_Medical_Education_An_Ethical_Imperative [Accessed: July 20, 2023]

[3] Smith R. The long history of games in military training. Simulated Games. 2010;**41**:6-19. Available from: https://apps.dtic.mil/sti/pdfs/ADA550307.pdf [Accessed: June 15, 2023]

[4] Connoly P. The Art of Medieval Warfare: From Rome to Constantinople. Rio de Janeiro: Zahar; 1998

[5] File: The Operations Room at RAF Fighter Command's No. 10 Group Headquarters, Rudloe Manor (RAF Box), Wiltshire, showing WAAF plotters and duty officers at work, 1943. Available from: https://commons.wikimedia.org/wiki/File:The_Operations_Room_at_RAF_Fighter_Command%27s_No._10_Group_Headquarters,_Rudloe_Manor_(RAF_Box),_Wiltshire,_showing_WAAF_plotters_and_duty_officers_at_work,_1943._CH11887.jpg [Accessed: June 15, 2023]

[6] Chris B. Science for war and peace: Military use has helped advance science, but science's role in the quest for peace is critical. Science Culture. 2022;**74**(4):1-6. Available from: http://cienciaecultura.bvs.br/scielo.php?script=sci_arttext&pid=S0009-67252022000400020&lng=en [Accessed: June 18, 2023]

[7] Brazil. Air force agency. In: Peccini J. Flight Simulator of the C-105 Amazonas of the Brazilian Air Force is Homologated by ANAC. Brasilia: Brazilian Air Force; 2016. Available from: https://www.fab.mil.br/noticias/mostra/28285/CERTIFICA%C3%87%C3%83O%20-%20Simulador%20de%20voo%20do%20C-105%20Amazonas%20da%20For%C3%A7a%20A%C3%A9rea%20Brazilian%20%C3%A9%20approved%20by%20ANAC [Accessed: November 11, 2023]

[8] Santos CA, Neto JP, Silva JN. 10 books, 10 regions, 10 games to learn and have fun. Norprint. 2008. Available from: http://jnsilva.ludicum.org/hm2008_9/1grecia.pdf [Accessed: June 18, 2023]

[9] Rehder R, Abd-El-Barr M, Hooten K, Weinstock P, Madsen JR, Cohen AR. The role of simulation in neurosurgery. Child's Nervous System. 2016;**32**(1):43-54. DOI: 10.1007/s00381-015-2923-z. Epub 2015 Oct 5. Available from: https://pubmed.ncbi.nlm.nih.gov/26438547/ [Accessed: June 18, 2023]

[10] Coelho G, Vieira T. History of surgical simulation and its application in neurosurgery. Scientia Medica. 2018;**28**(1):13-19. Available from: https://revistaseletronicas.pucrs.br/ojs/index.php/scientiamedica/article/view/29688/16668 [Accessed: June 18, 2023]

[11] Persaud TVN. A history of anatomy: The post-vesalian era. In: Thomas CC, editor. Illinois: Springfield; 1997

[12] Bradley P. The history of simulation in medical education and possible future directions. Medical Education. 2006;**40**:254-262. Available from:

https://pubmed.ncbi.nlm.nih.gov/16483328/ [Accessed: June 18, 2023]

[13] Owen H. Early use of simulation in medical education. Simulation in Healthcare. 2012;7(2):102-116. Available from: https://pubmed.ncbi.nlm.nih.gov/22374231/ [Accessed: July 16, 2023]

[14] Bates AW. Dr Kahn's museum: Obscene anatomy in Victorian London. Journal of the Royal Society of Medicine. 2006;**99**:618Y624. Available from: https://www.ncbi.nlm.nih.gov/pmc/articles/PMC1676337/ [Accessed: July 27, 2023]

[15] Cooper JB, Taqueti VR. A brief history of the development of mannequin simulators for clinical education and training. Postgraduate Medical Journal. 2004;**13**(1):11-18. Available from: https://www.ncbi.nlm.nih.gov/pmc/articles/PMC1765785/ [Accessed: July 26, 2023]

[16] Singh et al. History of simulation in medicine: From Resusci Annie to the Ann Myers medical center. Neurosurgery. 2013;**73**(4):9-14

[17] Barreto DC, Silva KGN, Moreira SSCR, Silva TS, Magro MCS. Realistic simulation as a teaching strategy for the nursing undergraduate course: Integrative review. Bahia Journal of Nursing, Salvador. 2014;**28**(2):208-214. Available from: https://www.hindawi.com/journals/nrp/2012/765212/ [Accessed: July 21, 2023]

[18] Santos Filho JAM. Human Placenta as a Training Model for Brain Aneurysm Surgeries [thesis]. Brazil: Federal University of Minas Gerais; 2015. 71 f. Available from: https://periodicos.ufba.br/index.php/enfermagem/article/view/8476/8874 [Accessed: July 21, 2023]

[19] Silva AR, Miyazaki AH, Caridade CD, Tassi E. The Advent of Realistic On-Site Simulations for Complex Surgical Cases: A Strategy to Ensure Excellence in Patient Safety. Ribeirão Preto: HC Quality Magazine; 2022. pp. 79-85. Available from: https://www.hcrp.usp.br/revistaqualidadehc/uploads/Artigos/454/454.pdf [Accessed: July 21, 2023]

[20] Silva AR. Surgical Planning for the Process of Separation of Conjoined Craniopagus Twins. Ensuring Quality and Excellence in the First Stage. Ribeirão Preto: HC Quality Magazine; 2022. pp. 9-16. Available from: https://www.hcrp.usp.br/revistaqualidadehc/uploads/Artigos/452/452.pdf [Accessed: July 21, 2023]

[21] Caselato GCR. Use of Realistic Simulators in Pediatric Neurosurgery [thesis]. Brazil: University of Sao Paulo; 2019. 129 f. Available from: https://www.teses.usp.br/teses/disponiveis/5/5138/tde-01072019-144748/publico/GiselleCoelhoResendeCaselato.pdf [Accessed: July 21, 2023]

[22] Carneiro MMG, Kobashikawa. Virtual Reality and its Applications in the Medical Area. São Paulo: Pet-Si Group Newspaper; 2019. Available from: http://www.each.usp.br/petsi/jornal/?p=2628 [Accessed: July 21, 2023]

[23] Kolbe M, Grande B, Spahn DR. Briefing and debriefing during simulation-based training and beyond: Content, structure, attitude and setting. Best Practice & Research. Clinical Anaesthesiology. 2015;**29**(1):87-96. DOI: 10.1016/j.bpa.2015.01.002. Epub 2015 Jan 28. Available from: https://pubmed.ncbi.nlm.nih.gov/25902470/ [Accessed: July 21, 2023]

Section 3

Pediatric Neuro-Rehabilitation

Chapter 5

Application of the International Classification Functioning, Disability, and Health (ICF) as Clinical Reasoning Tool in Pediatric Neurorehabilitation

Hanan Demyati

Abstract

The clinical reasoning model is a theoretical framework that facilitates the transformation of information into practical knowledge within the context of clinical practice. It serves as a valuable resource for healthcare professionals, offering a structured approach for the assessment and development of treatment plans. Biomedical disability models often influence clinical reasoning models in pediatric neurorehabilitation, emphasizing diagnostic reasoning and using a shared vocabulary and language to guide thinking and communication during information gathering, assumption formulation, and care action planning. This method prioritizes physical symptoms over psychological, social, cultural, and environmental factors of a given condition. This idea assumes that the health condition or pathology is the sole fundamental factor contributing to any form of physical dysfunction and that the reduction of the disease will lead to a restoration of the previous state of "normalcy". The International Classification of Functioning, Disability, and Health (ICF) framework can be used as a clinical reasoning tool as it guides cognitive processes and decision-making based on the interdependent relationships between the three primary components and contextual factors. The ICF framework recognizes that changes in the child's environmental and psychological context, activity and social involvement, and pathology can affect child outcomes without emphasizing changes in pathology.

Keywords: clinical reasoning, neurorehabilitation, ICF, pediatric, WHO-ICF

1. Introduction

Pediatric neurorehabilitation is heavily impacted by biomedical model, which is based on acute care medicine. Consider how we treat sudden severe chest pain: a history is taken, the child is evaluated, other options are ruled out to make the appropriate diagnosis, the right treatment is found, the child is intervened, and the condition is monitored after treatment. This approach focuses on fixing to imply that a specific diagnosis will result in suitable treatment. In pediatric neurorehabilitation, body mechanics and biopsychosocial factors are considered. Heterogeneous groups in the same health condition as the treatment may address signs and symptoms underlying biomedical aspects of the condition, but since the intervention is obvious, the evidence to support or refute it is not enough [1].

This way of thinking has several limitations toward fixing, which refers to the expectation that an appropriate diagnosis will lead to the right interventions. A common diagnosis, Cerebral Palsy (CP) and Autism Spectrum Disorder (ASD), seems specific in pediatric neurology, while the heterogeneous nature of those disorders can affect children's development for a number of biological reasons with a wide range of impacts. Some of our "treatments" may address biomedical aspects of the condition. For instance, the utilization of botulinum toxin to manage spasticity and anticonvulsants to treat seizure disorders has been observed. However, due to the restricted comprehension and complexity nature of the underlying biomedical processes associated with illnesses such as CP and ASD, even when the biological "impairments" of these disorders can be changed, there are generally few links between bodily alterations and functional outcomes [2, 3]. Development is fast, yet many of our treatments are slow. It is difficult to find causal links between interventions and results due to natural changes influenced by growth and development.

Health is "the ability to adapt and to self-manage" [4]. WHO provided a set of concepts about how we could think about health in 2001 [5]. The International Classification of Functioning, Disability, and Health (ICF) framework is a conceptual framework used to record the positive and negative aspects of every person's functioning and puts every person in a context: functioning and disability are results of the interaction between the health conditions of the person and their environment (in **Figure 1**). The ICF framework provides a standard language for the definition and measurement of people's health and function [5].

The clinical reasoning model is a theoretical framework that facilitates the transformation of information into practical knowledge in the context of therapeutic practice. It serves as a valuable resource for therapists, offering a structured approach for both assessment and treatment planning. This method is executed by using a coherent sequence of activities [6].

The reciprocal interactions between the three core ICF components and environmental factors can influence clinical reasoning and decision-making. The ICF framework allows changes in the patient's environmental and personal context,

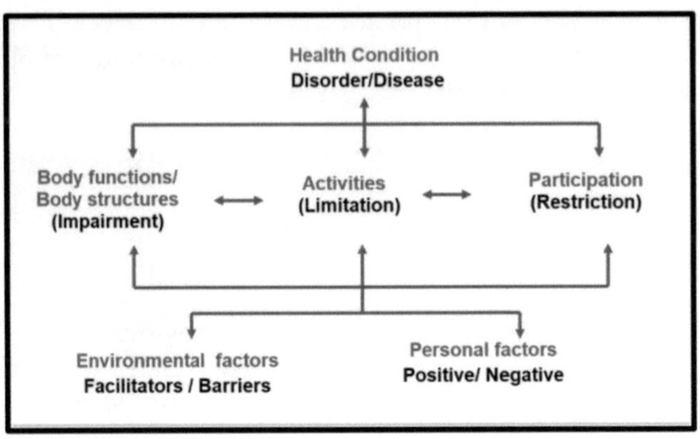

Figure 1.
International classification of functioning, disability, and health (copied from WHO [5]).

activity and social participation, and pathology to affect patient outcomes. Improved outcomes without pathological changes are a useful clinical reasoning tool for pediatric neurorehabilitation. The ICF framework allows all health issues to be considered in a border social-ecological setting, which might turn the paradigm upside down. This shows that any section of the framework may have influenced others in this dynamic system [7, 8].

2. The international classification functioning, disability, and health (ICF) model

The International Classification of Functioning, Disability, and Health (ICF) "are functional frameworks that classify health outcomes; they can be used to describe the functioning of all people, not only persons with a health condition(s)." The ICF model is derived from a framework developed by the World Health Organization (WHO) (see **Figure 1**) [9].

This framework presents an individual's functioning and disability as consequences resulting from the interplay between health problems and other contextual factors, including both environmental and personal factors. The term "functioning" encompasses the entirety of bodily functions, activities, and participation in many living circumstances, including work, family, and leisure. The term "disability" encompasses a range of conditions, encompassing impairments in bodily function and structure, limitations in activities, and restrictions in participation [9].

The ICF model encompasses body functions and structures, as well as activities and participation. A significant innovation offered by the ICF model, the concept of a child's environmental and personal/social context are conceptualized and implemented. The consideration of the child's needs is situated within the framework of the family, taking into account how the nature and types of participation undergo significant transformations from dependent ties during infancy to intricate and more independent life circumstances during adolescence [10]. This innovation also addresses the notion of developmental changes in participation through the imitation of actions and behaviors. The ICF model acknowledges that variations in the environment and the timing of developmental milestones may indicate delays in development rather than functional impairments or limitations [9, 10].

The ICF is founded upon an integration of social and medical theories of disability and places emphasis on the constituents of health rather than the outcomes of illness [9]. The several dimensions of the ICF framework integrate biological, psychological, social, and environmental factors that contribute to child functioning [10]. Research findings have indicated that just the process of diagnosing a child does not serve as an accurate guide for determining the level of treatment provided or the functional results experienced by the patient [9]. The utilization of a medical diagnostic as an individual instrument may result in the omission of crucial information required for effective healthcare planning and management [11].

According to the data presented in **Figure 1**, the ICF framework categorizes health conditions into three distinct health outcomes: bodily function and structure, activities, and participation. Disease, disorder, or injury might potentially lead to the reduction of three different health outcomes: impairment, activity limitations, and participation restrictions. The interplay among the three components is subject to the influence of contextual factors, which can be categorized into two components: environmental factors and personal factors [9].

The "body" domain (body structure and body function) covers physical and mental functions, sensory responses, multiorgan system structure and function, movement, and reproduction. The "activities and participation" domain evaluates the patient's capacity to learn, apply knowledge, complete general tasks, communicate, and care for themselves. The ICF also described two types of contextual factors, namely environmental and personal factors. Environmental domains include patient-assistance items and technologies, community services, and relationships, support, and care outside the clinical setting. Each component has a hierarchy of categories and codes in the ICF. Personal factors such as age, sex, education, social class, culture, past experiences, personal character traits, lifestyle, coping style, and occupation are not coded [10, 11].

3. Pediatric neurorehabilitation services

Pediatric neurorehabilitation services include a variety of therapeutic disciplines, such as rehabilitation medicine, physiotherapy, occupational therapy, speech therapy, orthotics and prosthetics, nutrition, psychology, and social services. These services are characterized by their interdisciplinary nature. The presence of divergent governance and policy frameworks among health professionals presents challenges for implementing uniform standards for working practices within the healthcare system. The presence of diversity may influence the quality of services provided to such patients by healthcare professionals [12].

Pediatric neurology affects the child's psychological, social, and emotional well-being as well as their physical health. This can affect children's daily physical functioning, including body structure and function and task performance. These tasks include their everyday activities, what they desire to do in their environment, and personal characteristics that help or hinder their functional activities (e.g., at home, in the community, or at school) [13]. Thus, it is important to consider social and family circumstances in pediatric neurorehabilitation.

Healthcare, education, and social services can struggle to support neurologically manifested children and their families. This condition is complicated, so a model like the ICF that considers bodily impairments, personal effects, and environmental effects is needed to manage pediatric neurorehabilitation holistically.

4. Clinical reasoning model in pediatric neurorehabilitation

Clinical reasoning is important as it promotes knowledge acquisition by utilizing simple phrases to explain complicated relationships [12]. The clinical reasoning models utilized in the field of neurorehabilitation are frequently inspired by the biomedical model of disability. As a result, therapists might prefer diagnostic reasoning that aligns with the principles of the biomedical model [13, 14]. The biomedical model applies standard terminology and discourse in the various stages of treatment decision-making, including initial consultation, data collection, hypothesis formulation, and care planning. However, it primarily concentrates on the physical symptoms of a condition and does not adequately consider the psychological, social, cultural, or environmental dimensions [15]. The biomedical paradigm is based on two fundamental assumptions. Firstly, it posits that disease or disorder is the primary and only factor responsible for all physical dysfunction. Secondly, it asserts that the elimination or reduction of the disease would lead to a restoration of the individual's state to what is considered "normal" [16].

The models considered significant to the practice of pediatric neurorehabilitation include analytical, non-analytical, and hypothetico-deductive reasoning. The analytical model predominantly focuses on a systematic approach to assessment prior to decision-making, whereas the nonanalytical model includes a more spontaneous process that is influenced by the recognition of similar earlier cases [17]. Hypothetico-deductive reasoning involves the formulation and evaluation of diagnostic hypotheses by analytical testing methods, such as patient history and physical examination. These methods are employed to either validate or disapprove of solutions that have been developed through nonanalytical means [18].

4.1 Analytical clinical reasoning model

Theoretical frameworks for clinical reasoning suggest the existence of a sequential set of analytical procedures utilized to establish a correlation between a patient's symptoms and the ultimate diagnosis [19]. This method uses analytical reasoning in a more planned way by sticking to a set of distinct steps: careful observation, data collection, a physical exam, coming up with hypotheses, and finally diagnostic testing to confirm these hypotheses [20]. Therapists who adopt a biomedical clinical reasoning approach in pediatric neurorehabilitation may prioritize the development of a recovery strategy and the attainment of a diagnosis as the ultimate objectives.

4.2 Nonanalytical clinical reasoning model

Nonanalytical clinical reasoning refers to a cognitive process when individuals are able to arrive at a conclusion without relying on formal analytical methods, instead drawing upon their past interactions and experiences [18, 21]. The automation of this process is frequently noted and seen as an indicator of heightened clinical proficiency. This phenomenon can be attributed to the disparity in prior clinical experience between novices and individuals with higher degrees of expertise, as supported by earlier research [21]. This methodology enables expeditious decision-making, although some scholars contend that it may engender erroneous inferences among less seasoned practitioners. This approach allows for quick decisions to be made by less experienced professionals, and there is a risk of inappropriate conclusions being drawn.

4.3 Hypothetico-deductive clinical reasoning model

The present paradigm is dependent upon the collection of data from the patient, which is then utilized to build a hypothesis. This hypothesis is initially developed by the therapist and then subjected to testing. The confirmation or rejection of the hypothesis depends on the patient's response to treatment, necessitating the need for periodic examinations [22]. Practitioners across diverse therapeutic fields commonly employ this approach [19, 23]. The initial phase involves the therapist being equipped beforehand with a comprehensive and elaborate patient history, encompassing the patient's motivations for seeking rehabilitation treatments. Subsequently, the therapist proceeds to administer an examination technique employing several tests and assessments. Following the conclusion of the examination, the therapist proceeds to formulate several hypotheses pertaining to "evaluation, diagnosis, and prognosis." These hypotheses are developed by synthesizing and analyzing the data gathered throughout the examination, ultimately serving as a foundation for further assessment and prognostication. The therapist may employ a collaborative reasoning approach, drawing upon the patient's knowledge base, in order to attain a comprehensive grasp of the issue during the therapeutic session. During the process of hypothesis formation, the therapist may introduce generic questions and afterward reflect on the issues expressed by the patient. Ultimately, the therapist arrives at a definitive diagnosis or formulates a comprehensive plan for implementing a specific intervention [23].

Empirical data support the paradigms in rehabilitative treatment. Doody and McAteer [18] employed a qualitative approach and utilized the hypothetico-deductive model to examine the clinical reasoning abilities of expert and novice physiotherapists in the context of outpatient orthopedic care. A group of 10 seasoned doctors and 10 students were observed and recorded via audio while they conducted a comprehensive examination and administered treatment to an actual patient who had not been encountered previously. The findings indicated that every participant employed a hypothetico-deductive reasoning process. However, both individuals with expertise in the field and those with limited experience extended their analysis beyond the first diagnostic phase to incorporate a thoughtful approach to treatment. Specifically, manual therapy treatment was employed as a means to conduct more hypothesis testing. Furthermore, alongside the application of hypothetico-deductive reasoning, the professionals also employed a nonanalytical model, as anticipated, due to their extensive clinical expertise [18].

This model demonstrates a high level of development and serves as a valuable tool in the field of pediatric neurorehabilitation. It effectively integrates decision-making processes with corresponding actions and closely monitors the dynamic changes that occur throughout the patient's treatment journey. Kenyon [23] utilized this particular model as an instructional tool for providing clinical reasoning skills to students specializing in pediatric physiotherapy. However, it was noted that students exhibited a proclivity for providing an inaccurate portrayal of their actions and thoughts during the diagnostic procedure. However, the authors merely provided a reconstructed conceptualization of the appropriate approach to resolving the issue [23].

The therapists mostly based their decision-making process on subjective results obtained from physical examination rather than relying on objective testing. Consequently, they expressed a lack of confidence in the effectiveness of practical establishment testing. Hence, based on empirical observations, it appears that pediatric neurorehabilitation relies on a combination of analytical thinking, non-analytical reasoning, and hypothetico-deductive reasoning, as indicated by previous studies [22–25]. The clinical reasoning models in question likely originate from the framework of biomedical knowledge. Consequently, therapists in the field of pediatric neurorehabilitation often make the assumption that an intervention involving the manipulation of bodily functions will yield the intended outcomes in terms of the patient's physical performance and ability to engage in activities [22]. For instance, there is a common assumption that enhancing the muscular strength of an ambulant child (body function) will influence the child's capacity to walk with optimal efficiency (related to activity).

In the field of pediatric neurorehabilitation, it is crucial for therapists to apply a clinical reasoning model that acknowledges the significance of the biomedical model while also offering a structured approach to recognizing and addressing both biomedical and psychosocial factors. The ICF model facilitates the formulation of a hypothesis by taking into account the interplay between several aspects, such as bodily structure, function, activities, and participation, as well as environmental and personal factors, for every individual child.

5. Personal factors in the ICF framework

Personal factors (PFs), known as background knowledge about a person's life and way of living, have not been categorized by the WHO. Examples of personal factors include assets, coping methods, education, and behavioral patterns [8]. The facilitation of comprehension about the cognitive processes of children and their parents, including their evaluation and understanding of their own situations, aspirations, and coping mechanisms in their everyday lives, can be enhanced by the identification of these factors pertaining to functioning. The decision-making process regarding the choice of rehabilitation programs, measures, and other forms of support is contingent upon the effect of PFs and their respective interpretations [24].

Numerous studies have consistently demonstrated the significant function and special significance of PFs in the context of rehabilitation processes. Patient- and family-centered care emphasizes the importance of prioritizing the needs and preferences of individuals and their families during various healthcare processes. Moreover, by comprehensively comprehending and incorporating PFs into the evaluation of a client's functioning, professionals in neurorehabilitation can enhance their grasp of effective strategies to bolster child and parent commitment. PFs would enable therapists to engage in systematic documentation and optimize time management [24, 26]. In the meantime, it is advisable to utilize the ICF framework as a tool for organizing information and ideas associated with functioning, even in cases where PFs have not been officially defined within the categorical framework.

6. Roles of personal factors in pediatric neurorehabilitation

Personal factors (PFs) play an essential role in pediatric neurorehabilitation; asking and understanding about PFs promotes respect for values, beliefs, experience, and circumstances and the inclusion of client-defined families. PF assessment is crucial for pediatric neurorehabilitation planning and functioning documentation. Rehabilitation programs include multiple phases; motivation is personal, and it has been shown to predict exercise intervention adherence. Additionally, different clients value different things, which affect commitment. Considering how different PFs affect commitment might help professionals encourage empowerment and strengths [24, 26]. The rehabilitation process combines two theoretical frameworks: treatment theory shows how to change a factor, and enablement theory recognizes that functioning is complex and determined by multiple factors and models of these complex interrelationships. Understanding child PF variation is necessary to apply enabling theory to pediatric neurorehabilitation. The PFs provide crucial information on functioning throughout a child's rehabilitation. In clinical practice, the ICF organizes and codes functioning, and environmental and child PFs can affect health, functioning, and the neurorehabilitation process [27, 28].

7. Environmental factors in the ICF framework

The classification of environmental factors was developed to include significant elements of the physical, social, and attitudinal environments in which individuals live and engage in their daily activities. The factors consisted of both immediate factors, such as products and technology for mobility, as well as more distant factors, such as societal attitudes, systems, and policies. These factors have the potential to influence an individual's functioning. Additionally, there are factors that necessitate interventions targeted at the individual, such as the provision of accessible environments, as well as interventions aimed at society, such as the development and implementation of inclusive policies [8].

The term "disability" can be used to describe various situations. Firstly, it can refer to an individual who solely experiences a physical issue at the bodily level, known as an impairment, without any limitations in their activities or restrictions in their participation. For example, this could include a person with severe scarring on their face who does not encounter any difficulties in their daily activities or engagement in society. Secondly, disability can represent individuals who face challenges in functioning across all three levels: the body (impairments), the person (activity limitations), and society (participation restrictions). Thirdly, disability may involve individuals who have both an impairment and an activity limitation but do not experience any participation restrictions. Fourthly, disability can refer to individuals who encounter activity limitations and participation restrictions but do not have any impairments. Lastly, disability can also apply to individuals who do not have any impairments or activity limitations but face participation restrictions in their daily lives [29].

An illustrative case of an individual encountering impairments, limitations in activities, and restrictions in participation would involve a child with spina bifida. This child, regrettably, lacks access to essential services such as orthotic and prosthetic services, which are crucial for their well-being. Additionally, due to the absence of assistive technology in the form of an orthosis, the child faces difficulties in mobility. Furthermore, their ability to attend school is hindered by an inaccessible educational environment and the presence of negative attitudes toward their condition. To gain a comprehensive understanding of an individual's experience of disability, it is necessary to delineate the various dimensions of functioning alongside an examination of the environmental and personal elements that contribute to this experience. The alteration of contextual elements might lead to a modification in the outcome, consequently impacting the experience of impairment. The ICF model offers a conceptual framework that enables the description of the various elements involved in an interaction.

8. Roles of environmental factors in pediatric neurorehabilitation

In the relationship between environmental factors and other components of functioning in the ICF model, disability arises from the interplay between an individual's health condition and the surrounding contextual elements in which the individual is situated. This relationship is further analyzed in terms of the components of functioning and the three viewpoints of body, person, and society. At the social, bodily impairments, and individual activity restriction levels, it is clear that the consequences are influenced by the interaction of an individual's health state and many contextual factors [30].

The child who utilizes a wheelchair and is currently not enrolled in an educational institution does not require any modifications to their physical condition in order to access educational opportunities. In order to enhance a child's engagement in education, it is imperative to address both the accessibility of the school and the prevailing attitudes inside the education system. The education student diagnosed with epilepsy does not necessarily have to abandon their pursuit of training. It is imperative to critically examine the perspectives held by education authorities in order to identify a more efficacious strategy for effectively addressing the potential incidence of a seizure during instructional sessions.

The ICF model offers a comprehensive framework for categorizing environmental influences and their impact on individuals with health conditions. The ICF model serves as the initial step in advancing the comprehension of the influence of the environment on impairment. The application of the ICF model within the context of pediatric neurorehabilitation has the potential to facilitate the active involvement of families in the process of defining goals. This approach also enables therapists to be more adaptable to the specific requirements of the family and to effectively communicate information in a manner that is meaningful and beneficial to them. Moreover, applying the ICF model in the context of pediatric neurorehabilitation could enhance a therapist's engagement with both the child and their family. It has the potential to facilitate the establishment of attainable objectives and facilitate progression from one level of care to another, taking into account the child's level of functioning, disability, and health while also considering the child's environment and personal factors.

9. Clinical reasoning in pediatric neurorehabilitation

The therapist's level of knowledge, cognitive abilities, and metacognitive skills have a significant impact on the clinical reasoning process because they enable them to effectively recognize and resolve problems in situations that are ambiguous or uncertain [31].

The clinical reasoning process persists throughout the child's neurorehabilitation course of continuing child management. Reassessment serves the purpose of either providing support for the hypotheses and chosen course of action or indicating the need for revision or production of hypotheses, as well as further data gathering and problem clarification. This may involve an additional examination or a referral for consultation with other specialists. During a therapeutic session, clinicians engage in the ongoing process of interpreting child and parent reactions in order to inform their clinical judgments. Additionally, therapists regularly evaluate treatment outcomes to assess the validity of their management hypotheses [32].

Child and parent thinking regarding their difficulties is of equal importance to the therapist's thinking. Children and their families typically enter their interaction with a therapist with preconceived notions about the nature of their disorder, which are influenced by personal experiences and guidance from healthcare professionals, as well as input from their social network. Previous research has demonstrated that patients' comprehension of their clinical condition has a significant influence on their pain tolerance, impairment levels, and ultimate outcome [32, 33]. The presence of a child's or parent's beliefs and emotions that hinder their management and recovery might have a detrimental impact on their engagement in the management process, their self-efficacy, and ultimately, their overall outcome. On the other hand, research has demonstrated that patients who are included in the decision-making process exhibit a higher level of accountability for their own treatment and are more likely to have improved outcomes. By engaging in a collaborative reasoning process with their therapists, patients can maximize their self-efficacy and level of responsibility for their management [34].

Therapists specializing in pediatric neurorehabilitation are required to thoroughly evaluate and take into account all conceivable aspects that may have an impact on a child's overall well-being. Therapists are commonly associated with a primary emphasis on the physical aspects of health. However, in line with the modern biopsychosocial perspective on health and disability, it is essential for therapists to recognize that addressing a child's well-being necessitates a comprehensive assessment of environmental and psychosocial factors that can impact health. This approach should be implemented within the boundaries of the therapists' professional training and expertise. A successful approach to addressing this matter necessitates a comprehensive perspective on health and disability as well as a thorough understanding of evaluation and management principles, including knowledge of appropriate referral pathways. Additionally, it demands the acquisition of skills to effectively address all potential elements that may contribute to the issue at hand.

Furthermore, the ability to engage in clinical reasoning is essential in determining the relevance of these potential contributing factors to the specific patient, enabling the healthcare provider to make proper clinical judgments that would ultimately enhance the patient's overall healthcare outcomes [35]. The ICF model offers a standardized language and framework that facilitates communication regarding health and healthcare across many professional disciplines and scientific fields. The conceptual framework of the ICF emphasizes the absence of a direct cause-and-effect relationship between a particular health condition and the resulting functional outcomes. Additionally, it recognizes contextual elements as significant determinants of outcomes. The ICF model offers a comprehensive framework and organizational system for gathering and categorizing clinical, behavioral, and contextual data. This framework has the potential to have a beneficial impact on the processes of assessment, intervention design, and outcome evaluation [36, 37]. This facilitates the establishment of a comprehensive clinical and contextual profile for a pediatric patient with a neurological health condition and offers systematic guidance for the integrated provision of services to children and their families who need to be included in their rehabilitation management.

Most common pediatric neurological disorders have a reciprocal relationship with their body functions and structures, their ability to conduct functional tasks, and their subsequent engagement in familial, occupational, and recreational responsibilities. The physical well-being, activities, participation, and health of individuals can be impacted in either a positive or negative manner by a range of factors. These factors encompass both environmental elements and various factors that contribute to the shaping of individuals' behaviors and experiences. These factors include social attitudes, architectural characteristics, legal and social structures, climate, and terrain. Gender, age, psychological traits (e.g., thoughts, beliefs, and coping styles), health and illness behaviors, social circumstances, education, and past and present experiences are also playing a significant role [38].

10. Application of the ICF as clinical reasoning tool in pediatric neurorehabilitation

Therapists in pediatric neurorehabilitation typically use a degree of routine in their evaluation process. Based on their expertise in ICF knowledge and their clinical practice, the therapists have determined the specific categories of information that have been considered highly valuable for the identification of problems and the making of management decisions, as shown in **Figure 2**. These categories include environmental data, subjective and objective attributes of the patient's impairments

DOI: http://dx.doi.org/10.5772/intechopen.1003078

(such as location, behavior, and history of symptoms), as well as specific evaluations of functioning, structure, and cognition.

In addition to these established procedures, individualized investigations and examinations are customized to accommodate the individual manifestations of each child. The development of tailored inquiries and tests for each individual child is prompted by the formulation of first hypotheses. The cognitive process known as "hypothesis testing" ideally involves the systematic exploration of both confirming and disconfirming evidence. The obtained data are further analyzed to determine their alignment with previously collected data and relevant theories.

The interpretation of routine inquiries, tests, and spontaneous information provided by child/family will be conducted within the framework of initial hypotheses. Through this process, the therapist gains a progressive comprehension of the child's neurological disorder. The initial hypothesis will undergo modifications, and further hypotheses will be taken into consideration. The process of generating and testing hypotheses persists until an adequate amount of information is acquired to enable a therapist to formulate a diagnosis pertaining to the physical and psychosocial manifestations. This diagnosis also considers the suitability of therapist involvement and/or referral to other healthcare professionals, as well as the implementation of rehabilitation management strategies.

The clinical reasoning involved in the assessment and management using the ICF component in child and family contexts necessitates the careful study of the cognitive processes employed by the therapist, child, and family, as well as the collaborative nature of decision-making among them. **Figure 2** depicts an ICF model of clinical reasoning as a collaborative process involving patients, as proposed in **Figure 2**. Within the context of pediatric neurorehabilitation settings, the therapist's cognitive processes are initiated by the initial data and cues acquired, such as the referral information and observations made of the patient. The initial data presented will elicit a variety of impressions or provisional judgments. Although not commonly recognized as such, these early interpretations can be regarded as hypotheses since they are

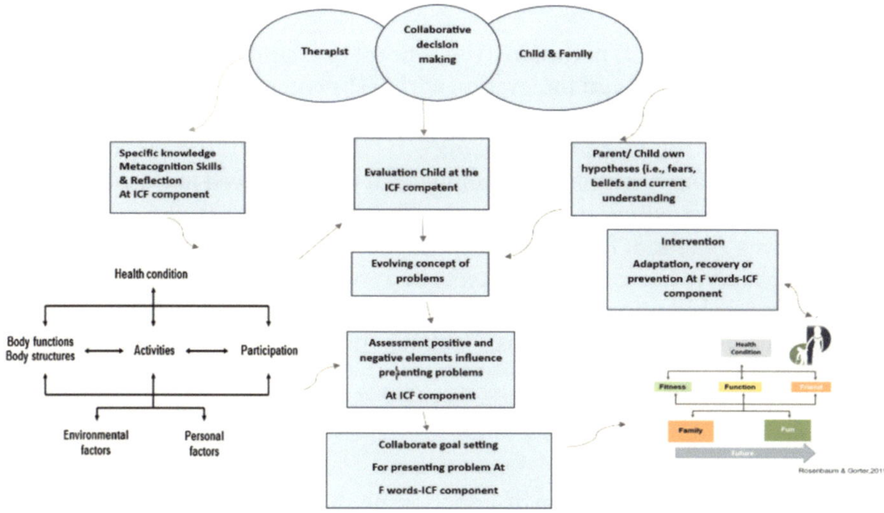

Figure 2.
ICF model of clinical reasoning as collaborative process between therapist in pediatric neurorehabilitation and child & family.

not definitive or conclusive choices. However, these first impressions are evaluated in light of additional information (data) that may either corroborate or contradict them. While there are similarities between this procedure and hypothesis testing, it is important to note that not all therapists may possess a comprehensive understanding of the ICF model or be aware of this process or their thinking in general. The process of hypothesis formation encompasses the integration of specific data interpretations or inductions with the synthesis of many hints or deductions [36–39].

The use of the six F-word concepts at the clinical level has the potential to enable service providers to effectively incorporate the ICF framework into the development of child-family-neurorehabilitation team goal setting (**Figure 2**). This approach would involve the inclusion of an individual's strengths in order to customize interventions. There are six fundamental factors that play an important role in the goal-setting process in pediatric neurorehabilitation [1]:

The first F-word, "function," pertains to the activities performed by individuals, encompassing their roles, jobs, occupations, and tasks. Hence, it is imperative to promote child's engagement in functional practice, regardless of the level of perfection attained.

The second F-word: Family serves as a fundamental component of external contextual influences inside child lives. Hence, the implementation of a family-centered approach within rehabilitation services has the potential to significantly enhance therapy outcomes and foster improved collaboration among healthcare practitioners. Collaborating with the family to ascertain their objectives can significantly enhance therapy outcomes and facilitate the family's access to resources to make well-informed decisions.

The third F-word: Fitness, the importance of physical fitness has been largely overlooked until recently. However, evidence indicates that individuals with chronic illnesses exhibit lower levels of fitness than what is considered optimal. While it is widely acknowledged that engaging in an exercise program can yield numerous advantages in terms of maintaining physical activity levels, it is imperative to incorporate physical training into rehabilitation.

The fourth F-word: Fun refers to activities that child finds enjoyable and meaningful in their daily lives.

The fifth F-word: Friend, pertains to the concept of friendship, which aims to enhance child engagement and integration within the community. Social factors have a crucial role in the well-being of a child, and it is imperative to take into account the quality of friendships as a facilitating factor.

The six F-words: Future, child, and family need to be involved in the plan of care and the interventions, which are only decided for them by the health provider.

By addressing function, fitness, family, fun, friends, and constantly reminding therapists in pediatric neurorehabilitation to be aware of the importance of children and families in rehabilitation services. It is crucial to involve child and their relatives in the decision-making process rather than making unilateral decisions on their behalf.

11. Conclusion

The International Classification of Functioning, Impairment, and Health (ICF) serves as a valuable instrument in enhancing comprehension of health and impairment within the context of pediatric neurorehabilitation. The utilization of this tool facilitates the enhancement of clinical reasoning among healthcare professionals by including a greater amount of information that surpasses the limitations of a mere list of diagnoses. Neurorehabilitation personnel must possess an awareness of and familiarity with the personal and environmental elements pertaining to their patients in order to have a comprehensive understanding of their values, desires, and objectives. The incorporation of this element is seen as crucial for the implementation of evidence-based practice within the field of pediatric neurorehabilitation.

The understanding of the impact of the environment and personal factors on disability has experienced a substantial transformation from the ICF framework in pediatric neurorehabilitation. The ICF recognizes the environment as a distinct and essential element within its framework. The ICF's conceptual framework necessitates the inclusion and clarification of environmental elements in order to fully comprehend disability. The conceptualization of intervention has similarly seen a shift in focus. This paradigm shift includes interventions aimed at both individuals and society, with an emphasis on removing barriers and cultivating facilitators.

Conflict of interest

The author declares no conflict of interest.

Author details

Hanan Demyati
Prince Sultan Armed Forces Hospital, Madinah, Saudi Arabia

*Address all correspondence to: tomsunny54@gmail.com

References

[1] Rosenbaum P, Gorter JW. The 'F-words' in childhood disability: I swear this is how we should think! Child: Care, Health and Development (John Wiley & Sons Ltd). 2011;**38**(4):283-289

[2] Verschuren O, Ada L, Maltais DB, Gorter JW, Scianni A, Ketelaar M. Muscle strengthening in children and adolescents with spastic cerebral palsy: Considerations for future resistance training protocols. Physical Therapy. 2011;**91**:1130-1139

[3] Wright FV, Rosenbaum PL, Goldsmith CH, Law M, Fehlings DL. How do changes in body functions and structures, activity, and participation relate in children with cerebral palsy? Developmental Medicine and Child Neurology. 2008;**50**(4):283-289. DOI: 10.1111/j.1469-8749.2008.02037.x

[4] Huber EO, Tobler A, Gloor-Juzi T, Grill E, Gubler-Gut B. The ICF as a way to specify goals and to assess the outcome of physiotherapeutic interventions in the acute hospital. Journal of Rehabilitation Medicine. 2011;**43**(2):174-177. DOI: 10.2340/16501977-0629

[5] World Health Organization. Towards a common language for functioning, disability and health ICF. In: International Classification. Vol. 1149. 2002. pp. 1-22. Available from: https://cdn.who.int/media/docs/default-source/classification/icf/icfbeginnersguide.pdf

[6] Banning M. Clinical reasoning and its application to nursing: Concepts and research studies. Nurse Education in Practice. 2008;**8**(3):177-183. DOI: 10.1016/j.nepr.2007.06.004

[7] Kostanjsek N. Use of the international classification of functioning, disability and health (ICF) as a conceptual framework and common language for disability statistics and health information systems. BMC Public Health. 2011;**11**(Suppl. 4):S3. DOI: 10.1186/1471-2458-11-S4-S3

[8] Demyati H. Exploring the utility of the ICF-CY (international classification functioning disability and health children and youth version) framework as a clinical reasoning tool for physiotherapists who treat children with cerebral palsy [PhD thesis]. United Kingdom: Univerity of Strthclyde; 2017. Available from: https://stax.strath.ac.uk/concern/theses/g732d910q

[9] World Health Organization. International Classification of Functioning, Disability and Health: Children & Youth Version. Vol. 1. Geneva: World Health Organization; 2007. DOI: 10.1017/CBO9781107415324.004

[10] World Health Organization. International Classification of Functioning, Disability and Health (ICF). Geneva: World Health Organization; 2001

[11] dos Santos AN, Neves A, Pavão SL, de Campos AC, Rocha NACF. International classification of functioning, disability and health in children with cerebral palsy. Disability and Rehabilitation. 2012;**34**(12):1053-1058. DOI: 10.3109/09638288.2011.631678

[12] Darrah J. Using the ICF as a framework for clinical decision making in pediatric physical therapy. Advances in Physiotherapy. 2008;**10**(3):146-151. DOI: 10.1080/14038190802242046

[13] Cruz EB, Moore A, Cross V. Clinical reasoning and patient-centred care in musculoskeletal physiotherapy

in Portugal - A qualitative study. Manual Therapy. 2012;**17**(3):246-250. DOI: 10.1016/j.math.2012.02.007

[14] Jones M, Jensen GM, Edwards I. Clinical reasoning in physiotherapy. In: Higgs J, Jones M, Loftus S, editors. Clinical Reasoning in the Health Professionals. 3rd ed. Philadelphia: Elsevier; 2008. pp. 163-174

[15] Wade DT, Halligan PW. Do biomedical models of illness make for good healthcare systems? British Medical Journal. 2004;**329**(7479):1398-1401. DOI: 10.1136/bmj.329.7479.1398

[16] Marcum J. Biomechanical and phenomenological models of the body, the meaning of illness and quality of care. Medicine, Health Care and Philosophy. 2005;7(311e20):311-320. DOI: 10.1007/s11019-004-9033-0

[17] Eva KW, Hatala RM, LeBlanc VR, Brooks LR. Teaching from the clinical reasoning literature: Combined reasoning strategies help novice diagnosticians overcome misleading information. Medical Education. 2007;**41**(12):1152-1158. DOI: 10.1111/j.1365-2923.2007.02923.x

[18] Doody C, McAteer M. Clinical reasoning of expert and novice physiotherapists in an outpatient orthopaedic setting. Physiotherapy. 2002;**88**(5):258-268. DOI: 10.1016/S0031-9406(05)61417-4

[19] Tan S, Ladyshewsky R, Gardner P. Using blogging to promote clinical reasoning and metacognition in undergraduate physiotherapy fieldwork programs. Australasian Journal of Educational Technology. 2010;**26**(3):355-368 [Cited 2023 August 2]

[20] Carraccio CL, Benson BJ, Nixon LJ, Derstine PL. From the educational bench to the clinical bedside: Translating the Dreyfus developmental model to the learning of clinical skills. Academic Medicine. 2008;**83**(8):761-767

[21] Norman GR. Research in clinical reasoning: Past history and current trends. Medical Education. 2005;**39**(4):418-427

[22] Case K, Harrison K, Roskell C. Differences in the clinical reasoning process of expert and novice cardiorespiratory physiotherapists. Physiotherapy. 2000;**86**(1):14-21. DOI: 10.1016/S0031-9406(05)61321-1 [Cited 2023 August 2]

[23] Kenyon LK. The hypothesis-oriented pediatric-focused algorithm: A framework for clinical reasoning in pediatric physical therapist practice. Physical Therapy. 2012;**93**(3):413-420. DOI: 10.2522/ptj.20120080

[24] Karhula M, Saukkonen S, et al. ICF personal factors strengthen commitment to person-centered rehabilitation - A scoping review. Frontiers in Rehabilitation Sciences. 2021;**2**(709682):1-11. Available from: www.frontiersin.org

[25] May S, Withers S, Reeve S, Greasley A. Limited clinical reasoning skills used by novice physiotherapists when involved in the assessment and management of patients with shoulder problems: A qualitative study. The Journal of Manual & Manipulative Therapy. 2010;**18**(2):84-88. DOI: 10.1179/106698110X12640740712770

[26] Geyh S, Schwegler U, Peter C, Müller R. Representing and organizing information to describe the lived experience of health from a personal factors perspective in the light of the international classification of functioning, disability and health

(ICF): A discussion paper. Disability and Rehabilitation. 2019;**41**:1727-1738. DOI: 10.1080/09638288.2018.1445302

[27] Lee JY, Ready EA, Davis EN, Doyle PC. Purposefulness as a critical factor in functioning, disability and health. Clinical Rehabilitation. 2017;**31**:1005-1018. DOI: 10.1177/0269215516672274

[28] Whyte J. Contributions of treatment theory and enablement theory to rehabilitation research and practice. Archives of Physical Medicine and Rehabilitation. 2014;**95**:S17-23.e2. DOI: 10.1016/j.apmr.2013.02.029

[29] Schneidet M, Hurst R, et al. The role of environment in the international classification of functioning, disability and health (ICF). Disability and Rehabilitation. 2003;**25**(11-12):588-595

[30] Arocha JF, Patel V. Methods in the study of clinical reasoning. In: Higgs J, Jones M, Loftus S, editors. Clinical Reasoning in the Health Professions. 3rd ed. Philadelphia: Elsevier; 2008

[31] Edwards I, Jones M. Movement in our thinking and our practice. Manual Therapy. 2013;**18**(2):93-95. DOI: 10.1016/j.math.2012.10.002

[32] Edwards I, Jones M, Hillier S. The interpretation of experience and its relationship to body movement: A clinical reasoning perspective. Manual Therapy. 2006;**11**(1):2-10. DOI: 10.1016/j.math.2005.10.0

[33] Edwards I, Jones M, Carr J, Jensen GM. Clinical reasoning strategies in physical therapy. Physical Therapy. 2004;**84**(4):312-330. DOI: 10.1093/ptj/84.4.312

[34] Rothstein JM, Echternach JL. Hypothesis-oriented algorithm for clinicians. A method for evaluation and treatment planning. Physical Therapy. 1986;**66**(9):1388-1394

[35] Jette AM, Haley SM, Kooyoomjian JT. Are the ICF activity and participation dimensions distinct? Journal of Rehabilitation Medicine. 2003;**35**:145-149

[36] Edwards I, Jones M, Higgs J, Trede F, Jensen G. What is collaborative reasoning? Advances in Physiotherapy. 2004;**6**(2):70-83. DOI: 10.1080/14038190410018938

[37] Bruyère SM, Peterson DB. The international classification of functioning, disability and health: Contemporary literature overview of literature. Rehabilitation Psychology. 2005;**50**(2):1-21

[38] Martinuzzi A, De Polo G, Bortolot S, Pradal M. Pediatric neurorehabilitation and the ICF. NeuroRehabilitation. 2015;**36**(1):31-36. DOI: 10.3233/NRE-141188

[39] Leonardi M, Bickenbach J, Raggi A, Sala M, Guzzon P, Valsecchi MR, et al. Training on the international classification of functioning, disability and health (ICF): The ICF-DIN basic and the ICF-DIN advanced course developed by the disability Italian network. Journal of Headache and Pain. 2005;**6**(3):159-164. DOI: 10.1007/s10194-005-0173-2

Chapter 6

Idiopathic Intracranial Hypertension

Maja Kostic, Elizabeth Colvin, Huynh Duy, Sarah Ro, Carolyn Quinsey, Inga Shevtsova and Sriram Machineni

Abstract

Idiopathic intracranial hypertension (IIH), also known as pseudotumor cerebri, is a condition marked by increased cerebrospinal (CSF) pressure in the absence of secondary causes, such as brain tumors, venous sinus thrombosis, and meningitis. The exact cause of IIH is unknown, but the rise in intracranial pressure (ICP) is a defining characteristic leading to the clinical presentation of headaches, transient visual obscurations, pulsatile tinnitus, and retrobulbar pain. This text aims to discuss IIH and the effectiveness of a multi-disciplinary approach, emphasizing collaboration by neuro-ophthalmology, neurology, neurosurgery, radiology, oculoplastic, and weight loss teams to achieve clinical remission of IIH. Literature was reviewed to discuss aspects of IIH in the pediatric population, and our clinical experience was utilized to provide recommendations regarding the importance of a multi-disciplinary team. This chapter explores IIH in the pediatric population regarding its demographics, clinical manifestations, potential underlying pathophysiology, diagnostic steps, and the importance of a multi-disciplinary approach to management, as it is the most optimal. This allows patients to receive comprehensive care that will address more aspects of IIH while also maintaining long-term goals and remission.

Keywords: idiopathic intracranial hypertension, neuro-ophthalmology, Pediatrics, multi-disciplinary management, elevated intracranial hypertension

1. Introduction

Idiopathic intracranial hypertension (IIH), also known as pseudotumor cerebri, is a condition marked by increased cerebrospinal (CSF) pressure in the absence of secondary causes, such as brain tumors, venous sinus thrombosis, and meningitis [1]. The exact cause of IIH is unknown, but the rise in intracranial pressure (ICP) is a defining characteristic [2] leading to the clinical presentation of headaches, transient visual obscurations, pulsatile tinnitus, and retrobulbar pain [3]. Other symptoms include dizziness, neck, and back pain [1]. IIH patients commonly present with papilledema, vision loss, double vision, cranial nerve deficits, or nonspecific neurologic signs [4]. IIH is present in the adult and pediatric populations, impacting vision and quality of life.

Although symptoms of IIH can be debilitating, one of the priorities of care is to prevent any permanent vision loss. Lowering intracranial pressure becomes the focus once the risk of vision loss is mitigated. Currently, insufficient integration of multiple disciplines prevents early detection in some cases. Many IIH patients require neuro-ophthalmologic examination for proper diagnosis [5] but may instead be dismissed from primary care or emergency departments, allowing IIH to go undetected and worsen. While several investigators have reported on the importance of the multidisciplinary management approach of IIH, studies providing evidence of the superiority of multidisciplinary over monodisciplinary management are lacking. Due to the various presentations and categorization of IIH as a diagnosis of exclusion, swift diagnosis, and management of IIH in the pediatric population necessitates a multi-disciplinary approach. This text aims to discuss IIH and the effectiveness of a multi-disciplinary approach, emphasizing collaboration by neuro-ophthalmology, neurology, neurosurgery, radiology, oculoplastic and weight loss teams to achieve clinical remission of IIH.

2. Demographics

IIH is regarded as a diagnosis of exclusion. Therefore, clinical presentation can be a defining indication of the underlying disorder. IIH has an incidence of 1–2 per 100,000 in the general population 4 with an incidence of 0.63–0.9 per 100,000 in the pediatric population (defined as <18 years old) [6–8]. In adults, IIH is disproportionately found in overweight women of childbearing age, in whom as much as 4–21 per 100,000 people are affected [4]. Although more predominant in the adult population, IIH is present in the pediatric population with differing demographics [9]. Pubescent status has been shown to play a role in the gender predilection of IIH in the pediatric population. Aylward et al. demonstrated that in the pre-pubescent population, there is nearly a 1:1 ratio of female to male incidence of IIH [8, 10]. However, female pubescent adolescents were more likely to present with IIH as compared to pubescent males 8.

3. Clinical presentation of IIH

Suspicion of IIH should be raised based on clinical complaints. Patients typically report headaches, transient visual obscurations, pulsatile tinnitus, and retrobulbar pain [3]. Headache is the most commonly described symptom associated with IIH, with one-quarter of patients reporting a constant, daily headache [1]. Pulsatile tinnitus may accompany the headache, which is described as a whooshing, whistling, or humming noise heard in the ear. It is believed to be caused by turbulent pulsatile blood flow that is perceived through the auditory system [1]. Neither headache nor pulsatile tinnitus are specific for IIH as they are clinically too broad, but they are clinical clues when combined with additional visual findings.

Visual symptoms include a wide range of deficits and are the main source of chronic morbidity in IIH [1, 11]. Visual symptoms may include transient visual obscurations, which are short (seconds to minutes) vision changes that can be described as fogginess, black, white, or gray-out, and episodes of brief visual sparkles or flashes different from a visual migraine aura [1, 12]. Often, papilledema presents as one of the cardinal signs of IIH [13]. Central vision loss is rare as the majority of vision loss in IIH begins in the periphery [1]. Constant or intermittent horizontal diplopia, which resolves with occlusion of either eye, may occur due to unilateral or bilateral cranial nerve VI (abducens) palsy. The palsy results as a false localizing sign of high ICP due to increased tension on cranial nerve VI. Early detection of IIH allows for early treatment to prevent intracranial pressure escalation, papilledema worsening, and loss of vision [1].

The typical clinical presentation of IIH involves a young, potentially overweight, post-pubescent female who complains of headaches and recent vision changes. A thorough investigation into current medications is required when a potential IIH patient presents as tetracycline usage has been shown to cause IIH [14, 15]. There is much debate regarding the link between hormonal oral contraceptives (OCP) and IIH. Contreras-Martin et al. showed that there is an association between IIH in women and pubescents taking OCPs; however, this has been refuted by Kilgore et al. [14, 16]. Therefore, we recommend a detailed history of the type of OCP (estrogen-containing versus non-estrogen-containing), how long the patient has taken the medication (i.e, was it recently started?), and the patient's willingness to stop the OCP. With this information, the clinician should assess how likely the onset of IIH is correlated with OCP usage and if it is medically indicated for the patient to stop hormonal treatment. Further investigations are needed to definitively conclude if patients taking OCPs are at an increased risk of IIH.

IIH is correlated with numerous metabolic conditions, including obesity, polycystic ovarian syndrome (PCOS), and weight gain [17]. Therefore, questions regarding recent weight gain or rapid changes in weight can give a clinical clue as to whether the patient may be suffering from IIH. As pediatric rates of obesity continue to rise, there is an expected increase in the prevalence of IIH. When an overweight pediatric patient presents with recent onset vision changes, suspicion should be raised for IIH.

4. Pathogenesis: a multitude of theories

There are many theories regarding the underlying pathogenesis of IIH in adults and pediatric patients; however, not one theory is precise enough or all-encompassing. It is understood that the elevation in ICP is a main characteristic, but there are several mechanisms that may be responsible for the increase, as described by the following:

- Increased CSF volume secondary to increased production or resistance to CSF outflow.
- Loss of cerebral autoregulation resulting in elevated cerebral arterial pressure.
- Increased cerebral venous pressure leading to increased CSF volume and decreased CSF outflow.
- Obesity-related increased intracranial venous pressure.
- Altered sodium and water retention mechanisms.
- Abnormalities of vitamin A metabolism and others 2.

4.1 Popular theories: reduction in CSF absorption and transverse sinus stenosis

CSF reabsorption by arachnoid granulations may be reduced in IIH. This reduction may be attributed to either an increase in CSF outflow resistance or a reduction in the pressure gradient between the subarachnoid space and the superior sagittal sinus, leading to elevated ICP [18]. Outflow resistance of CSF is known to be elevated in posthemorrhagic hydrocephalus, malignant meningitis, and with high CSF protein in Guillain-Barré syndrome [2]. The reduction in CSF reabsorption may also be due to anatomical abnormalities in the cerebral venous sinus system, which are commonly seen in patients with IIH. This theory was explored by Ahmed et al., who utilized a Dural stent to improve papilledema and IIH symptoms. This resulted in 49 of the 52 patients being cured of all reported IIH symptoms [19].

4.2 Popular theories: obesity

In addition to the elevation of ICP, obesity is a consistent risk factor for the development of IIH. The risk of IIH increases as a function of body mass index (BMI) and weight gain over the following year. In addition, the risk of IIH-induced vision loss increases with increased BMI, the highest risk being a BMI >40 kg/m [20]. Fat distribution might play a significant role in IIH as truncal fat mass is correlated with LP pressure [21]. Central obesity increases intra-abdominal pressure, pleural pressure, cardiac filling pressure, and central venous pressure. Therefore, central obesity may lead to increased intracranial venous pressure, causing IIH [22]. Obesity has a link to IIH due to the resolution of symptoms with weight loss, preferentially adiposity from the truncal region [21]. Adipokine leptin, which regulated satiety in the hypothalamus, was found to be elevated in the serum and CSF of patients with IIH; however, further investigation is necessary to clarify if this cytokine plays a direct role in the dysregulation of ICP [23].

5. Diagnosis

After a patient's clinical presentation raises suspicion for IIH, certain measures should be taken to confirm the diagnosis. Currently, the Modified Dandy Criteria is the accepted diagnostic criteria for IIH [1, 13]. The Modified Dandy Criteria, as seen in **Table 1**, is composed of five criteria to separate IIH from secondary causes of elevated ICP.

Papilledema, or optic nerve swelling, is a characteristic finding on examination of a patient with suspected elevated intracranial hypertension. Per the Modified Dandy criteria in **Table 1**, a patient may be diagnosed with IIH if Frisen Grade II papilledema is found with additional diagnostic criteria. The Frisen grading scale is explored below in **Figure 1**.

After a clinical examination, evaluation of suspected IIH should always start with neuroimaging to rule out any secondary causes of elevated intracranial pressure. A gadolinium-enhanced MRI and venography are the imaging modality of choice for neuroimaging. A number of radiographic features suggestive of IIH can be seen via neuroimaging, including transverse sinus stenosis, empty sella, distension of the perioptic subarachnoid space, vertical tortuosity of the intra-orbital optic nerve, intraocular protrusion or gadolinium enhancement of the prelaminar optic nerve, and posterior scleral flattening, all of which are shown in **Figure 2** [17, 25].

1. Signs and symptoms of increased ICP
2. Absence of localizing findings on neurologic examination
3. Absence of deformity, displacement, or obstruction of ventricular system with otherwise normal neurodiagnostic studies, except for: a. Evidence of increased CSF pressure (greater than 20 cm water) b. Abnormal neuroimaging apart from empty sella turcica c. Optic nerve sheath with filled-out CSF spaces d. Smooth-walled non-flow-related venous sinus stenosis or collapse
4. Awake and alert
5. No other causes of increased ICP present with CSF opening pressure of 20–25 cm H_2O, required at least one of the following: a. Pulse-synchronous tinnitus (pulsatile tinnitus) b. Cranial nerve VI palsy c. Frisen Grade II papilledema d. Echography for drusen negative and no other disc anomalies mimicking disc edema present e. MRV (Magnetic Resonance Venography) with lateral sinus collapse/stenosis, preferably using ATECO technique f. Partially empty sella on coronal or sagittal views and optic nerve sheaths with filled-out CSF spaces next to the globe on T2 weighted axial scans

Table 1.
Modified dandy criteria.

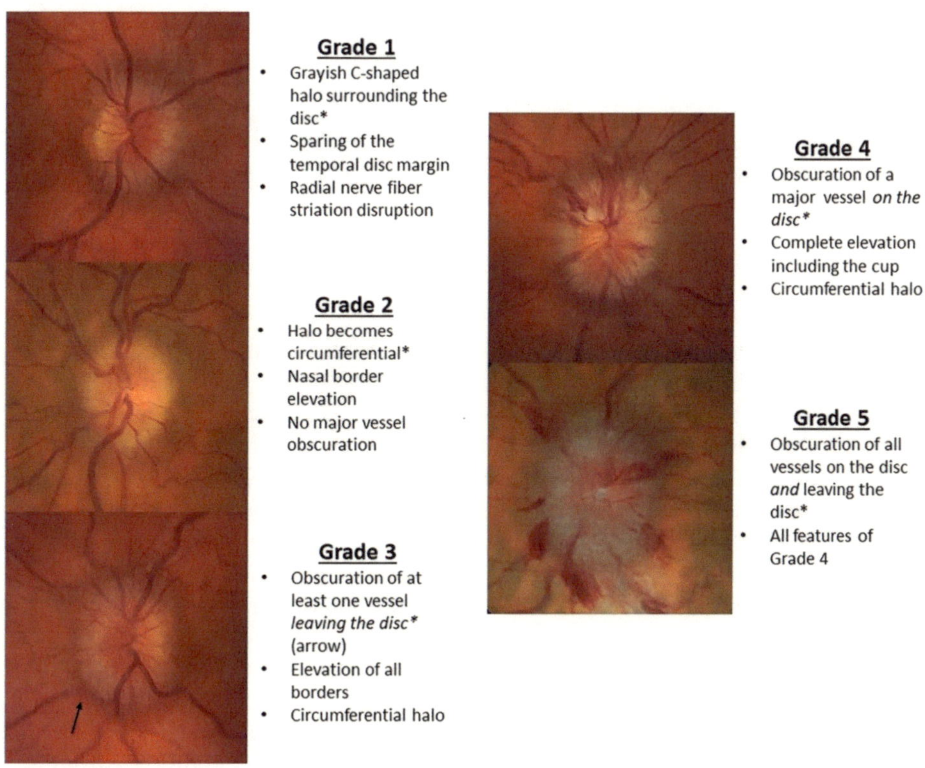

Figure 1.
Frisen grading scale of papilledema with characteristic findings on examination [24].

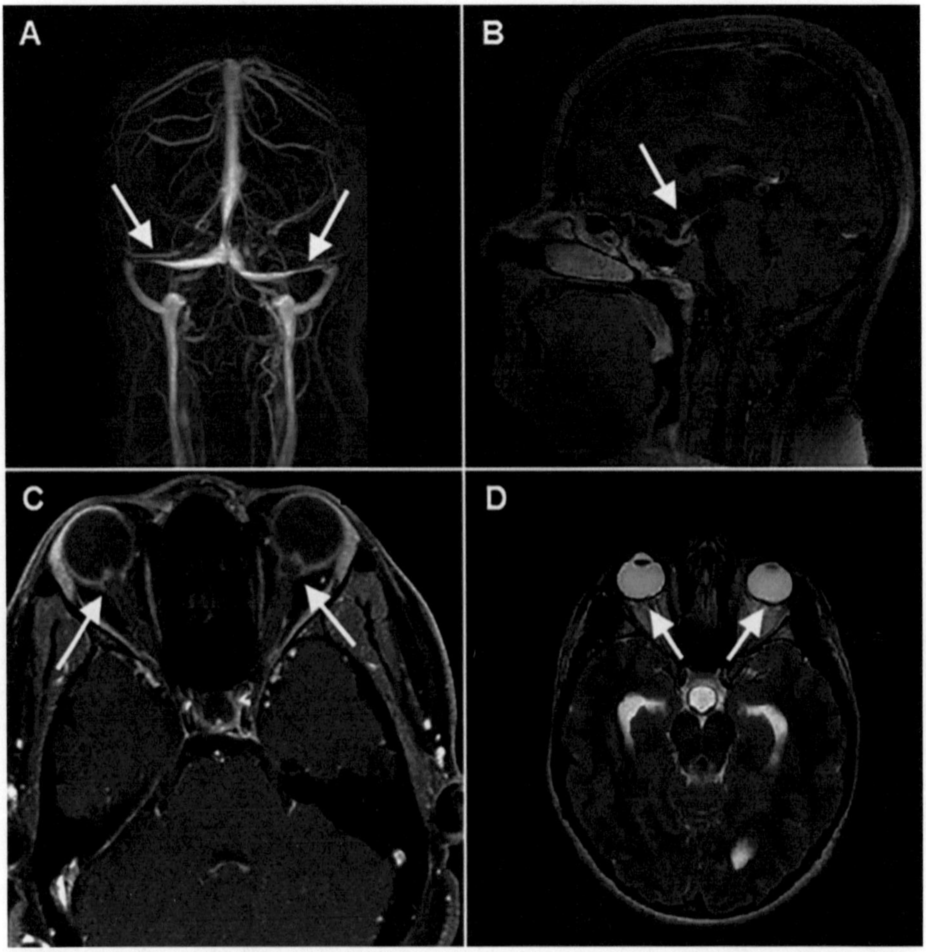

Figure 2.
Common radiographic features suggestive of IIH on magnetic resonance imaging and venography. (A) Bilateral transverse sinus stenosis; (B) empty sella; (C) optic nerve head edema; (D) posterior scleral flattening [17, 25].

Following neuroimaging, a lumbar puncture can help identify an elevated opening pressure, which is defined as greater than 20 cm water per the Modified Dandy Criteria [25]. The overall goal of the lumbar puncture is to confirm if there is an elevated ICP [8]. However, there is variability within pediatric patients and their opening pressures. Therefore, some patients may be susceptible to IIH at a lower threshold than others. If the clinical manifestations are indicative of IIH but the opening pressure is within a normal range, we recommend pursuing treatment based on the clinical presentation outlined in the Modified Dandy criteria [26].

Additional imaging may include Optical coherence tomography (OCT) and automated perimetry. These tests not only provide further evidence of optic nerve involvement but also allow for better monitoring of edema of the retinal nerve fiber layer (RNFL) and retinal pigment epithelium and Bruch's membrane as well as visual field over time [27]. Visual field (VF) testing, as seen in **Figure 3** can allow for monitoring of progressive peripheral vision loss [28]. **Figure 4** details the differences between a non-edemic nerve, as seen on fundus photography, versus an edematous nerve and how edema is manifested on an OCT [27].

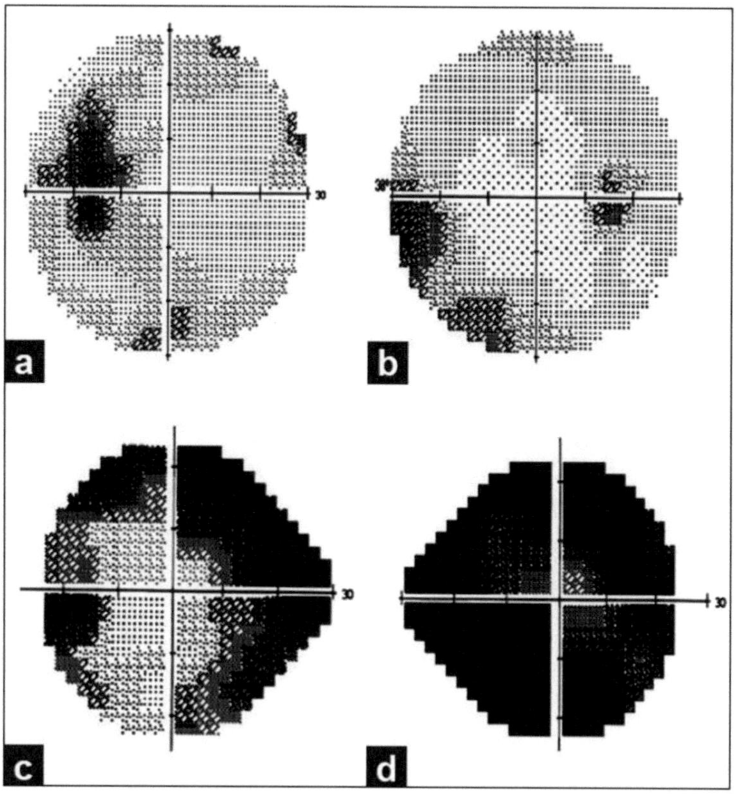

Figure 3.
Visual field defects in idiopathic intracranial hypertension. (a) Enlarged blind spot. (b) Nasal step. (c) Biarcuate scotoma. (d) Severe visual field constriction [28].

6. Treatment and management

We believe a multi-disciplinary approach to IIH treatment and management provides the best outcomes for patients. In a non-multidisciplinary setting, barriers to expedited care can cause irreversible blindness. Coordination of multiple specialties involved in IIH can potentially improve successful weight loss, allow fast-track referrals to specialty clinics, and increase long-term remission of IIH for these patients. Each discipline, as outlined in **Figure 5**, has a unique role in expediting the treatment and continued management of a patient with IIH. Each discipline within the IIH team must be approachable and accessible, understanding the gravity of the diagnosis. At our institution, we have established an IIH team that encompasses these disciplines, and their roles will be further explored below.

6.1 Neuro-ophthalmology

Any patient with diagnosed or highly suspected IIH must be seen by a neuro-ophthalmologist. Treatment (surgical versus non-surgical interventions) varies depending on the extent of papilledema and vision loss at the time of presentation. The underlying goal is to avoid surgical intervention and minimize vision loss while treating the symptoms of IIH. Pediatric patients typically begin with non-surgical interventions, which include acetazolamide or topiramate to help reduce ICP. In office

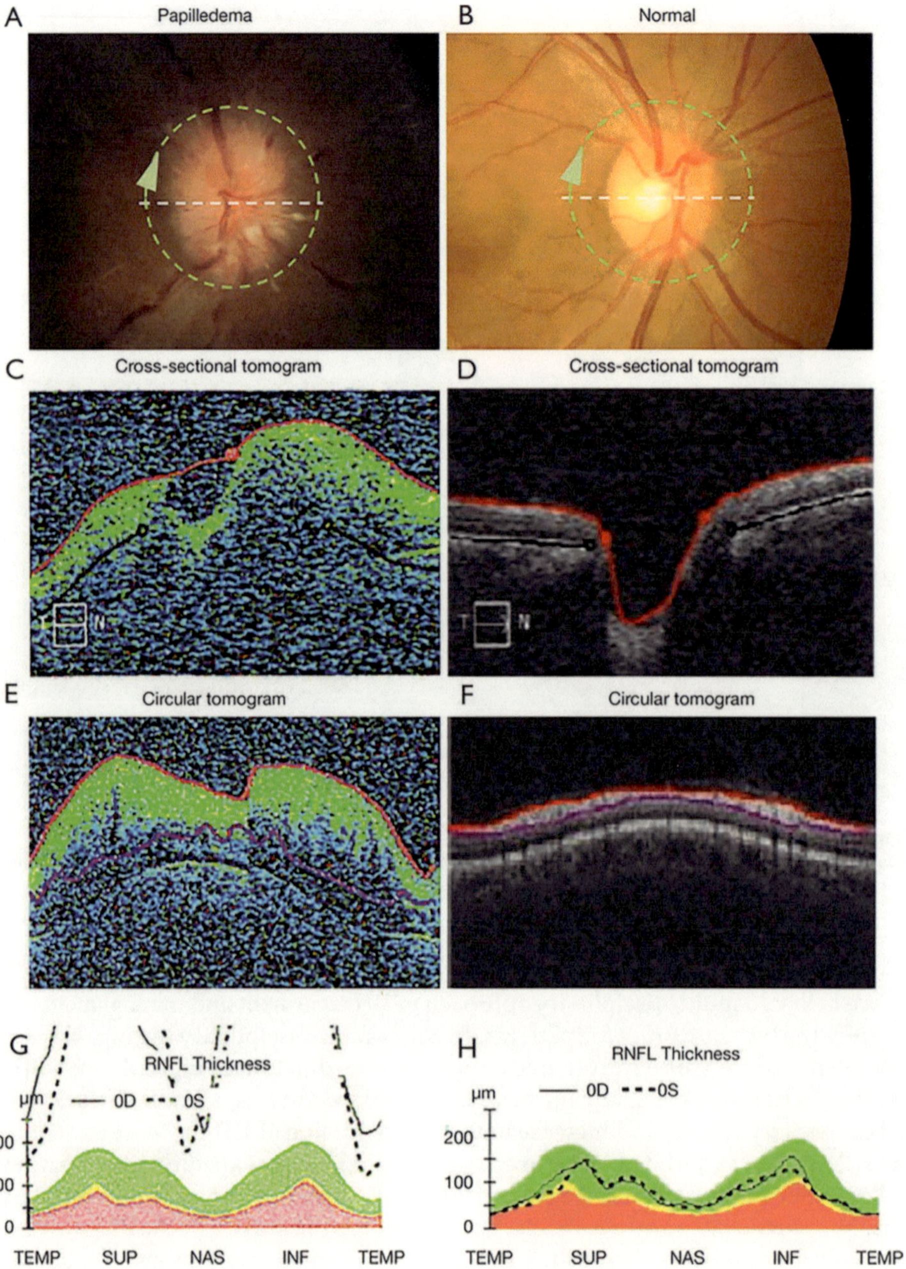

Figure 4.

Panel of images demonstrates comparison between papilledema and normal optic disc by fundus photography and SD-OCT of RNFL. (A) Fundus photography shows marked swelling of optic disc with obscuration of peripapillary major retinal vessels in papilledema compares to (B) normal optic disc with sharp margin. Also depicting in fundus photography are (white dashed line in A, B) plane of cross-sectional tomogram of RNFL and (green circular dashed line in A, B) plane of circular tomogram of peripapillary RNFL. (C) Cross-sectional and (E) circular tomogram of swelling optic disc by SD-OCT demonstrates marked thickening of RNFL, area between red and purple line, compares to (D, F) tomograms from normal optic disc. (G, H) comparison of RNFL thickness to normal range for patient age (green area). (H) Measurement of RNFL is within normal range for age. On the contrary, (G) swelling optic disc RNFL thickness is well above normal range. However, validity of RNFL thickness measurement can be limited by poor automated segmentation in marked swelling optic disc. RNFL, retinal nerve fiber layer; SD-OCT, spectral-domain optical coherence tomography. Figure and caption from Malhotra et al. [27].

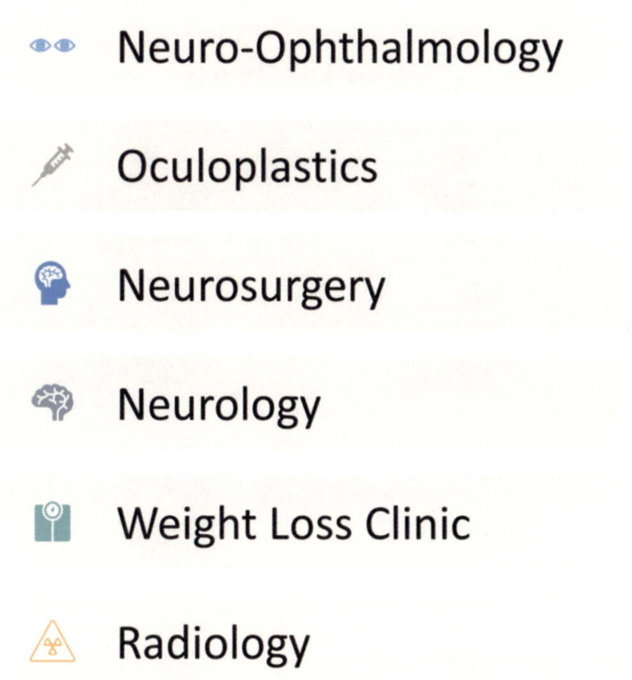

Figure 5.
Diagram of all disciplines we incorporate into the management of a patient with IIH.

imaging, including fundus photos, OCT, retinal nerve fiber layer (RNFL), ganglion cell layer (GCC), and VF are all taken at initial presentation to establish a baseline, especially if the patient has never been evaluated before. An immediate referral to radiology is placed to ensure an MRI is conducted within 48 hours of presentation to rule out any secondary causes of the ICP.

As early as the first presentation with IIH, weight management is discussed. We utilize a healthy eating poster, seen in **Figure 6**, that outlines what unhealthy food choices are and healthy replacement options. A referral to a weight loss clinic is placed, and the patients will subsequently see the same poster to ensure consistency in resources for weight loss.

Pediatric patients in our clinic will then be followed for varying durations depending on the severity of symptoms and interventions pursued. Any pediatric patient who presents with Frisen grades II–IV papilledema is seen every 2–4 weeks. If a pediatric patient presents with Frisen Grade V papilledema, they are immediately hospitalized for further consultation with neurosurgery.

6.2 Neurosurgery

Surgical interventions like optic nerve sheath fenestration, CSF shunting, or venous sinus stenting are reserved for severe cases of IIH with immediate risk of permanent vision loss [29] or instances where full medical management is unsuccessful/not tolerated. There are several surgical options for individuals with IIH, but surgical management varies between adults versus pediatric patients. Making the decision to pursue surgical management is a very delicate decision that must incorporate collaboration with the entire IIH team.

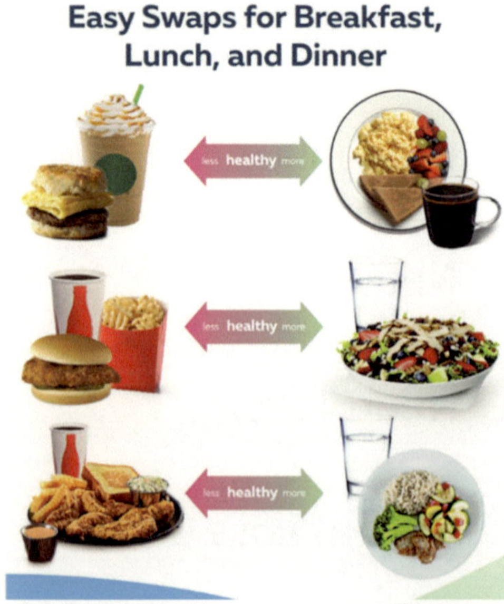

Figure 6.
Healthy food poster that we utilize in clinic.

In pediatric patients who do pursue surgical intervention, ventricular peritoneal shunt is the standard surgical treatment. This is most often placed in the frontal location since these patients often have slit or small ventricles, and placement and revision are more straightforward with frontal vs. occipital placement. There do not exist guidelines for specific hardware such as programmable valves [30].

Shunt placement surgery is often well tolerated with a 1-night hospital stay. However, infection and hardware failure rates need to be a consideration [31]. Further, reliance on a VP shunt forever changes the patient's healthcare and can be a confounder factor that makes it difficult for patients to get care. Lastly, a plan should be in place for possible shunt failure and where the patient should be evaluated, as shunted IIH is often not well evaluated in the emergency room where other types of shunted hydrocephalus would be evaluated [32].

Venous stenting is not well studied in children and could be considered in a case-by-case patient anatomy and clinical context. Optic nerve sheath fenestration is a surgical procedure performed to decompress the optic nerve to alleviate papilledema. The procedure creates a window in the optic nerve sheath to release CSF from the subarachnoid space, subsequently decreasing the pressure on the optic nerve [33]. At our institution, optic nerve sheath fenestration is completed by the oculoplastic team in consultation with the neuro-ophthalmologist and neurosurgery team.

6.3 Weight loss clinic

Currently, the standard of care mostly focuses on weight loss counseling and medical therapy [34]. Patients under this management approach can sometimes be on acetazolamide for years with the prospect of continuing this for the rest of their lives. Reliance on medical therapy is common and has been shown to lower intracranial

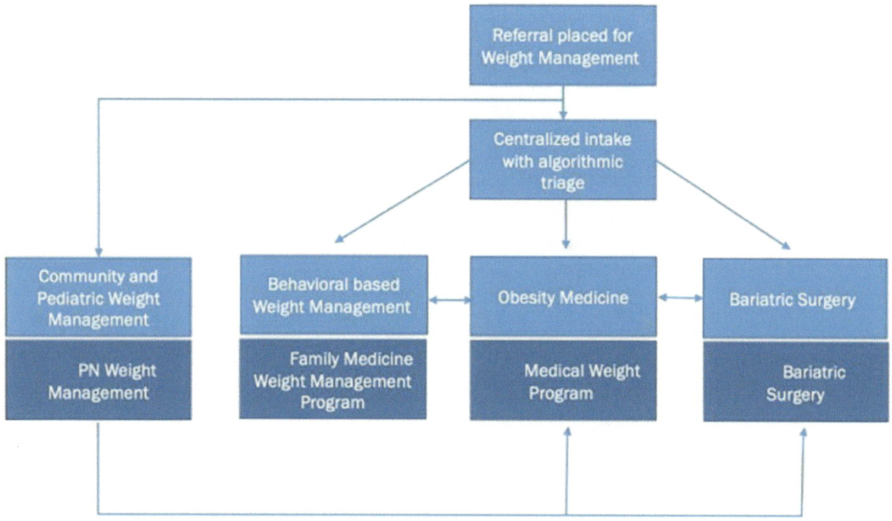

Figure 7.
Weight management algorithm.

pressure and relieve most symptoms [34]. While clinical remission is observed in successful weight loss, [35] most patients with IIH struggle to maintain a consistent weight loss plan. In addition, patients attempting self-directed weight loss are less likely to be successful and likely to recur with weight gain afterward [20]. Therefore, we believe the inclusion of a weight loss clinic can be vital for IIH patients to create a weight loss program, ensuring proper methods for weight loss and continued weight stability after remission. **Figure 7** is the algorithm that is utilized to structure weight loss management at our institution.

6.4 Radiology

An immediate referral to radiology is placed for magnetic resonance imaging of the brain and orbits with venography. Per our IIH team, radiology ensures the necessary imaging is completed within 48 hours of referral. With suspected IIH patients, radiologists must assess for transverse sinus stenosis, empty sella, optic nerve edema, and posterior scleral flattening. If any of these are found, neuro-ophthalmology is called to expedite the relay of findings.

6.5 Neurology

Neurology is incorporated into the IIH team in order to help treat residual headaches that are refractive to acetazolamide or topiramate treatment or that are consistent with an underlying migraine disorder. In addition, neurologists help conduct and manage a lumbar procedure in patients with suspected IIH.

7. Clinical education

We believe an important step to mitigating vision loss from IIH is incorporating clinical education across multiple disciplines for the earliest signs and symptoms

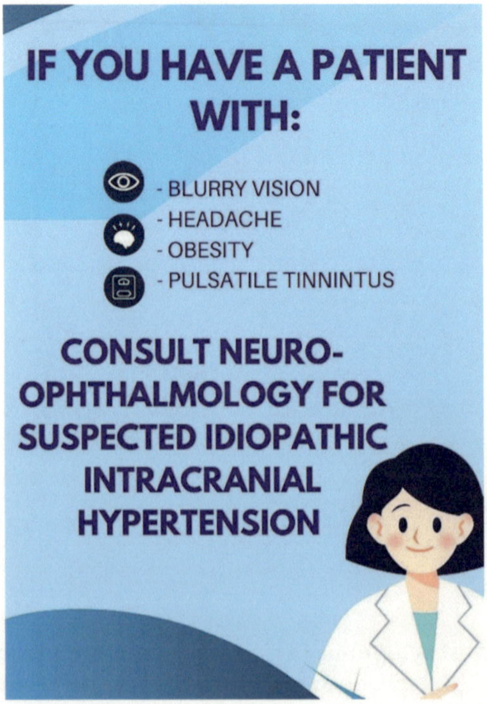

Figure 8.
Our poster that is utilized as an educational resource in various medicaldisciplines to raise awareness of IIH symptoms.

of IIH. We provide educational resources and tools for Emergency Room physicians, pediatricians, optometrists, neurologists, and primary care physicians at our institution. These educational resources attempt to mitigate the misdiagnosis of IIH as migraine symptoms. A major resource we utilize is **Figure 8**. Regardless of income or insurance status, anyone with IIH symptoms should not succumb to vision loss. We stand by a united goal to treat preventable blindness for all social groups through a multi-disciplinary team that helps expedite treatment and maintain vision.

8. Conclusion

This chapter explores IIH in the pediatric population regarding its demographics, clinical manifestations, potential underlying pathophysiology, diagnostic steps, and the importance of a multi-disciplinary approach to management, as it is the most optimal. This allows patients to receive comprehensive care that will address more aspects of IIH while also maintaining long-term goals and remission.

9. Case presentation

This is an example of one of our patients and our clinical approach to a patient with IIH:

Case 1 is a 15-year-old female with PMH of pre-diabetes, hypertriglyceridemia, eosinophilic esophagitis, class II Obesity (BMI 120% of 95th percentile, BMI

DOI: http://dx.doi.org/10.5772/intechopen.1003180

33.4 kg/m^2) who was referred by her optometrist with severe headaches, blurred vision, and papilledema. On exam, her BCVA was 20/20 in both eyes and color vision was full. She has a maternal great-aunt who had IIH and has had a long history of consuming ultra-processed foods, daily sweetened beverages, and a sedentary lifestyle. OCT RNFL were 124 μm the right eye and 144 μm in the left eye. MRI of the brain was unremarkable. The patient did not want a lumbar puncture done at the time. She was started on acetazolamide 500 mg daily. Weight loss was recommended, and she started with a registered dietician and a pediatric weight management physician. Her headaches and blurred vision resolved. Her papilledema resolved to within normal limits after 3 months of acetazolamide. Her symptoms resolved after 6 months of therapy, and her acetazolamide was switched to topiramate[1]. In 1 year, her BMI went from 33.4 kg/m^2 to 30.2 kg/m^2, and lost a total of 15 lbs (**Figures 9** and **10**).

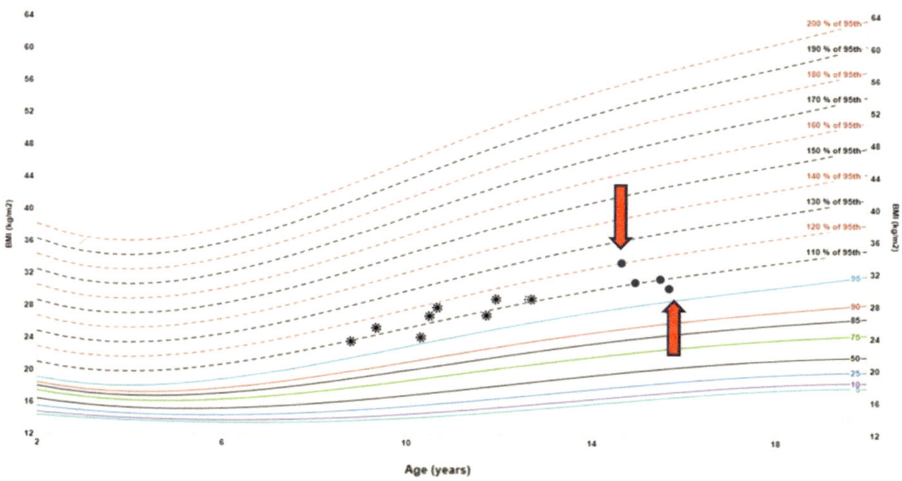

Figure 9.
Growth chart of BMI over time for Case 1.

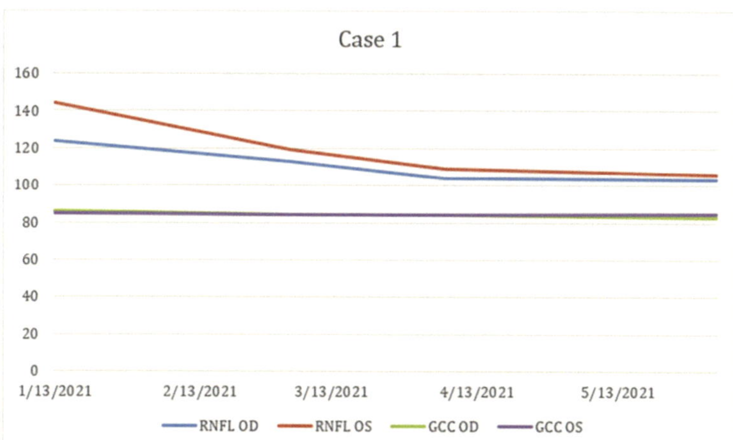

Figure 10.
OCT RNFL and GCC trends for Case 1.

Author details

Maja Kostic[1,2]*, Elizabeth Colvin[3], Huynh Duy[4], Sarah Ro[5], Carolyn Quinsey[6], Inga Shevtsova[7] and Sriram Machineni[8]

1 Department of Ophthalmology, University of North Carolina, Chapel Hill, NC, United States

2 Bascom Palmer Eye Institute, University of Miami, Miami, FL, United States

3 Campbell University, School of Osteopathic Medicine, Lillington, NC, United States

4 The Brody School of Medicine at East Carolina University, Greenville, NC, United States

5 Department of Family Medicine at the University of North Carolina, Chapel Hill, NC, United States

6 Department of Neurosurgery at the University of North Carolina, Chapel Hill, NC, United States

7 Department of Internal Medicine, Billings Clinic, Billings, Montana, United States

8 Albert Einstein College of Medicine, Bronx, NY, United States

*Address all correspondence to: mkostic@miami.edu

References

[1] Ahmad SR, Moss HE. Update on the diagnosis and treatment of idiopathic intracranial hypertension. Seminars in Neurology. 2019;**39**(6):682-691. DOI: 10.1055/s-0039-1698744

[2] Johanson CE, Duncan JA3, Klinge PM, Brinker T, Stopa EG, Silverberg GD. Multiplicity of cerebrospinal fluid functions: New challenges in health and disease. Cerebrospinal Fluid Research. 2008;**5**:10-10. DOI: 10.1186/1743-8454-5-10

[3] Giuseffi V, Wall M, Siegel PZ, Rojas PB. Symptoms and disease associations in idiopathic intracranial hypertension (pseudotumor cerebri): A case-control study. Neurology. 1991;**41**(2 (Pt 1):239-244. DOI: 10.1212/wnl.41.2_part_1.239

[4] Kilgore KP, Lee MS, Leavitt JA, et al. Re-evaluating the incidence of idiopathic intracranial hypertension in an era of increasing obesity. Ophthalmology. 2017;**124**(5):697-700. DOI: 10.1016/j.ophtha.2017.01.006

[5] Degnan AJ, Levy LM. Pseudotumor cerebri: Brief review of clinical syndrome and imaging findings. American Journal of Neuroradiology. 2011;**32**(11): 1986-1993. DOI: 10.3174/ajnr.A2404

[6] Gillson N, Jones C, Reem RE, Rogers DL, Zumberge N, Aylward SC. Incidence and demographics of pediatric intracranial hypertension. Pediatric Neurology. 2017;**73**:42-47. DOI: 10.1016/j.pediatrneurol.2017.04.021

[7] Gordon K. Pediatric pseudotumor cerebri: Descriptive epidemiology. Canadian Journal of Neurological Sciences. 1997;**24**(3):219-221. DOI: 10.1017/s031716710002182x

[8] Gaier ED, Heidary G. Pediatric idiopathic intracranial hypertension. Seminars in Neurology. 2019;**39**(6): 704-710. DOI: 10.1055/s-0039-1698743

[9] Brara SM, Koebnick C, Porter AH, Langer-Gould A. Pediatric idiopathic intracranial hypertension and extreme childhood obesity. The Journal of Pediatrics. 2012;**161**(4):602-607. DOI: 10.1016/j.jpeds.2012.03.047

[10] Aylward SC, Waslo CS, Au JN, Tanne E. Manifestations of pediatric intracranial hypertension from the intracranial hypertension registry. Pediatric Neurology. 2016;**61**:76-82. DOI: 10.1016/j.pediatrneurol.2016.04.007

[11] Corbett JJ, Savino PJ, Thompson HS, et al. Visual loss in pseudotumor cerebri. Follow-up of 57 patients from five to 41 years and a profile of 14 patients with permanent severe visual loss. Archives of Neurology. 1982;**39**(8):461-474. DOI: 10.1001/archneur.1982.00510200003001

[12] Friedman DI. Headaches due to low and high intracranial pressure. Continuum (Minneap Minn). 2018;**24** (4, Headache):1066-1091. DOI: 10.1212/CON.0000000000000623

[13] Wall M, Corbett JJ. Revised diagnostic criteria for the pseudotumor cerebri syndrome in adults and children. Neurology. 2014;**83**(2):198-199. DOI: 10.1212/01.wnl.0000452039.32455.3e

[14] Kilgore KP, Lee MS, Leavitt JA, Frank RD, McClelland CM, Chen JJ. A population-based, case-control evaluation of the association between hormonal contraceptives and idiopathic intracranial hypertension. American Journal of Ophthalmology.

2019;**197**:74-79. DOI: 10.1016/j.ajo.2018.09.014

[15] Walters BN, Gubbay SS. Tetracycline and benign intracranial hypertension: Report of five cases. British Medical Journal (Clinical Research Edition). 1981;**282**(6257):19-20. DOI: 10.1136/bmj.282.6257.19

[16] Contreras-Martin Y, Bueno-Perdomo JH. Idiopathic intracranial hypertension: Descriptive analysis in our setting. Neurologia. 2015;**30**(2):106-110. DOI: 10.1016/j.nrl.2013.08.009

[17] Wang MTM, Bhatti MT, Danesh-Meyer HV. Idiopathic intracranial hypertension: Pathophysiology, diagnosis and management. Journal of Clinical Neuroscience. 2022;**95**:172-179. DOI: 10.1016/j.jocn.2021.11.029

[18] Mollan SP, Ali F, Hassan-Smith G, Botfield H, Friedman DI, Sinclair AJ. Evolving evidence in adult idiopathic intracranial hypertension: Pathophysiology and management. Journal of Neurology, Neurosurgery and Psychiatry. 2016;**87**(9):982-992. DOI: 10.1136/jnnp-2015-311302

[19] Ahmed RM, Wilkinson M, Parker GD, et al. Transverse sinus stenting for idiopathic intracranial hypertension: A review of 52 patients and of model predictions. American Journal of Ophthalmology. 2011;**32**(8):1408-1414. DOI: 10.3174/ajnr.A2575

[20] Subramaniam S, Fletcher WA. Obesity and weight loss in idiopathic intracranial hypertension: A narrative review. Journal of Neuroophthalmology. 2017;**37**(2):197-205. DOI: 10.1097/WNO.0000000000000448

[21] Hornby C, Botfield H, O'Reilly MW, et al. Evaluating the fat distribution in idiopathic intracranial hypertension using dual-energy X-ray absorptiometry scanning. Neuroophthalmology. 2017;**42**(2):99-104. DOI: 10.1080/01658107.2017.1334218

[22] Sun WYL, Switzer NJ, Dang JT, et al. Idiopathic intracranial hypertension and bariatric surgery: A systematic review. Canadian Journal of Surgery. 2020;**63**(2):E123-E128. DOI: 10.1503/cjs.016616

[23] Hornby C, Mollan SP, Botfield H, O'Reilly MW, Sinclair AJ. Metabolic concepts in idiopathic intracranial hypertension and their potential for therapeutic intervention. Journal of Neuroophthalmology. 2018;**38**(4):522-530. DOI: 10.1097/WNO.0000000000000684

[24] Swiston C, Seay M. Case Report of Idiopathic Intracranial Hypertension and Frisen Scale Papilledema Grading. Utah: Moran CORE; 2018. Available from: https://morancore.utah.edu/section-05-neuro-ophthalmology/idiopathic-intracranial-hypertension-iih-and-papilledema-grading/

[25] Friedman DI, Liu GT, Digre KB. Revised diagnostic criteria for the pseudotumor cerebri syndrome in adults and children. Neurology. 2013;**81**(13):1159-1165. DOI: 10.1212/WNL.0b013e3182a55f17

[26] Suh SY, Kim S. IIH with normal CSF pressures? Indian Journal of Ophthalmology. 2013;**61**(11):681-682. DOI: 10.4103/0301-4738.119416

[27] Malhotra K, Padungkiatsagul T, Moss HE. Optical coherence tomography use in idiopathic intracranial hypertension. Annals of Eye Science. 2020;**5**:3-10. DOI: 10.21037/aes.2019.12.06

[28] Kedar S, Ghate D, Corbett JJ. Visual fields in neuro-ophthalmology.

Indian Journal of Ophthalmology. 2011;**59**(2):103-109. DOI: 10.4103/0301-4738.77013

[29] Higgins JNP, Cousins C, Owler BK, Sarkies N, Pickard JD. Idiopathic intracranial hypertension: 12 cases treated by venous sinus stenting. Journal of Neurology, Neurosurgery, Psychiatry. 2003;**74**(12):1662-1666. DOI: 10.1136/jnnp.74.12.1662

[30] Hanak BW, Bonow RH, Harris CA, Browd SR. Cerebrospinal fluid shunting complications in children. Pediatric Neurosurgery. 2017;**52**(6):381-400. DOI: 10.1159/000452840

[31] Kestle JRW, Riva-Cambrin J, Wellons JC, et al. A standardized protocol to reduce cerebrospinal fluid shunt infection: The hydrocephalus clinical research network quality improvement initiative. Journal of Neurosurgery Pediatrics. 2011;**8**(1):22-29. DOI: 10.3171/2011.4.PEDS10551

[32] Greener DL, Akarca D, Durnford AJ, Ewbank F, Buckland GR, Hempenstall J. Idiopathic intracranial hypertension: Shunt failure and the role of obesity. World Neurosurgery. 2020;**137**:e83-e88. DOI: 10.1016/j.wneu.2020.01.040

[33] Adesina O, Patel BC. Optic nerve decompression. In: StatPearls. Treasure Island, FL: StatPearls Publishing; 2023. Available from: https://www.ncbi.nlm.nih.gov/books/NBK538300/

[34] Wall M, Kupersmith MJ, Kieburtz KD, et al. The idiopathic intracranial hypertension treatment trial: Clinical profile at baseline. JAMA Neurology. 2014;**71**(6):693-701. DOI: 10.1001/jamaneurol.2014.133

[35] Ang JL, Teo KZ, Fraser CL. Weight loss in idiopathic intracranial hypertension: A retrospective review of outcomes in the clinical setting. Journal of Neuroophthalmology. 2021;**41**(4):e458-e463. DOI: 10.1097/WNO.0000000000001107

Section 4

Novel Therapeutic Approaches for Toddlers and Children with Early Trauma

Chapter 7

Trauma Informed Farm Animal Assisted Neurotherapy and Green Care Farming for Neurodiverse Conditions

Susan D. Rich, Briana R. Hickey and Elizabeth K. Kaprielian

Abstract

Farm animal assisted therapy is a novel way of interacting with neurodiverse children/adolescents, particularly those with early childhood trauma, and may help rewire brain circuits through entrainment with the gentle sounds and rhythms of a farm. This chapter will explore farm animal assisted therapy as a type of neurotherapy using a backdrop of Dream Catcher Meadows, a sanctuary for orphaned, injured and rescued farm animals whose personal stories help with bonding and attachment in neurodiverse and traumatized children and teens. Farms provide rich opportunities for language development, executive functions, sensory desensitization, skill development, fine/gross motor development, and parent-child bonding. The author provides historical and clinical perspectives to explain how farm animal assisted neurotherapy and green care farming provided within a comprehensive array of school, home, and community interventions can help neurodiverse children and teens develop a sense of community, meaning and purpose as well as adaptive functions for success in life. A range of techniques model empathy, compassion, theory of mind concepts, social communication/perception, and self-regulation through mindfulness, interspecies bonding, and entrainment. The history of Dream Catcher Meadows and case discussions from clinical practice elaborate therapeutic perspectives, augmented by session scenarios and non-clinical photographs.

Keywords: neurodiversity, prenatal alcohol exposure, neurodevelopmental disorders, adverse childhood experiences, trauma-informed therapy, farm animal assisted therapy, neurotherapy, neurophenotype, autism spectrum, green care, farming for health

1. Introduction: neurodevelopmental conditions vs. mental illness

Neurodevelopmental disorder associated with prenatal alcohol exposure (ND-PAE) [1] and related neurodevelopmental conditions (e.g., autism spectrum disorder) are complex, heterogeneous neurophenotypes that have few well-researched treatments outside of comprehensive institutional-based and multidisciplinary models [2, 3]. One in 20 American youth have Fetal Alcohol Spectrum

Disorder (FASD), also known as Neurodevelopmental Disorder associated with Prenatal Alcohol Exposure (ND-PAE; ICD-10 F88). According to the National Institutes of Health, FASD/ND-PAE is the leading, preventable cause of birth defects and developmental disabilities [4]. Approximately 1 in 58 Americans are estimated to have Autistic Disorder (ICD-10 F84.0). Individuals with ND-PAE/FASD can have comorbid autism, which has a higher neurophenotypic expression with prenatal alcohol exposure [5]. Severe and persistent mental illness (SMI) is more prevalent in individuals with FASD/ND-PAE [6] and autism [7], worsened by a history of adverse childhood experiences (ACEs). Thus, neurodevelopmental disorders (i.e., atypical neurophenotypes) can be precursors for SMI, including schizophrenia spectrum [8] and personality disorders (PDs) [9]. In modern psychiatry dominated by psychopharmacology, clinicians often resort to a plethora of antipsychotics and stimulants, which can have metabolic and growth effects in pediatric populations [10].

For children and adolescents with relatively higher functioning (i.e., mild or no intellectual disability), their symptoms may go relatively unnoticed by clinicians (i.e., pediatricians or primary care providers). In the classroom and home, their externalizing behaviors are often seen as willful, oppositional or defiant rather than involuntary reactions (internal dysregulation) to stress, trauma, anxiety or sensory sensitivities. For many of these children, social communication issues, sensory disintegration, executive dysfunctions, and emotional dysregulation (**Figure 1**) make it difficult for them to adapt to the expectations and pressures of school, home and the community, leading to vulnerability to psychosis during transition years (ages 17 to 24). Normal developmental resiliency factors (friendships, recreational activities, family ties, self-care, hobbies, etc.) are more elusive for neurodiverse individuals who may become more socially disenfranchised, reclusive, oppositional, defiant, noncompliant, and isolated from peer groups during adolescent years. The COVID-19 pandemic compounded the social

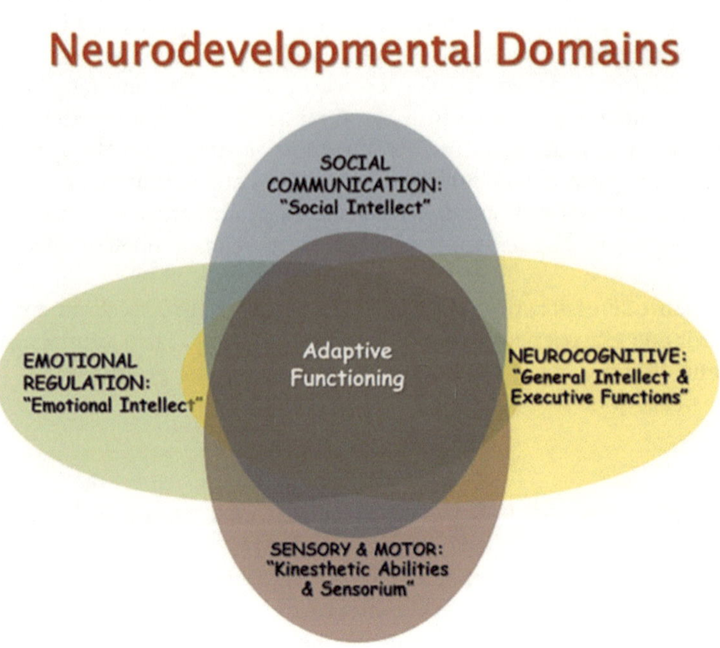

Figure 1.
Neurodevelopmental domains.

isolation, which was complicated by a relative growth in virtual social connections, subsequently making the transition back to "real world" school quite challenging.

There are multiple, complex etiologies for neurodevelopmental conditions, including epigenetic, genetic issues, preconceptional, prenatal and early life experiences, as well as evidence for alterations in the gut-brain microbiota [11]. Early and comprehensive intervention and treatment improves prognosis in children with an accurate neurodiverse diagnosis [12]. Traditional psychiatric and psychologically-based therapeutic approaches (i.e., talk therapy, play therapy, insight-oriented therapy, psychodynamic psychotherapy) may be inadequate or inappropriate [13] due to difficulties with insight, attachment-related transference problems, or metacognitive skills. For an individual to achieve a relatively comfortable, happy life, one must master Maslow's hierarchy - a difficult feat in today's world, especially for neurodiverse individuals. As Victor Frankl and Abraham Maslow taught, having meaning in one's life helps overcome almost any difficulty and is one of the keys to resiliency.

Theory of mind – being able to interpret the thoughts and feelings of another person, or 'mind reading,' was coined in 1978 by Premack and Woodruff. Being able to accurately interpret the meaning of facial expressions or implicit language is an important trait for human social communication. Many children with neurodiverse conditions are unable to use theory of mind to understand what others may be thinking in their minds and may appear callous and unemotional in their social interactions, seeming to lack empathy and have maladaptive social behaviors. These social challenges can lead to parent-child relational issues, interpersonal relationships, and existential crises as young people with neurodevelopmental issues transition into young adulthood. They often have significant difficulty with adaptive functions (i.e., conceptual, social and practical skills) important for development of successful school performance, friendships, and employment. Neurodevelopmental issues are often overlooked in individuals with relatively average intellectual functioning without significant speech and language issues, although they have significant deficits in social, conceptual and practical (i.e., adaptive) functions.

Neuroatypical individuals often lack the requisite adaptive functions and social supports to achieve Maslow's hierarchy (i.e., food/clothing/shelter; safety/security; love/belonging/sense of community; and meaning/purpose) on their own. Neurotypical peers in mainstreamed public school settings are often are ill-equipped to respond to maladaptive social behaviors, which can cause the atypical youth to feel disenfranchised, alienated, and isolated from their classmates. Over the years between elementary and middle school, it becomes relatively difficult for them to feel part of a friend group outside of the virtual reality of online gaming. Thus, their sense of belonging and community are restricted by their social dysmaturity. In our modern day of functional societies disrupted by pandemics, school shootings, global warming/climate change [14], social media, social injustices, even neurotypical youth have difficulty finding a sense of fulfillment, meaning and purpose. Relatively high functioning (i.e., not intellectually disabled) individuals with psychiatric, neurologic, and other brain-related disorders have problems transitioning to meaningful vocations and purposeful lives.

2. History of psychiatric farms

Farm animal assisted therapy is an emerging therapy for complex patients, particularly individuals with neurodiverse conditions, adverse childhood experiences, and associated maladaptive attachment. A farm as a third place for "community" meets an individual's need for Maslow's connection/belonging and meaning/purpose to improve mental health [15]. There is historic precedence for farms in mental health treatment, although seemingly a relatively archaic cultural construct in our modern world. The earliest psychiatric "asylums" (aka, "sanctuaries") were on farms as a milieu for treatment of individuals with severe mental health, intellectual disability, and neurodevelopmental conditions. Examples of the original institutions situated on large pastoral farms included Spring Grove [16], Forest Haven [17, 18], (previously the District Training School for the Mentally Retarded) and Springfield State [19] Hospitals in Maryland and St. Elizabeth's Hospital [20] in Washington, DC.

An institutional mileau was defined as therapeutic if it met certain criteria as outlined in *Community as Doctor*: [21] "to provide the contexts and facilities for the kinds of social processes and interpersonal relations that will bring about the following effects on patients:

1. provide the patient with experiences that will minimize distortions of reality;

2. facilitate realistic and meaningful communicative exchange with others;

3. facilitate participation with others so that s/he derives greater satisfaction and security there from;

4. reduce anxiety and increase comfort;

5. increase self-esteem;

6. provide insight into the causes and manifestations of mental illness;

7. mobilize initiative and motivate the individual to realize potential for creativity and productivity." [22]

These tenants, largely based on Abraham Maslow's Hierarchy of Human Needs [23], provided the essence for treatment of patients on large sprawling farms where doctors, nurses, staff and administrators lived in a community with patients who also worked in most operational aspects of the farm – from the kitchen to groundskeeping, gardens, animal husbandry, and even the gift shop. While quite paternalistic, these farms had the potential to provide a short-term sense of community and purpose in a relatively safe milieu. While living and working on the farms' fields of blueberries and blackberries, orchards and gardens, patients may have improved their adaptive functions but, unfortunately, often were not integrated back into the community in the unlikely event of discharge.

Decreasing funding in the 1960s led to harsh treatment, abuse, and neglect of patients by ill-trained, poorly supervised staff [17]. Forest Haven, which was located in Laurel, Maryland and operated by the District of Columbia opened in 1925 and was closed on October 14, 1991 "by order of a federal judge after years of physical and sexual abuse, medical incompetence, 10 deaths from aspiration pneumonia, and hundreds of other deaths under suspicious circumstances" [24, 25]. Thus, state-run psychiatric "sanctuaries" became warehouses to hide away people with mental illness from mainstream western society where they were seen as ill-suited or "unfit" to conform with social norms. When Dr. Roger Peele took over as medical director of St. Elizabeth's in the mid-1970s, he approached the director of NIH to request money to pay the patients for their labor. A time limited grant of $1 million was allocated for patient salaries, which lasted approximately 1 year before the farm and gardens were dismantled due to lack of funding for paying patients minimum wage [26]. Truly for a program to be sustainable, there must be ongoing funding that is not tied to political beliefs or economic instability.

With the necessary deinstitutionalization of the state psychiatric hospitals, communities received time-limited federal funding for community-based programs in the mid-1970s [27]. Therapies that may have been used in the asylums, such as occupational therapy, physical therapy, speech/language therapy, recreational therapy, and art therapy were theoretically incorporated into community mental health, public or privately run allied health agencies, or corporate-owned residential treatment programs. Other programs, such as horticulture therapy, aqua therapy (swimming), and working with farm animals gradually disappeared from all but a few privately owned residential treatment centers. One of these, Green Chimneys in Brewster, NY, focuses on individuals with autism and intellectual disability who may have co-morbid mental health challenges. According to their website, "Founded in 1947 and headquartered on a farm and wildlife center in Brewster, NY, with a second campus in Carmel, NY, Green Chimneys is recognized as a worldwide leader in animal-assisted therapy and educational activities for children with special needs. Green Chimneys services include an accredited special education school on two campuses; residential treatment center; nature-based therapeutic programs; community-based support for youth and families; and public education and recreation opportunities for all ages. Each of our programs celebrates the dignity and worth of all living things. Green Chimneys is a pioneer in animal and nature-based therapy, striving to create a harmonious relationship among children, animals and the environment incorporating an array of educational, residential, recreational, and mental health services. Through innovative therapies and tools to teach critical life skills, we help youth reclaim their childhood, discover their self-worth and create a future for themselves as independent, contributing adults." Green Chimneys is a model program for other states to follow.

Over the past three decades since deinstitutionalization, large tracks of state-owned asylums have devolved into dilapidated, asbestos-contaminated dormitory buildings riddling expansive landscapes. Many states still own hundreds of acres of land with sprawling abandoned campuses standing as a reminder of the dystopian, patriarchal institutional mental health system. With the disbursement of neurodevelopmentally impaired and traumatized patients into local communities that lacked resources to address their complex needs, deinstitutionalization eventually led to a rise in imprisonment and homelessness of people with mental illness [28].

3. What is farm animal assisted therapy?

As the institutional farms were being dismantled, across Europe and North America, a new humanistic movement [29] arose from social psychology called "green care," "social farming," "care farming," "therapeutic farming," or "farming for health" [30]. These modalities emerged within nature immersive experiential approaches, such as wilderness therapy, horticulture therapy, and various types of animal assisted therapy (e.g., equine, pet, multi-species). Green care has been piloted as a way to improve social, recreational, and vocational functioning in mental health [31], dementia care [32], cognitive decline [33], trauma [34], parent-child relational (attachment) issues [35], autism [36] and other disabilities [37]. Farming for health provides social connections, meaningful activities, practical skill development, and the health benefits of nature. Therapeutic farming also has been proposed as a way to improve access to mental health care for rural communities [38]. Equine assisted psychotherapy [39] has been utilized with transitional age youth in both outpatient and residential treatment centers to improve attachment, resiliency, and trust and to regain emotional regulation. A resurgence of horticulture therapy [40] has led to community-based mental health programs operating urban, suburban [41], and rural gardens [42]. Examples of green care farms are Nourishing Hearts Wellness Care Farm in Ontario, Canada [43] (privately owned and operated by Julie Casey MSW) and The Farm at Penny Lane in North Carolina (operated by UNC Chapel Hill School of Medicine Department of Psychiatry) [44].

Farm animal assisted therapy combines "green care" and "animal assisted therapy" [45] to augment more traditional strategies, including psychoeducation, cognitive behavioral therapy, supportive, insight-oriented psychotherapy, and psychopharmacology practiced in the milieu of a farm. Farm animal assisted psychotherapy has been used internationally to improve child-parent bonds, reduce anxiety, improve social relatedness, increase adaptive functions, and reduce the barriers to access. The aim of both green care and farm animal assisted therapy is to provide a safe/secure environment with human-animal connections to promote a sense of belonging and community and activities that inspire self-esteem, meaning and purpose. The human-animal connection [46] began at the earliest points in humanity when the first animals were tamed and domesticated by humans – perhaps as early as the neolithic period. The canine was a beloved companion who gave warmth, helped hunt for prey, protected early modern humans from predators, and likely provided comfort through a unique human-animal bond. Mammals have a similar basal ganglia as humans – controlling a range of functions from emotions, to motor control, learned behaviors, and executive functions. It is not surprising that our family pets respond to our emotions, providing a sense of comfort, security, and companionship. In the safety and security of the farm, individuals find a sense of love and belonging with the animals, surrounded by nature, and may begin to feel a sense of meaning and purpose with more time interacting and learning about the animals.

Multisensory therapeutic approaches provided from hands-on experiences with gentle farm animals has the potential to improve emotional regulation, social communication, neurocognitive and sensory/motor issues common in both ND-PAE/FASD and ASD [47]. Interacting with gentle farm animals provides novel sights, sounds, smells, and textures; entrainment with the sounds and vibrations of animals; social connections with beings with healthy attachment behaviors; nonverbal cues; and emotional expression. The quiet yet multisensory environment of a farm provides hands on experiences to desensitize to touch, textures, sounds, smells, and other sensory inputs (i.e., bugs, soil, sunshine, water, crowing roosters, bleating goats, neighing horses, odiferous poo patties, or other common farm phenomena). Even chickens clucking and pecking at grain becomes an opportunity to explore social communication in an indirect, nonthreatening way (**Figure 2**).

Farm animal assisted therapy is a way for a licensed therapist or psychiatrist to interact with adults, teens and children with a wide range of neuropsychiatric and neurodevelopmental conditions who may have difficulty tolerating more traditional office-based or institutional settings (e.g., due to fluorescent lighting, people in the waiting room, noises coming from other offices, etc.). Children with neurodevelopmental issues benefit from multimodal therapy to assist with their sensory issues, dysmaturity, mood dysregulation, heightened arousal, impulsivity, attention deficits, hyperactivity, coordination and balance issues and other motor deficits, and speech and language problems. Children who

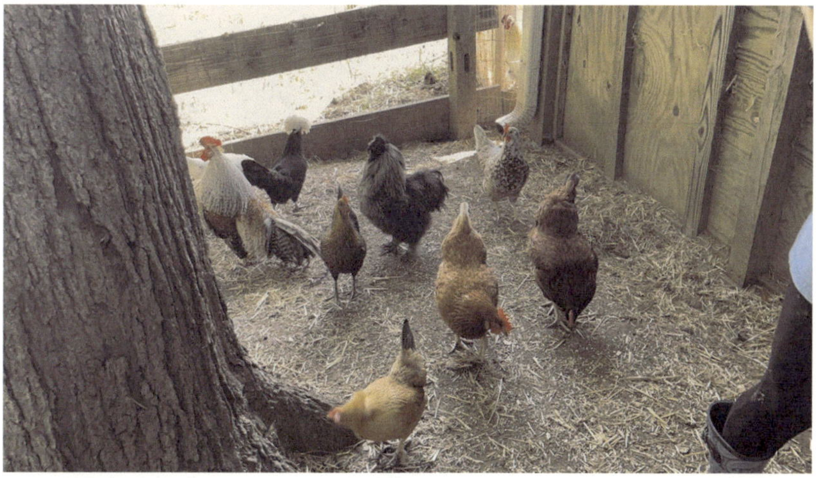

Figure 2.
Chickens clucking and pecking.

have difficulty picking up on social cues, have poor eye contact with peers and adults, and other social communication issues learn to interact with animals without fear of misunderstandings or maladaptive behaviors. Children become relaxed and are more easily able to overcome their insecurities and sensitivities while petting, grooming, playing with or hand-feeding animals sitting nearby. Like traditional play therapy, the therapist assesses, comments on, analyzes, and redirects a child's reactions during the therapy session to help move the patient past certain ways of viewing the world (e.g., anxious, suspicious, pessimistic, angry). Perspectives can be analyzed and reflected back in a more positive way to improve self-concept and perception about others. Cognitive distortions can be examined in a non-threatening way from the objective view of the animals, much like examining a storybook character or comic superhero.

Children with adverse childhood experiences (trauma) may have difficulty trusting a therapist or psychiatrist, becoming anxious, angry, or hyperaroused during therapy sessions. Gently raised farm animals provide unconditional love, bonding and attachment cues that are important in socialization of children with a variety of neurodevelopmental differences. Holding, touching and stroking the fur and feathers of animals allows a bond of attachment to form within a child or teen to improve trust and interpersonal connection with the therapist. Activities on the farm such as brushing the horses, feeding the chickens grain by hand, petting and massaging the pig, taking hay to the goats, and sitting quietly interacting with the juvenile emus provides social connections and builds trust with the animals and their bonded therapist. The animals offer opportunity to develop trust through contact with unconditionally loving and accepting beings who provide comfort, joy, and novelty while working with the trained therapist.

A highly anxious, traumatized patient who was adopted as a teen from an orphanage commented when she walked into the paddock with the goats for the first time (**Figure 3**): "I feel very uncomfortable that they [the 14 goats] are all looking at me ... I've got to get out of here!" It was an opportunity to explore the automatic thoughts that arise when people in a group turn to look at her (e.g., when she walks into a classroom after others are seated, when she raises her hand to speak in class, as she is walking around a crowded grocery or department store and makes eye contact with strangers). Using the goats' perspectives (i.e., non-biased, non-judgmental, neutral), we discussed and

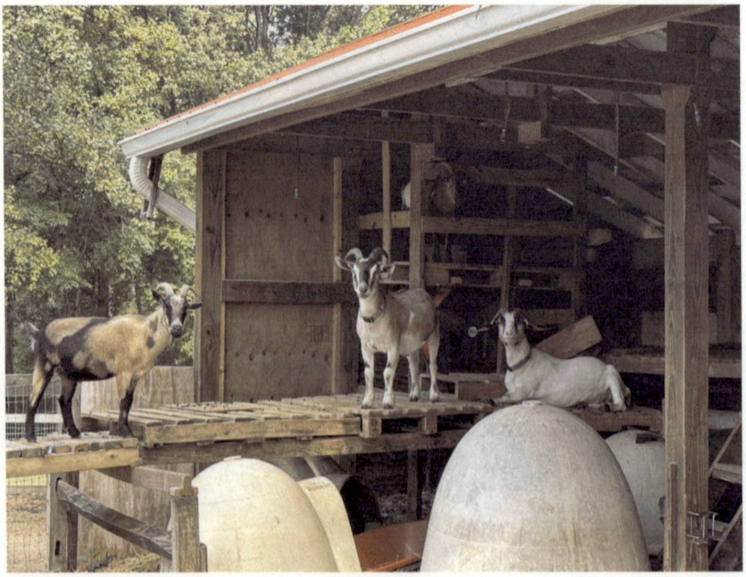

Figure 3.
Goats looking at a person can create arousal similar to a group of people.

analyzed her thought distortions and negative self-talk leading from feelings of social anxiety that trigger her "fight or flight" response. Resulting cognitive distortions (aka, misperceptions about the goats) cause her to assume she can "mind read" (i.e., "they do not like me ..., why are they looking at me? ... they think I'm weird"). This cross talk between her automatic thoughts and negative self-talk then spiral into paranoia in public settings, family gatherings, and peer groups. Insight into these areas of their maladaptive social perspectives can shift to positive self-talk using a cognitive behavioral approach.

Theory of mind is possible when one person is able to accurately interpret the intentions, thoughts or feelings of another by analyzing vocalizations, nonverbal cues, and context of a situation. By scattering grain for the chickens then discussing what hens might mean as they peck and cluck about the coop (**Figure 2**) allows the child a non-threatening, objective perspective to explore "what others might be thinking" to develop theory of mind. Listening to the various sounds the chickens make and analyzing their social behaviors as they "talk to each other" allows a therapist to ask the child open-ended questions like: "What do you think they are talking about? Why do you think that one just pecked the other one? How did that one know there was food over there with the others?" The way chickens (especially hens) behave in a coop hierarchy is not different than the way teen girls behave in the middle school social structure. Understanding that much of the behavior is primitively wired (brain stem based), one can begin to articulate and weave the concepts of "primitive drives" and "competition" into the therapy sessions. Ultimately, the goal is for the children to be more comfortable with nonverbal cue interpretation in their peers while remaining relatively calm.

3.1 Farm animal therapy: A naturalistic form of neurotherapy

Each farm animal has its own sounds, vibrations, and unique sensory experience for the child or teen. Interacting with gently raised farm animals through their unique

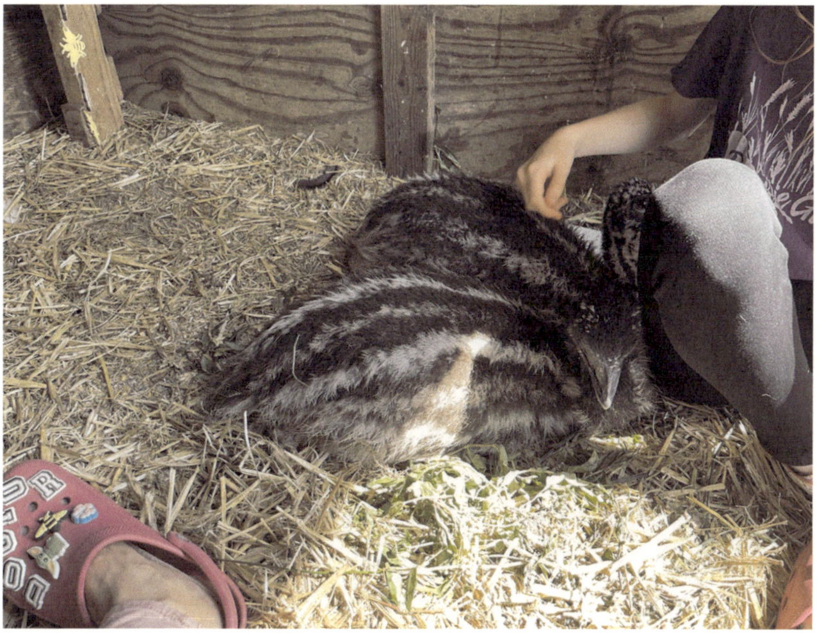

Figure 4.
Emus whistling.

sounds and rhythm's is a way to practice entrainment to re-establish one's resonant frequency. Individuals with misophonia or sound sensitivity can desensitize while immersed in the sounds of the farm - roosters crowing, goats bleating, emus whistling (**Figure 4**), horses whinnying (**Figure 5**), pigs squealing or grunting, dogs barking and cats meowing. Sound healing works through entrainment and resonant frequency. Entrainment is the "adjustment or moderation of one behavior either to synchronize or to be in rhythm with another behavior [48]." The natural process of a rhythm compels an organism to fall into synchrony with the rhythm (i.e., clapping our hands or tapping our feet while keeping cadence with music). Likewise, entrainment can be conveyed more subtly through sound therapy, which entrains brainwaves to a slower rhythm to relax the body and mind by downregulating sympathetic overdrive. Resonant frequency is the rate at which each object or being vibrates. "Think of the body like a symphony orchestra with all parts (muscles, bones, organs, cells, etc.) having their own frequencies which, when healthy, are all in perfect rhythm and harmony. When the body systems become compromised due to physical or emotional causes, certain frequencies are affected and literally become out of tune. Just as in an orchestra, when one instrument is out of tune, nothing sounds right! Everything is affected. With sound therapy, utilizing various instruments and tones, the body is gently brought back to its natural state of harmony" [49].

Neurotherapy involves 'rewiring' neurons to improve brain function in some way. Neurotherapy is defined as "any neurotechnology with a therapeutic application ... Common applications include mood disorder management, cognitive learning and performance improvement, and addiction or habit management ... Neurotherapy, while still very early in its development, has already shown efficacy in altering brain function to provide relief to patients suffering from a range of disorders" [50]. While working with farm animals is not technology, it is a therapy that may reset the nervous system of neurodiverse populations through frequency and resonance. A series of farm animal assisted neurotherapy sessions with gently raised goats, horses, pig, and chickens can help lower a child or teen's arousal, putting them in a calmer mood state and rewire brain circuits while engaging in activities on the farm. The process entrains the rhythms of children and adolescents with the rhythms of gently raised farm animals to provide moments of calm for recentering and practicing emotional regulation. The reassuring, caring, nurturing, accepting, validating and cocooning external world allows the child to externally regulate (i.e., external locus of control) in such a way that translates into internal regulation (i.e., internal locus of control) over time.

While neuroscience has not yet been applied to farm animal assisted therapy (i.e., examining brain waves or neural circuits before and after sessions), it is possible that this form of therapy can help "rewire" hyperaroused limbic circuits of children with conditions such as selective mutism, post traumatic stress disorder, reactive attachment disorder, and social anxiety disorder. For example, an anxious, sensory sensitive boy cautiously enters the emu enclosure with the juvenile brothers, reluctant to sit and

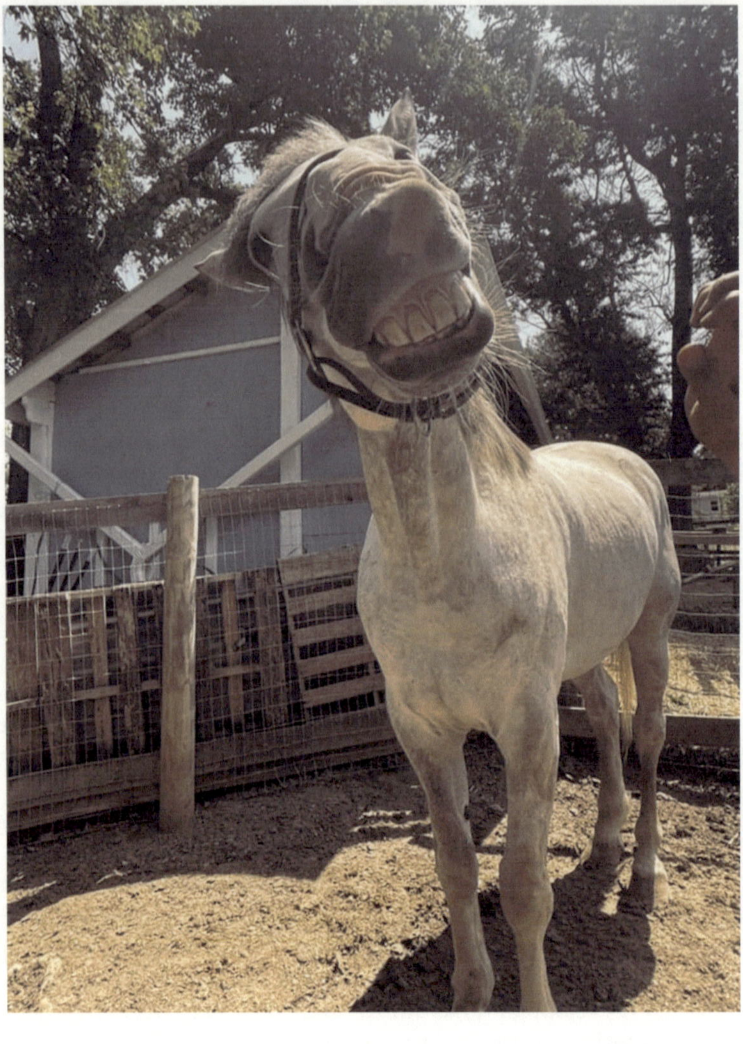

Figure 5.
Kingston Whinning.

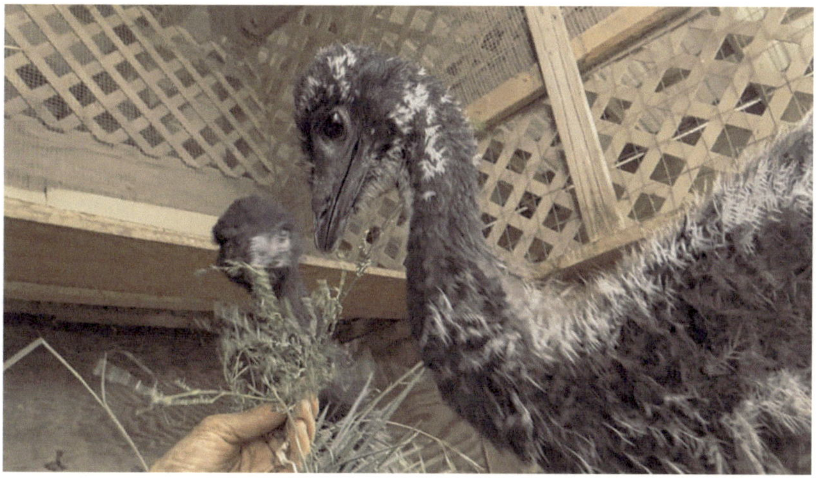

Figure 6.
Feeding emus grass.

engage due to uncertainty about the behaviors of the animals. The boy stood at the door frozen, asking - "Will they peck me? Will they like me? How will they know me?" He was visibly anxious, cautious, frozen in a state of fight/flight/freeze. The therapist gently encouraged and guided him to sit farther away from the animals to allow him to observe and be comfortable with their unusual mannerisms (baby emus have very little boundaries; will stare in a person's face; and peck at shoe strings, jewelry, and other dangling items). While his mother sat in the enclosure feeding the emus a bouquet of weeds and grass, the boy asked whether he could feed them, too. The therapist offered him a bouquet of grasses and weeds, which the emus began to pull and peck at. When the animals were seen to enjoy his mother's company and become comfortable enough to lie down next to her, the boy felt more comfortable to sit a bit closer in hopes of them falling to sleep by him, too. Before the session ended, he was regulated, calm and joyful – proud of being able to comfort and feed the emus. His arousal had lowered and he was no longer hyper-vigilant in dealing with the uncertainty of the situation. He then restated a few times that he was not coming back to the farm for a month because of his vacation and wondered whether the emus would remember him. The therapist reassured him that the emus are very friendly and would relate to him as well as they had this session. The process of the emus becoming comfortable in the environment (i.e., lying and sleeping next to the patient's mom) allowed the boy to calm and self-regulate enough to eventually feed them from his hand (**Figure 6**).

4. A child psychiatrist's journey into farm animal-assisted psychotherapy

The process of incorporating multiple species of furry and feathered co-therapists into a private practice setting situated adjacent to a small nonprofit green care farm animal sanctuary evolved from a vision of a farm for treatment of neurodevelopmental disorder associated with prenatal alcohol exposure (ND-PAE) [51]. Maryland's pristine horse farms inspired this vision to develop a therapeutic farm for children with prenatal alcohol exposure when I completed medical school and moved to the state in 2001. From a neurodevelopmental lens, these children often have adaptive functioning deficits disproportionate to their intellectual abilities, leading to problems with socialization, academic achievement, and vocational success. In 2008, I entered the realm of animal assisted psychotherapy by incorporating two guinea pigs into play therapy while working with a boy with severe reactive attachment disorder and Fetal Alcohol Syndrome. His mother said she had never seen him so relaxed as when he was laying on the rug in the middle of the office with one of our family's two guinea pigs, Buddy and Spike, on his chest. Through play therapy, Buddy worked in the mystical realm of the transitional space as a sentient "object" - "chattering" with the boy while I interpreted the guinea pig's side of the conversation. Over the next few years, both children and adults often requested the guinea pigs join their sessions, sometimes bringing their own celery, carrots, or apples as a treat to share.

After several different rescued guinea pigs had participated as co-therapists, I hatched chicks in the spring of 2013 with my son's Kindergarten class and my daughter's school science fair project. My patients candled the eggs with awe in a little dark space between the doors separating my waiting area and office from my kitchen and eagerly awaited their next visit to watch the little feathery friends grow into something special – a real life attachment object. The special attachment was highlighted when two little adopted 5-year-old twin boys called on a snow day from Kindergarten, worried about how the chickens were doing outside in their coop. Though their mother had said they had not ever asked how their frail, elderly grandparents were doing, the boys woke up excitedly concerned to call and find out about "Dr. Suess's chickens."

Having had pet cats and a family dog growing up and cats during my adult life, I had felt connected to animals, though the deep therapeutic benefits were only apparent when seeing it first-hand in my clinical practice. Success with guinea pigs and chickens led me to read more literature on pet therapy and animal assisted psychotherapy. Chickens were being used in memory care facilities [52] – patients would remember the day of the week "Clementine, the hen" visited but could not recognize family members who cared for them daily. The reading for me became liberating and validating to my clinical findings. In 2014, we adopted a 4-month-old kitten from the Humane Society and later that year, we got a golden doodle puppy from a Mennonite family in Western, MD. The cat, Elsa, remains shy and skittish from her first few months of life living in a small cage at the shelter, so she has never been very therapeutic. Even though she is not that affectionate, many children relate to her anxiety and social phobia and she has become a way to discuss etiology of their own shyness and social isolation. There was something magical and therapeutic in the human-animal bond between children and our golden doodle puppy, Copper, who interacted like he was one of us. He would sit patiently at the waiting area door, smiling and wagging waiting for the next child to come, then greeting them with kisses and hugs as though they were his favorite person on the planet. Difficult-to-reach adolescents were asking their parents when they were coming to see me and Copper again and younger children were upset to leave by the end of the sessions. The little boy who had called about the chickens during the snowstorm had misunderstood his new nanny driving to the nearby park for playtime before his session and became so enraged that she was purposefully not taking him to the session. By the time they finally arrived in the waiting area, she was disheveled and out of breath, relating how he refused to get out of the car at the playground, insisting he had to get to his appointment with Dr. Suess and Copper.

During July 2015, my office coordinator at the time, Donna, who was a long time equestrian, mentioned therapeutic riding and other types of equine therapy for kids with autism, knowing of my quest to find solutions for the children affected by prenatal alcohol exposure. I bought several books on the topic for her daughter who was volunteering at Great and Small [53] – a local hippotherapy equine facility in our county. Donna explained that my one-acre wooded property was not large enough for even a miniature horse but a friend of hers had a pet goat that was house trained and went everywhere with her. Of course, my curiosity about potentially using goats in therapy sparked a bit of reading. They are friendly, social, and form strong attachments with humans yet are smaller and easier to manage than horses. Goats may have been the first domesticated farm animal – used for their milk, hides, meat, and warmth in the colder climates. One of the most environmentally well-adapted species, the goat is able to survive in desert conditions, temperate rain forests, and high-altitude mountain ranges. Like domesticated dogs with their human packs, goats form social bonds, have a hierarchy of herd organization, and are both loyal and dependent on the shepherd. They learn routines, can be taught to respond to certain cues, and attach to their caregiver. The goat can become a beloved farm animal assisted therapist, particularly goats rescued from dairy farms which are taken away from mother's who are milked for profit and have no time for nursing.

The next afternoon, I read about a dairy farmer in West Virginia on Facebook looking to rehome twin baby goats and drove with my pre-teens in our Pruis V to pick them up. Dr. Tanya Fayen is a retired professor of comparative literature who now raises mixed breed pygmy and Nigerian dwarf dairy goats for people's backyards and homestead farms. She named the twin pair Romulus and Remus, born from a teen female goat by a dwarf buck who snuck in with her unintentionally. The male kid, Romey, had been rejected by their mother who had to be tied to a milking stand to nurse him (likely not ready for parenting). She would gently and lovingly nurture her daughter, Rosie, but pushed and butted her son away. Male goats on dairy farms are typically sold for meat, although Dr. Fayen attempts to rehome them as pets. The female kid, Rosie, inherited the fainting gene from her grandmother, Noli, who had been paralyzed by the other goats in the herd who did not understand her myotonic seizures during episodes of anxiety and arousal. Like elephants who nudge their herd mates to get up when they are lame, the goats on the dairy farm unintentionally beat poor Noli till her back broke. We took in Rosie so that the same fate would not befall her. I believed taking a bonded pair of siblings would improve bonding and attachment. (**Figure** 7) What we learned over the next few years was that Romey's early rejection by his birth mother made him have similar maladaptive attachment as a children with reactive attachment disorder. He, unlike our other goats, will headbutt caregivers as they attempt to put hay for him and he bullies some of the other goats. One teenaged girl with severe reactive attachment disorder and aggression toward her parents expressed insight as Romey was chasing her through the forest, "Maybe this is how my mom feels when I'm coming after her."

In 2016, I purchased a 6.43 acre residential farm in Potomac, MD for my home and psychiatric practice. My nonprofit, 7th Generation Foundation, Inc. was awarded 501c3 status later that year and leased 5.43 acres of the property for $0 to begin operating a green care farm animal sanctuary, Dream Catcher Meadows. Montgomery County, MD awarded two separate business permits (for the practice and farm) and my family, volunteers, and I eventually received agricultural status through the State of Maryland Department of Assessments and Taxation by selling $2500 in agricultural products and having the requisite number of animals per acre to qualify as a farm. The county allows the nonprofit to provide agricultural education and tourism programs as accessory uses of the farm. These programs provide community outreach and engagement for our farm animal sanctuary. Community organizations, civic groups, volunteers, and school children and their families benefit from the green care

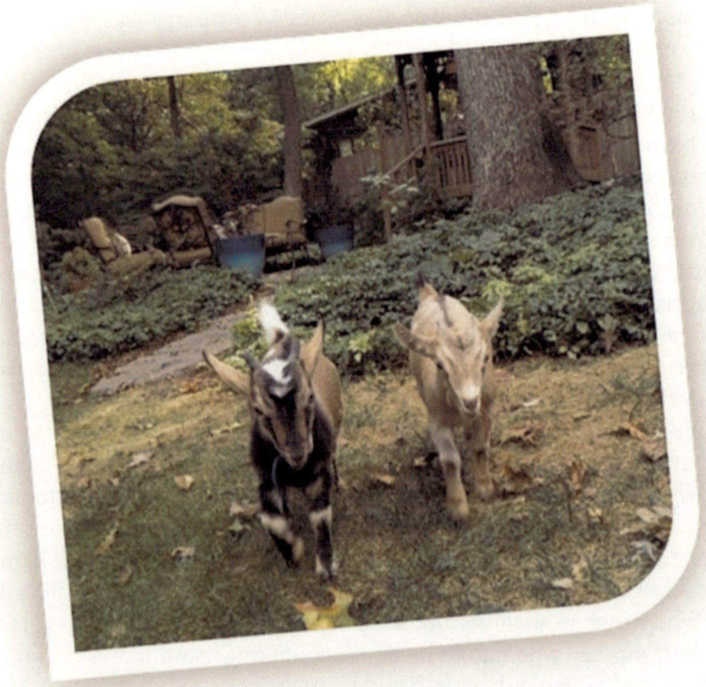

Figure 7.
Romey and Rosie.

opportunities. One of these programs, discussed later, is "Earthkeepers Kinder Farming," a social, farm educational, and recreational activity for children and families.

In 2018, we rehomed Romey and Rosie's disabled grandmother to the farm, Noli, who was only able to walk on her front two legs. Noli enjoyed being pulled around the farm and neighborhood in a small Radio Flyer wagon, sitting in the grass of the barnyard adjacent to the goat paddock, and lived out the next 9 months of her life being gently nurtured and loved by the 2-legged kids who visited. The children in my practice benefitted from spending time with and learning about the disabled, epileptic goat (Noli) and other disabled and injured animals. Over the years, we have rehomed a total of 16 goat kids – most of which were either rejected or orphaned by their birth moms, have minor birth defects, or would have been sold for meat due to being males on a dairy farm. Their stories have powerful meanings for the patients I treat – many of them adopted or with other adverse childhood experiences mirroring those of the animals. Our horse Kingston was rehomed to our farm after he was retired prematurely from fox hunting due to a navicular injury. These experiences seemed to help patients develop compassion and empathy for friends and family who are sick and injured in the process.

The earlier the kid is removed from his mother, the more of Maslow's Hierarchy he needs from the human caregiver (food/shelter, safety/security, love/belonging, and meaning/purpose). In addition to a few to several times a day bottle feeding and care, a baby goat needs safety/security (protection from predatory wildlife and older/larger farm animals), love/belonging (feeling part of a herd or family); and meaning and purpose (being taken out for walks with the therapist and children, climbing on structures, and being petted and groomed). By raising the baby animal with a strong human-animal connection, the animal learns to trust and remain calm even when

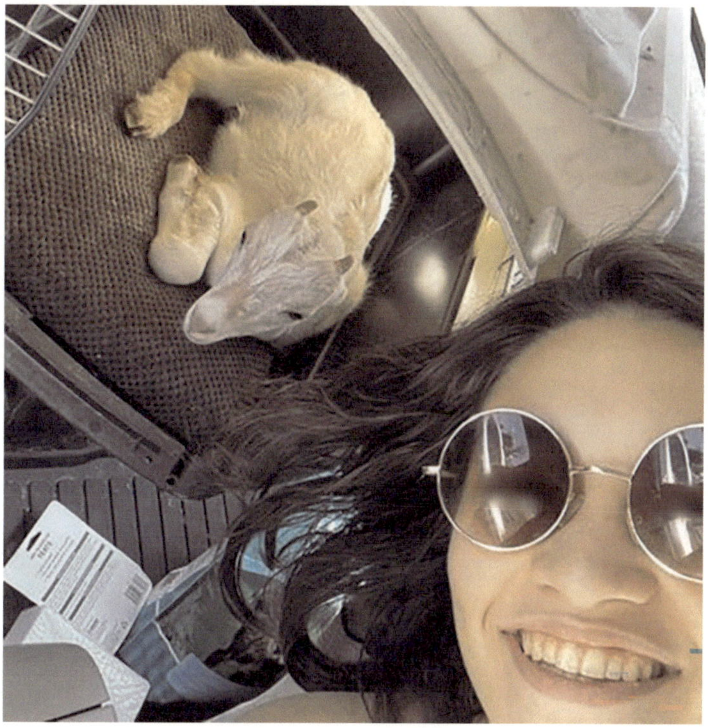

Figure 8.
The rescue of Rerun (selfie by co-author, BRH).

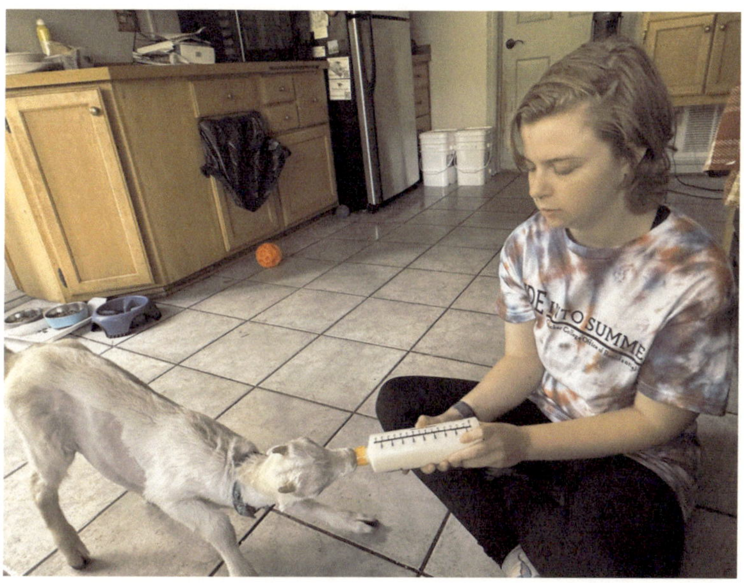

Figure 9.
Bottle feeding Rerun (photo of co-author., EKK).

children are less regulated. By taking in weanlings, spending quality time with them providing nurturing and care giving, the therapist imprints on the animal, which promotes the healthy attachment bonds in the therapy session between patient and co-therapist animal. We are currently hand raising a 4-week-old Lamancha male, Rerun (**Figures 8–10**), who came to us through a dairy farmer in Maryland. He is cryptorchid, had an umbilical and urachus infection, and severely malnourished and anemic (likely from an infestation of goat lice, which we washed off with the vet

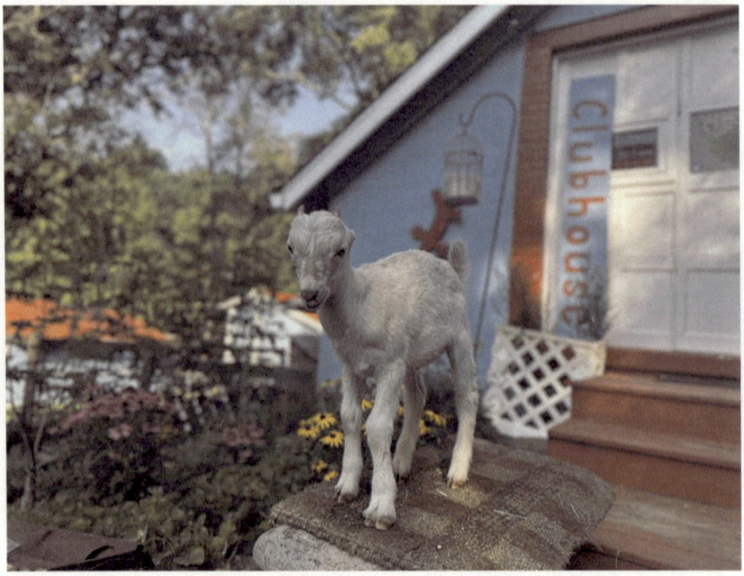

Figure 10.
Four week old Rerun.

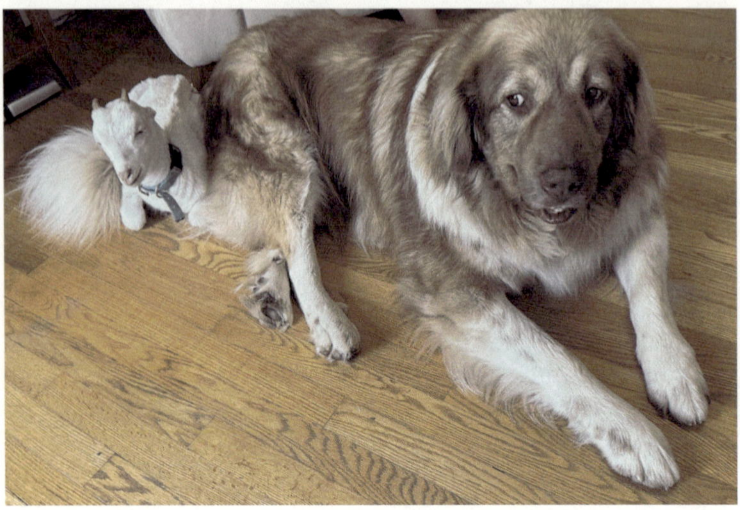

Figure 11.
Rurun and Clifford.

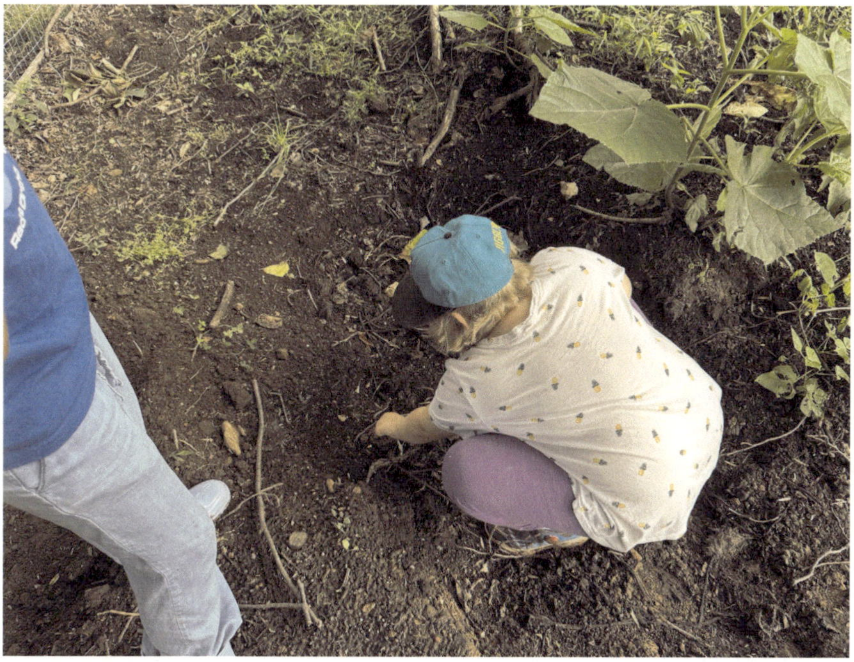

Figure 12.
Digging in compost soil.

recommended dish soap). He is under the care of the University of Pennsylvania Veterinary Medicine New Bolton Center and will return there for surgery to remove his non-descended testes. Like all the other bottle babies we have raised, he stays in the house in my bathroom at night, goes down to the barnyard in the morning during chores, and plays with the dogs and cats for socialization (**Figure 11**).

The approach of working with gentle, hand-raised animals works because the animals are bonded with or imprinted on me as their primary attachment figure. My children, our volunteers, and I have bottle fed several of our "baa-bies," who call me "maa-maa." I am their primary caregiver, so they know me and respond to me with similar attachment behaviors as children. The goats look into your eyes like dogs do, respond to emotions and facial expressions, provide nonverbal cues such as nudging and rubbing against your leg for attention, and provide a multi-sensory experience to offset anxious feelings brought on by traditional talk therapy.

5. Dream Catcher Meadows: A "Third Place" for OneHealth, Belonging, and Sustainability

A green care farm animal sanctuary can be a "real life" third place for neurodiverse individuals to learn about OneHealth while experiencing social, recreational and vocational activities. According to the Brookings Institute, "third places" play a strategic role "in strengthening our sense of community. Third places is a term coined by sociologist Ray Oldenburg and refers to places where people spend time between home ('first' place) and work ('second' place). They are locations where we exchange ideas, have a good time, and build relationships ... For young Americans, many third places are now virtual – from Facebook and chat rooms to group texts. But as Oldenburg notes, the most effective ones for building real community seem to be physical places where people can easily and routinely connect with each other: churches, parks, recreation centers, hairdressers, gyms and even fast-food restaurants." [54].

The OneHealth [55] approach to environmental sustainability includes an understanding of the inextricable link between human health, animal health, and the environment we all share. Abnormalities in gut flora has been linked to a variety of mental health [56], immunological, metabolic, neurological [57], and neurodevelopmental [58] conditions. Agriculture and crops have the potential to improve gut health in humans [59]. Activities on farms - digging in soil (**Figure 12**), planting produce, composting to create new soil, planting trees and plants, holding bugs (**Figure 13**), picking berries grooming and petting the animals, and cleaning water buckets, coops, sheds, and bedding – all can contribute to improved gut (and mental) health [60]. Up to 50% of our dopamine and 90% of our serotonin manufactured in our bodies is regulated by our gut microbiome in communication with our intestinal enterochromaffin cells [61]. Likewise, interspecies physical contact provides access to a wider range of microbes accessible through transfer of natural microbiota from fur or feathers to skin (**Figure 14**).

In contrast to the virtual world of videogames, the multi-sensory real-life world of a farm takes longer to take apart a pallet, clean and change water buckets, or to build a structure for goats or a pig (**Figure 15**). The process provides meaningful life skills, collaboration, teamwork, and socialization in real life. Our "In Real Life Friends on the Farm" program for 14 to 17 year old neurodiverse individuals included a project disassembling reclaimed, used pallets from the farm which we reassembled into small foot lockers the participants could use to store their work boots. Other projects with interns and volunteers repurpose reclaimed playground equipment pallets, fencing

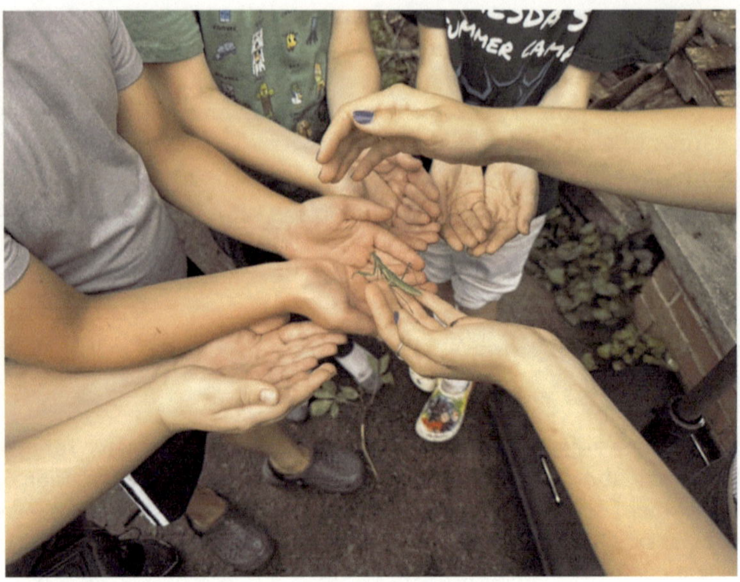

Figure 13.
Holding a praying mantis.

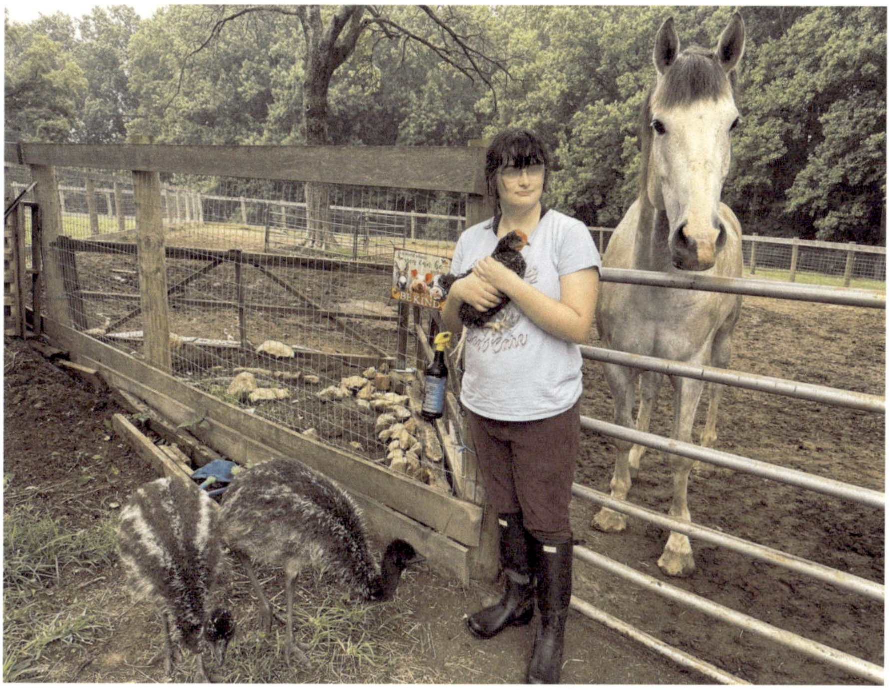

Figure 14.
Interspecies interactions.

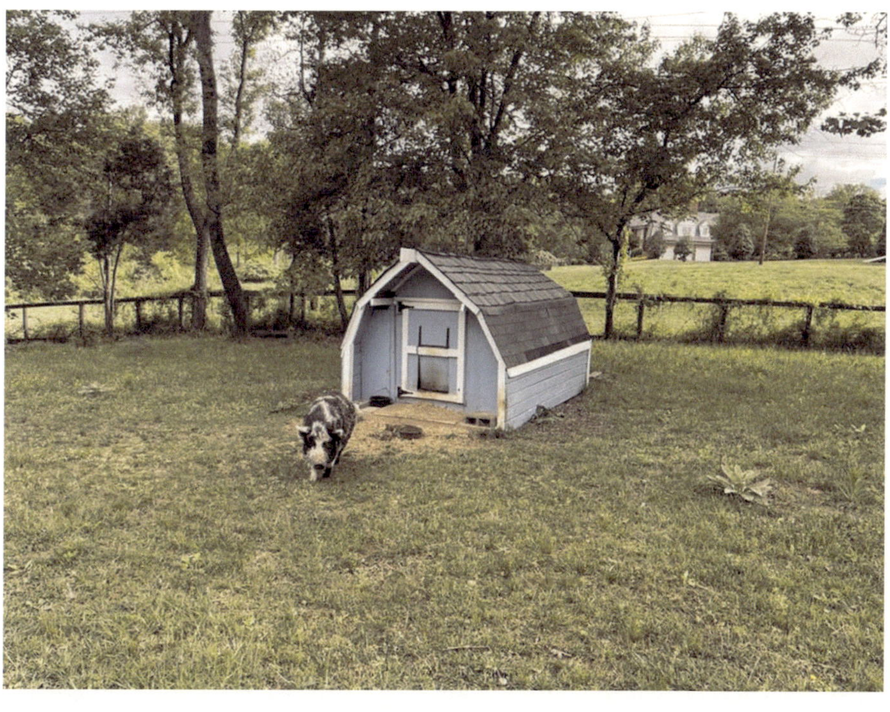

Figure 15.
Noah's house made from reclaimed materials.

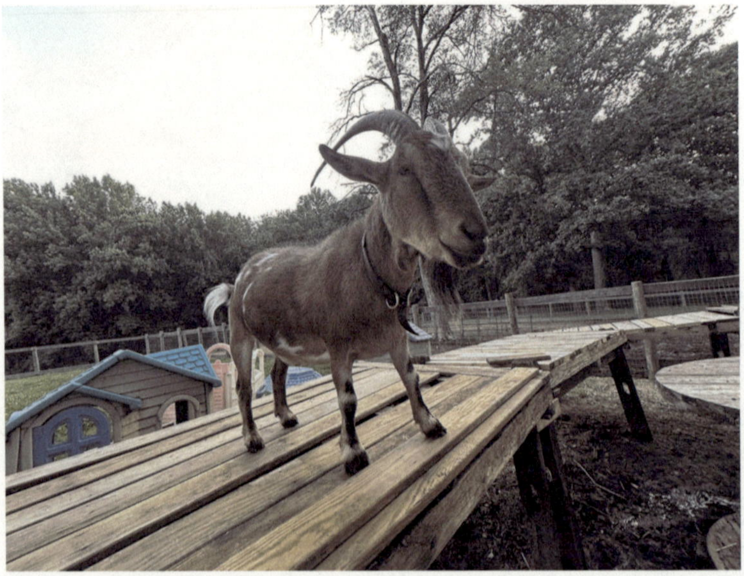

Figure 16.
Goat climbing structure made from reclaimed building materials and pallets.

materials, and salvaged wood into climbing bridges (**Figure 16**) and housing for the goats, chickens, and pig. Building these structures collaboratively allows the teens to become invested in the infrastructure of the farm and see the fruits of their volunteerism enjoyed by the animals. Thus, the farm provides a safe space for community organizations to bring groups of young adults with neurodevelopmental issues, for students to earn service learning hours, for children to gain social and recreational opportunities, and for high school students to learn life skills and improve adaptive functions (**Figure 17**). Even our weekend volunteers (**Figure 18**) enjoy activities on the farm–expressing relief from the stress of working in special needs classrooms, attending virtual high school, being sequestered during the pandemic, and re-entering the real world post-pandemic. An overview of the farm provides perspectives from local high school students and their parents who volunteered at the farm during the pandemic. (Video 1 available from: https://archive.org/details/mccmd-Dream_Catcher_Meadows and Video 2 available from: https://www.youtube.com/watch?v=vMWHxMEPiH8).

The operations of the farm can be both environmentally and financially sustainable by: transplanting and promoting growth of native species of plants; encouraging growth of volunteer fruiting seeds from compost soil; utilizing the natural fertilizers and soil conditioners; reclaiming building materials to reduce construction costs; minimizing contract labor costs by negotiating nonprofit fee rates with local businesses; collaborating with scouting and other nonprofit groups for volunteer experiences; working with teen and young adult volunteers to provide animal care (**Figures 19** and **20**); and obtaining grants for capital improvements to the infrastructure. Cost savings can be achieved by asking local contractors for nonprofit rates, purchasing reclaimed materials on Facebook Marketplace, and engaging community members who may be willing to donate unused building supplies. We have completed dumpster dives where lumber has been discarded, picked up foam board insulation and slat wall for our welcome center, and hauled pallets from the trash heap of local

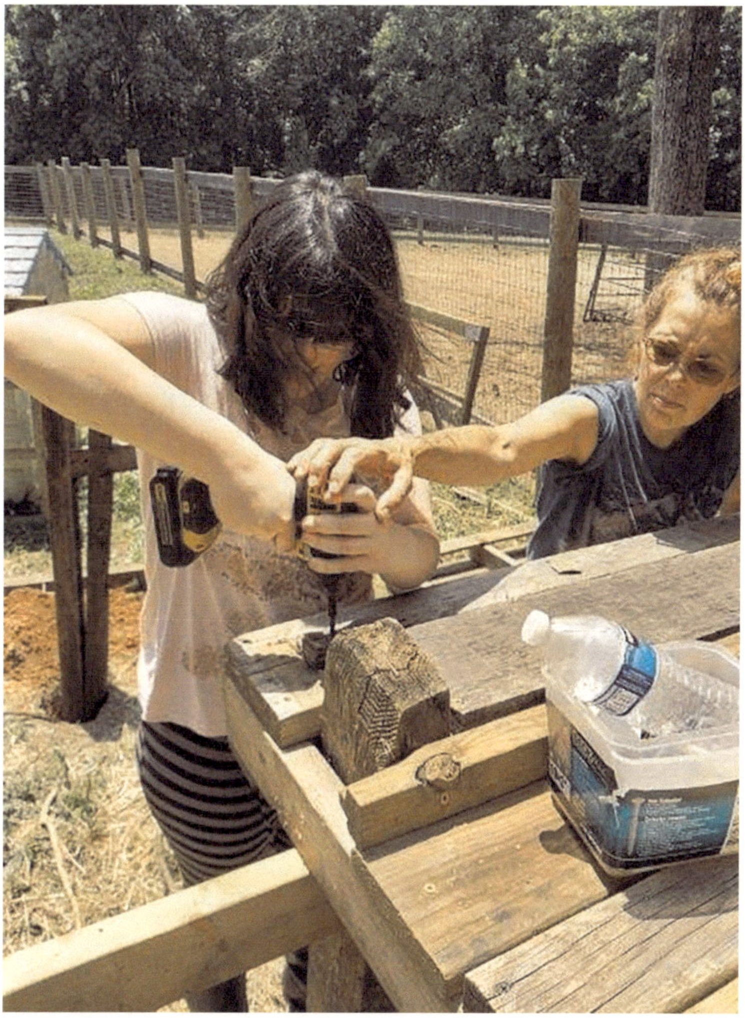

Figure 17.
Vocational skills development.

stores to reuse for the goat paddock. These lower cost or no cost options increase our ability to provide a healthier environment for the animals while improving our infrastructure more affordably. We have had recycled asphalt donated by a local road paving company, extending the driveway to the barn and registration booth. A local nonprofit food redistributor delivers excess and unusable produce, bread, and grain from their warehouse to the farm for our pig, chickens, horses and goats.
[Farm operations must include regular veterinary care of the animals, including recommended vaccinations and deworming of goats, horses and other livestock; hoof care; upkeep of the sheds, stalls, and coops; and maintenance of fencing and enclosures to ensure safety and hygiene of the animals and people.]

Environmental sustainability is enhanced through biodynamic approaches at the farm. We collect sustainable wood (fallen tree branches, limbs, and logs) for use in the wood stove, landscaping projects, and outdoor fireplace. Mowed grass can be used to supplement feed in the chicken coop, pulled weeds and vines are forage for the goats,

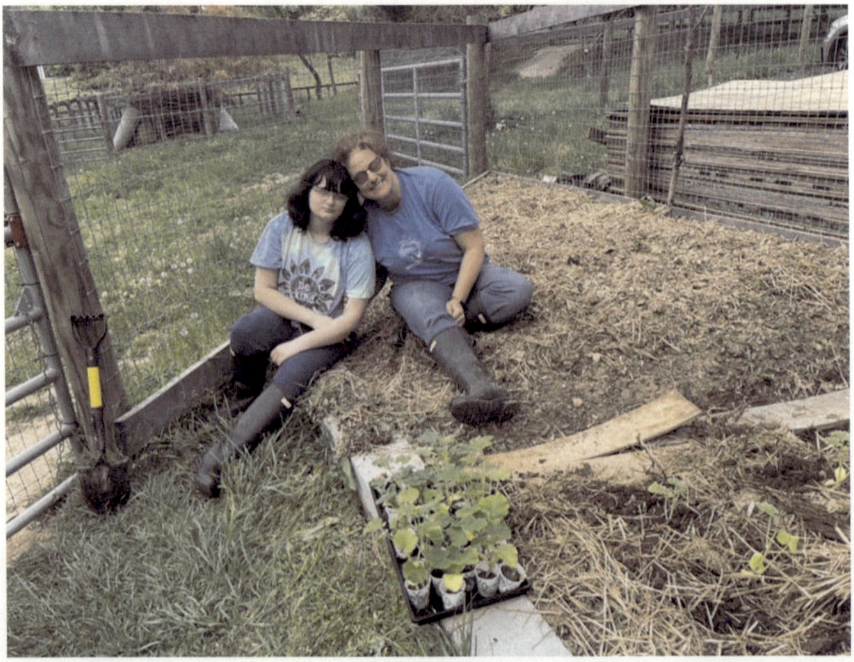

Figure 18.
Weekend volunteers.

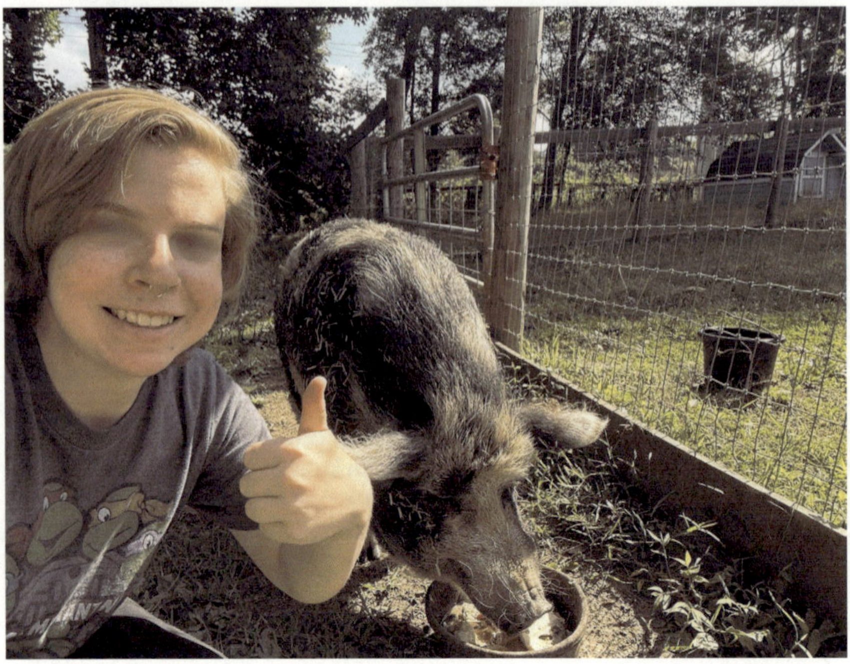

Figure 19.
One of our coauthors, EKK, feeding our rescued pig, Noah.

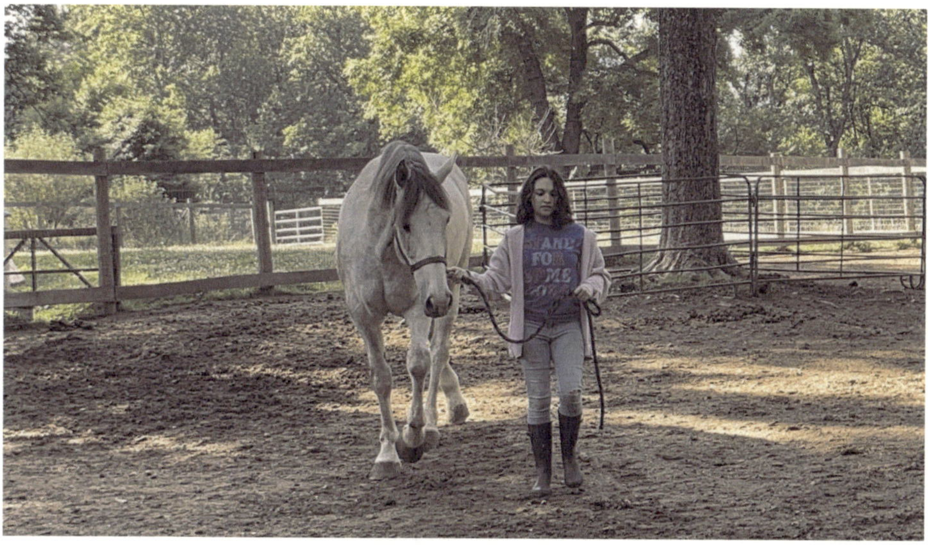

Figure 20.
One of our coauthors, BRH, ground training our horse, Kingston.

and donated produce can provide much needed nutrients to all the animals. Rotting produce in the compost will repopulate pumpkin plants, gourds, tomatoes, and other hearty species to prevent replanting year after year. Native species of bees are encouraged through building pollinator hotels rather than the more invasive species of honeybees, which were brought to North America by the European colonists. By carefully mowing out invasive (nonnative) species, transplanting baby volunteer native perennials, and allowing native species of grasses, trees and bushes to repopulate the open lawn, we ensure that the more hearty species more successfully return year after year. Biodynamic methods of waste redistribution include "fertilizing" the plants with goat pellets, enriching the soil around plants and bushes with horse manure (**Figure 21**), lasagna gardening techniques when building new flower beds, and in-ground composting of kitchen debris (coffee grounds, tea bags, egg shells, paper towels, paper plates, napkins, Kleenexes). (**Figure 22**) [Our practice of "in ground composting" produces a very rich, nearly black soil that we eventually hope to sell for financial sustainability of farm operations.] Sales of our goat manure, eggs, and produce helped secure the county's agricultural designation for purposes of taxation – another step toward financial sustainability.

By connecting with existing community organizations who provide volunteer opportunities for neurodiverse and neurotypical youth and young adults, operating costs (e.g., human resources, administrative costs) are minimized in order to maximize our reach in the community. We have had three Eagle Scouts complete projects for the farm, including building a bee hive, two mobile chicken coops, and a pollinator hotel with flower gardens. One Boy Scout is currently designing wooden benches for our barnyard area. We host agriculture education field trips and volunteer experiences in coordination with other local nonprofits serving neurotypical and neurodiverse young adults in day programs. We have hotsted both typical and special education schools and partial hospital programs for environmental/agricultural recreational and educational outings. We provide student service learning opportunities through our local school systems for middle and high school students to learn about sustainability

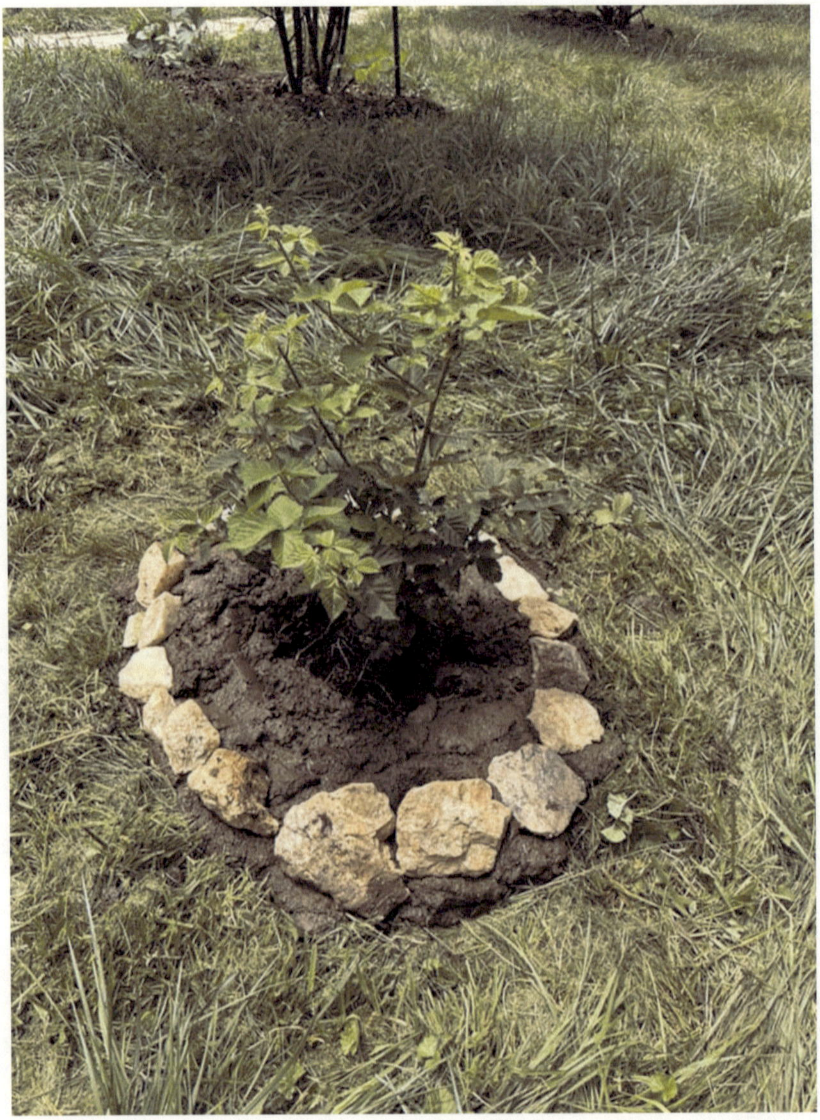

Figure 21.
Horse manure around bush.

and restorative agriculture while participating in projects on the farm. [Adult volunteers are background checked for the safety of younger children who may be participating in a group].

5.1 Green care farming: agricultural education groups offer social and recreational engagement

Green care farms create a community-based space for Maslow's elements of belonging and purpose through socialization and recreational activities that incorporate education about biodynamic agriculture. These activities are distinct from

DOI: http://dx.doi.org/10.5772/intechopen.1002513

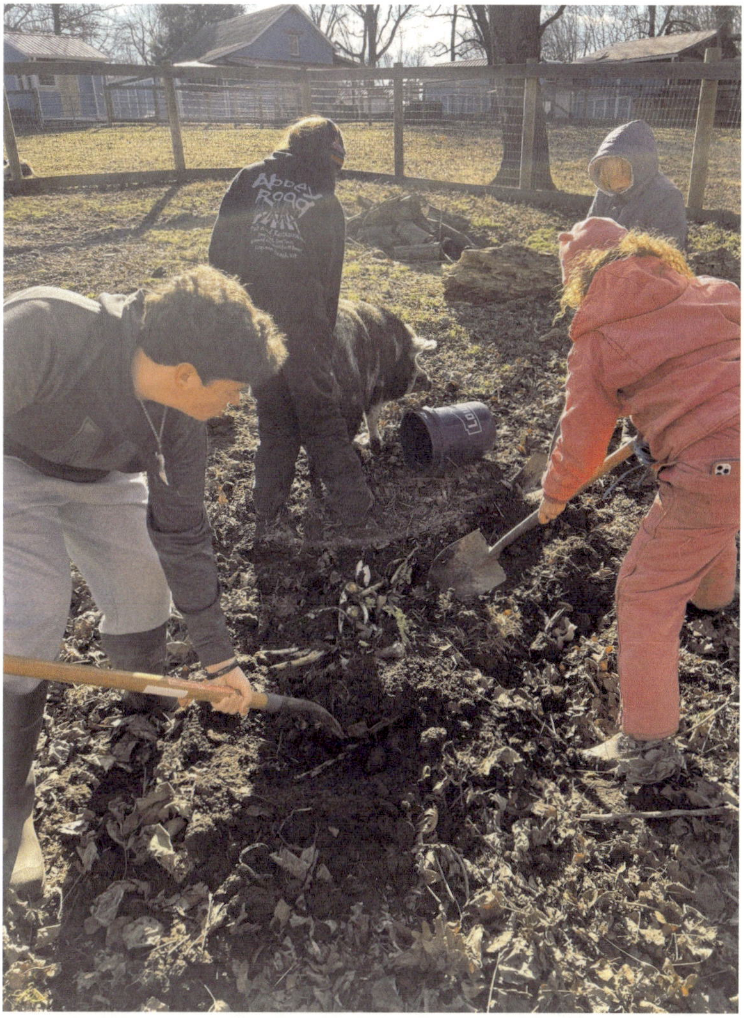

Figure 22.
Compost soil.

"therapy" and do not require a licensed mental health provider. Agricultural education and agricultural tourism have long been allowed on farms, with school children participating to learn about animals, the environment, and where their food comes from. Farm experiences facilitate a sense of community with meaning and purpose, particularly when a purposeful group project is introduced (e.g., building a lean-to structure for the animals, germinating and planting flowers for pollinators or pumpkins for animal feed, or burying compost). The children and teens enjoy walking through the pasture and forest with the goats and horses, practicing mindfulness while hand feeding the chickens, watching the antics of the orphaned pig, and helping socialize the baby emu brothers (our newest edition at Dream Catcher Meadows).

Inclusive group experiences on a green care farm provides a nature-immersive milieu for atypical and neurotypical peers to learn about environmental sustainability and restorative agriculture while caring for farm animals, engaging in recreational activities, and practicing healthy social skills. Our "In Real Life #IRL Friends on the Farm" program during the summer and fall of 2020 offered adopted 14 to17 year-olds

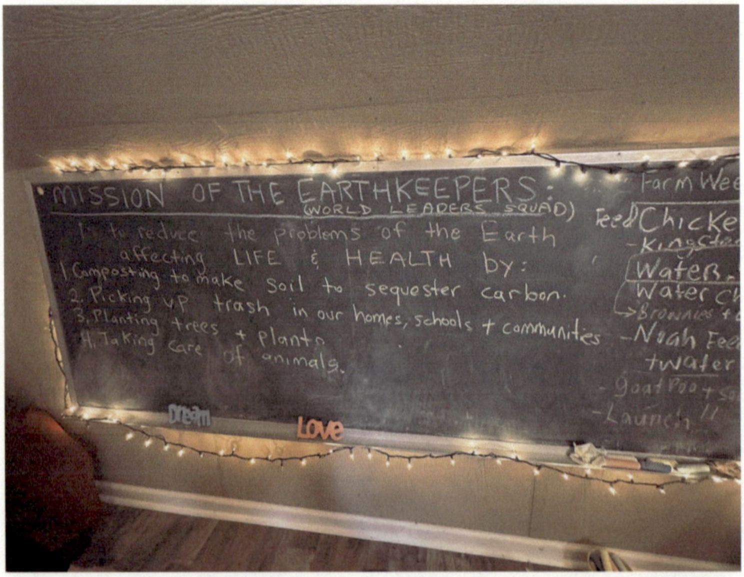
MISSION OF THE EARTHKEEPERS:
(WORLD LEADERS SQUAD)
to reduce the problems of the Earth
affecting LIFE & HEALTH by:
1. Composting to make soil to sequester carbon.
2. Picking up trash in our homes, schools + communities
3. Planting trees + plants
4. Taking care of animals.
Dream
Love

Figure 23.
Earthkeepers pledge.

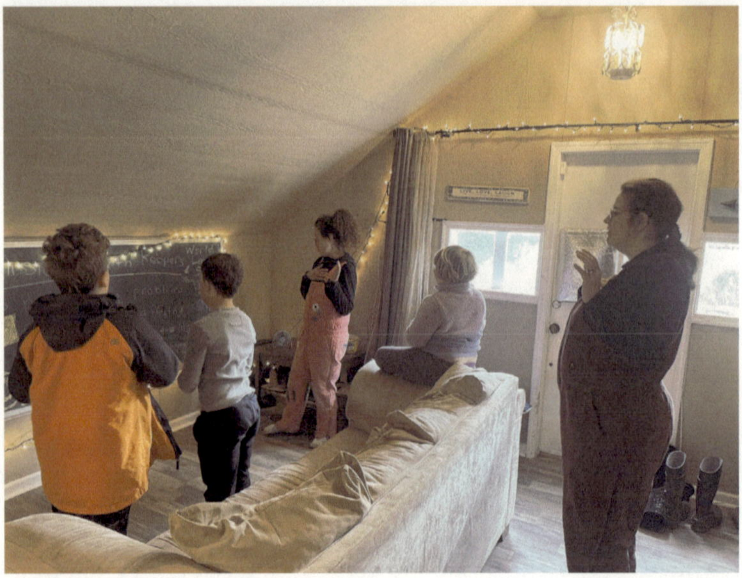

Figure 24.
Morning meeting and pledge.

with an outdoor social opportunity during the pandemic so that they could engage with peers, explore nature, and find meaningful (nonvirtual) experiences. During the summer of 2021, teens came for one-on-one experiences with a young engineer for the day to assist with building projects (i.e., an enclosed mini-barn for our pig made with reclaimed building supplies and 2 feet walls packed with straw stuffed inside feed bags, repairing goat structures and fencing, etc.). These experiences provided a sense

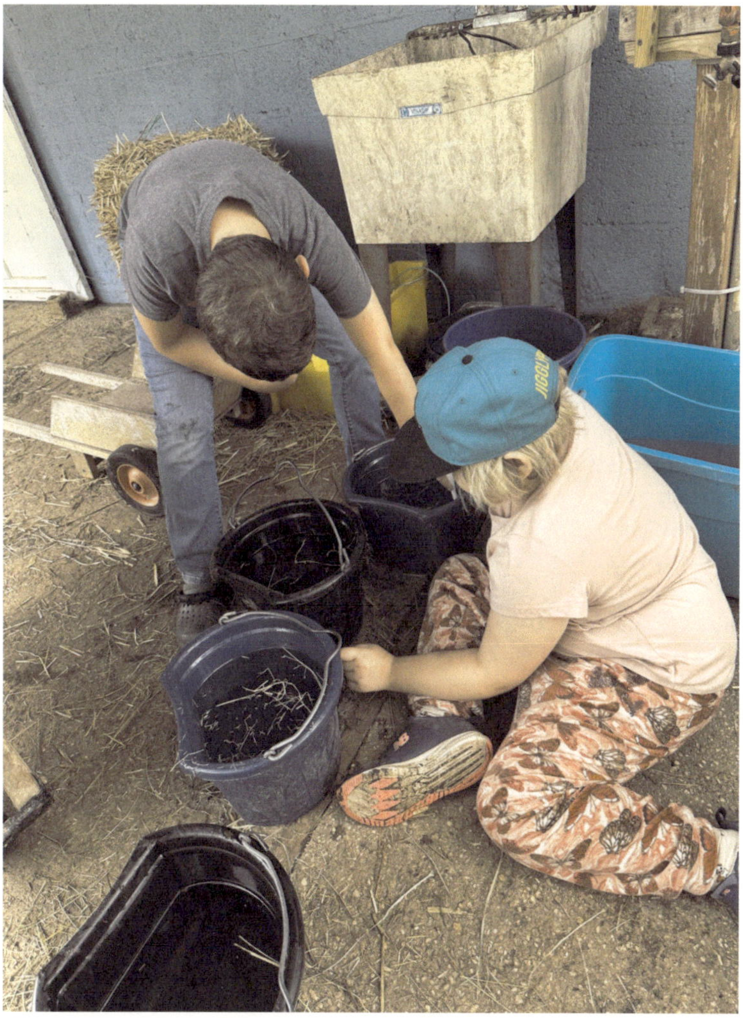

Figure 25.
Changing water buckets.

of community for overcoming isolation and boredom during the pandemic and offered a purposeful project-based activity.

More recently, our "Earthkeepers Kinder Farming" program for both neurotypical and neurodiverse 8 to 12-year-olds and their parents, provides a sense of meaning and purpose outside of the academic environment through farm experiences with peers. The two-hour weekend social group provides education about restorative agriculture, composting to sequester carbon, the concept of One Health (environmental health being inextricably linked to human health), the connection between the soil and the human gut microbiome, growing vegetables and other produce, and animal care. The aim is to provide the children with a sense of safety, belonging/community, and meaning and purpose. Parents likewise enjoy sharing responsibilities like feeding the horses their grain, sitting in mindfulness sessions with the baby emus and chickens, grooming the pig, and forest bathing. Sessions are typically co-facilitated with a college student and/or school teacher along with the green care farmer.

During the first session in March 2022, the children identified the most common worrisome problems of the earth from their school lectures and news reports (e.g., climate change/global warming, water pollution, landfills, decreasing biodiversity) to develop a consensus strategic plan, including a mission statement and realistic goals. They called out their concerns as the facilitator scribed on the chalkboard. The children then translated their problem statement into a mission statement to help solve some of the Earth's problems, including poor soil quality, trash in the oceans, global warming, and mistreatment of animals. Their pledge (recited at the beginning of each session) is: *"The mission of the Earthkeepers (The World Leaders Squad) is to reduce the problems of the Earth affecting life and health by: 1. Composting to make soil to sequester carbon; 2. Picking up trash in our homes, schools and communities; 3. Planting trees and plants; and 4. Taking care of animals."* (**Figure 23**).

A typical Saturday morning Earthkeepers social group would begin with a morning meeting in the clubhouse reciting the pledge (**Figure 24**) before enjoying a cup of hot chocolate and brownies or pancakes. During weekly or bi-weekly morning meetings, we discuss the strategies we are going to use to meet our eco-goals after feeding the chickens and pig, changing water buckets (**Figure 25**), taking the goats for a walk in the pasture and forest (**Figure 26**), letting the horses out to graze or grooming them. Some of the children will bring leftover food or slightly expired produce to feed the animals and/or waste from the kitchen to compost. Group participants decide what activities they would like to do and guide the group leader in the sequence of the 2-hour session. When we are developing our to do list for the day, one might call out: "I want to feed the chickens!" or "Please can I change the water buckets?" or "Can I feed Kingston [the horse] with my mom?" and the facilitator writes down their name next to the activity, with the adult or teen volunteer in charge of the activity.

After completing the morning animal care, the children will suggest the next activity: "Can we go to the mindfulness log now?" The mindfulness log is a very large fallen tree in the forest, adjacent to a neighbor's property with a large pond with fountains (**Figure 27**). We sit on the log quietly listening to the sounds of nature,

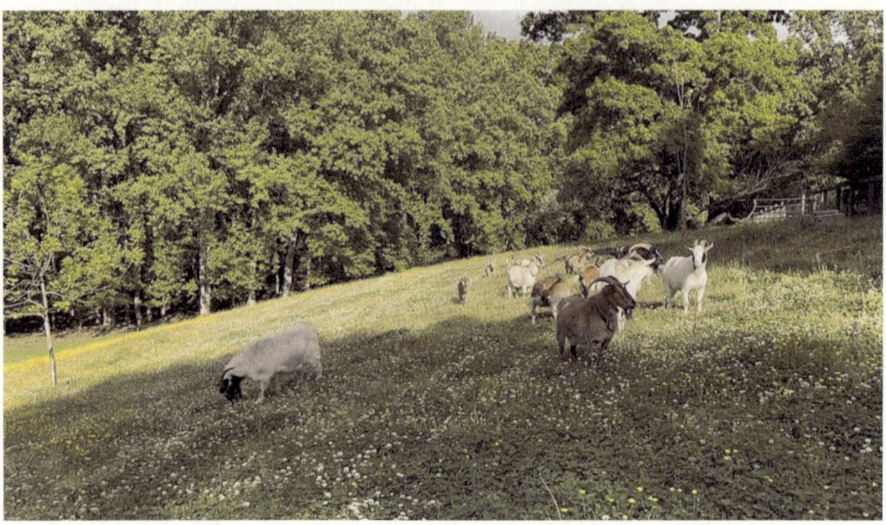

Figure 26.
Goats for walk in pasture.

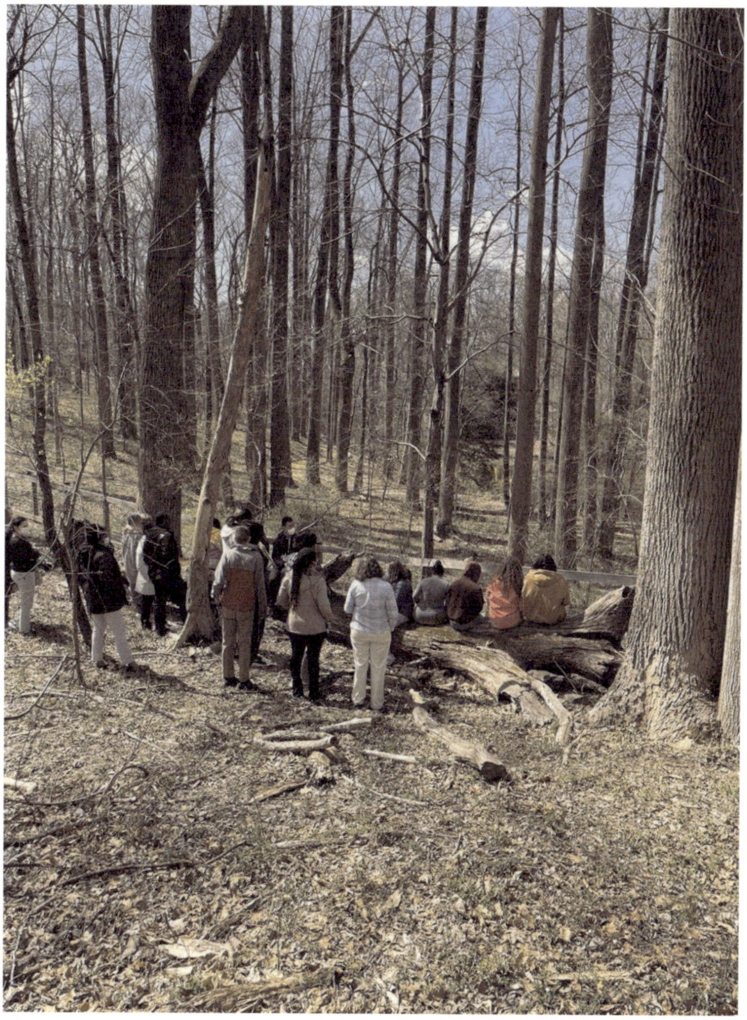

Figure 27.
Community civic group visits the mindfulness log.

smelling the decaying leaves, feeling the gentle breeze and hardness of the log beneath, and watching the green leaves contrasted against the blue sky. Another child might say, "Then can we roll down the hill?" The children attend seasonal sessions (spring, summer, fall, and winter), watching the birth and hibernation of life with the fluctuation of weather patterns. During the summer and fall, we pick wild wine berries, wild grapes, ground cherries, flowers, pumpkins, and decorative gourds. We also collect the freshly laid multi-colored chicken eggs (**Figure 28**), sending cartons home with the kids to compare to the store-bought variety. These multisensory experiences (sights, sounds, smells, textures, and flavors) provide sensory desensitization to help the children become more confident and regulated under a variety of environmental stimulating conditions.

Depending on the season, we plant and weed flower beds, transplant small seedlings and saplings, water plants, and prepare beds for the next growing season.

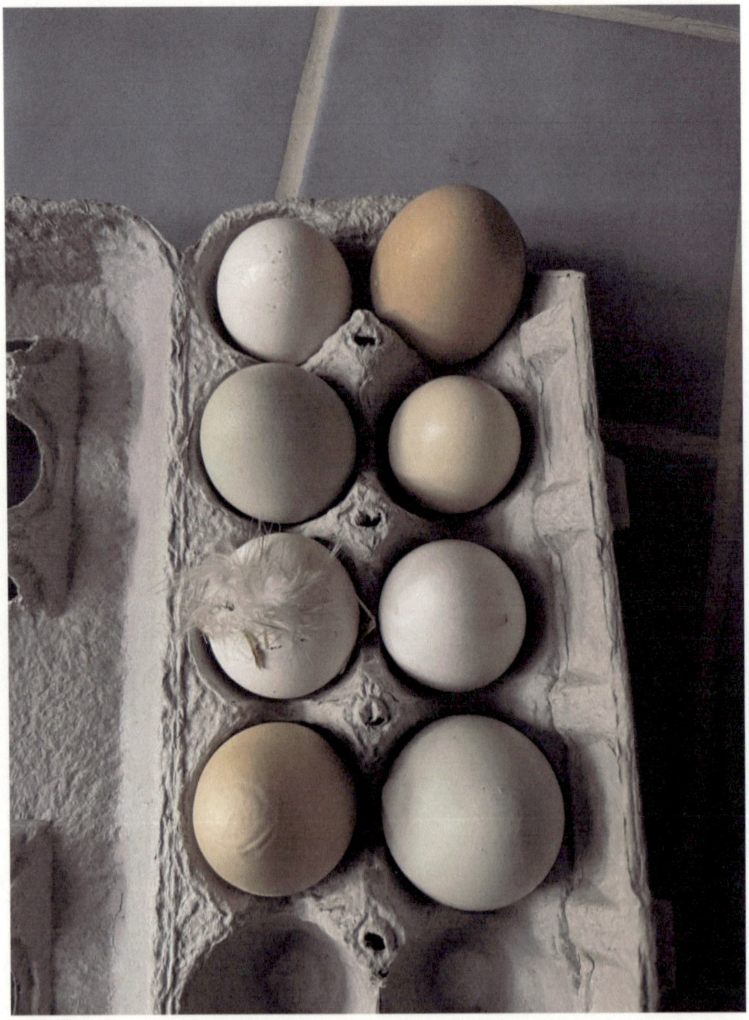

Figure 28.
Multicolored eggs.

Last fall, we harvested seeds from donated pumpkins that we fed to the chickens and pig, germinated and transplanted them to beds we made from the manure and muck collected from the horse paddock (**Figures 29** and **30**). An annual "Farm Week" includes making name plate door signs out of reclaimed lumber (**Figure 31**), participating in animal care, forest bathing with the goats (**Figure 32**), interacting with the horses (**Figure 33**), making and shooting off biodegradable rockets to reseed the pasture with seeds and goat poo (**Figures 34** and **35**), swimming in the pool (**Figure 36**), and learning about the medicine wheel approach to a holistic healthy lifestyle (**Figure 37**).

Three youngsters who had been coming to the farm for Earthkeepers social group activities and two of them for Farm Week were interviewed with their parents. Children commented that their favorite part about the experience was meeting new friends, belonging to a group, interacting with the animals, learning about nature, and feeling included. Here are some of their comments:

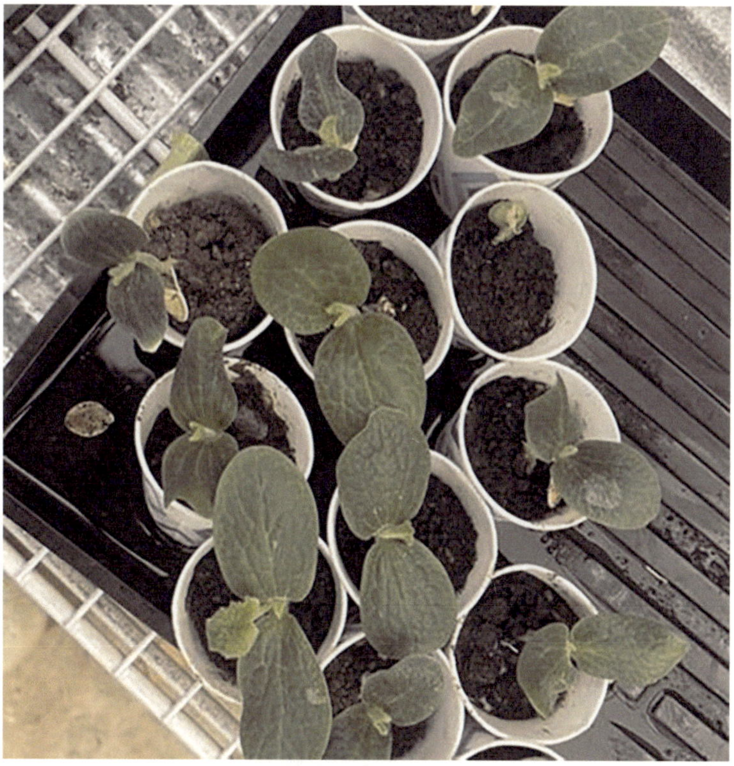

Figure 29.
Germinated pumpkin seeds.

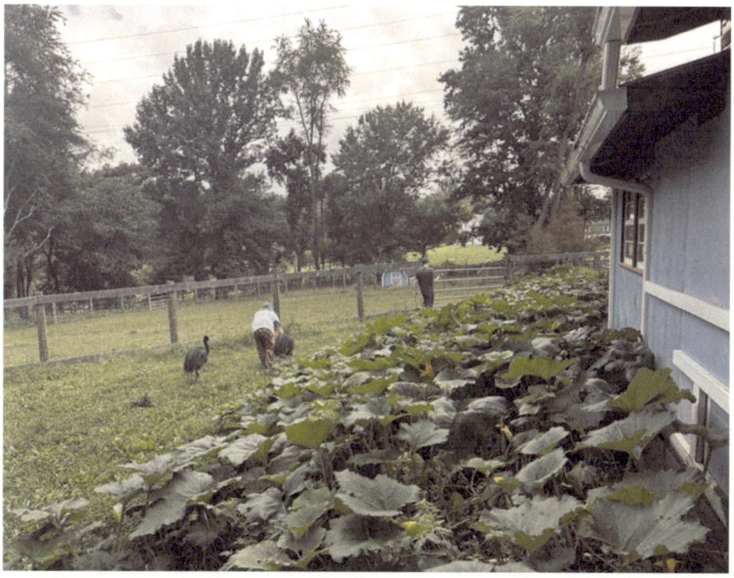

Figure 30.
Pumkin plants.

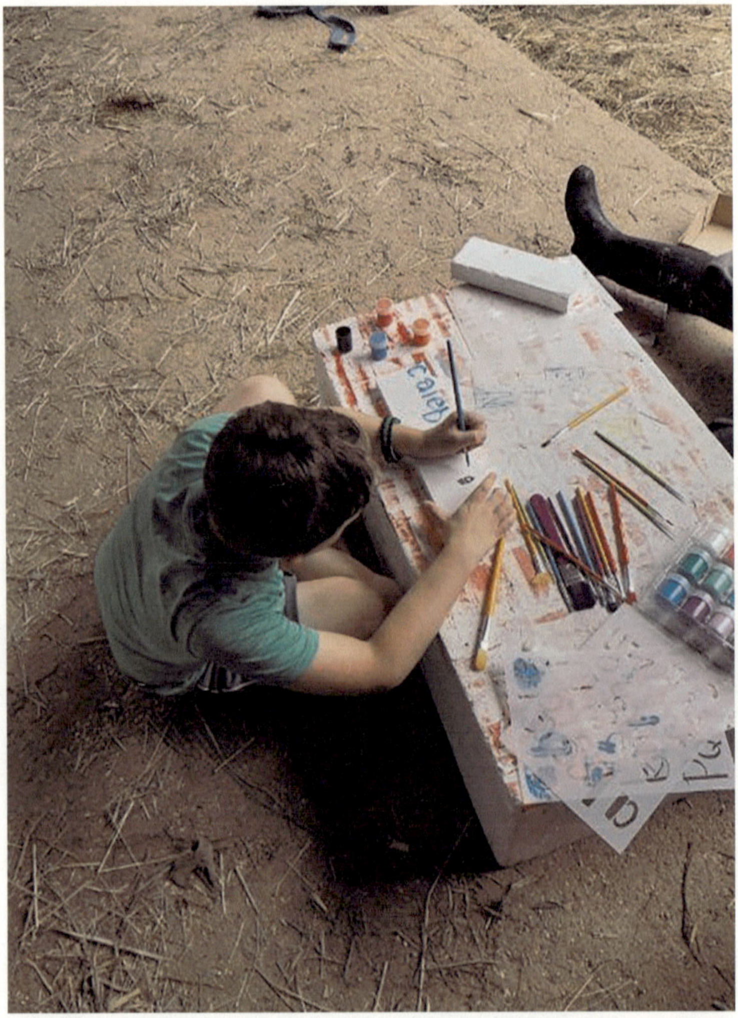

Figure 31.
Making name plate.

- "The farm is very nice. It really brings out the idea that anything we do can make a difference. When I first met my friends here, I said 'I'm pretty much set … anybody can be themselves and there's no criticism about what you do.'" Their parent added: "It's kind of like a magical oasis in the midst of a dry and barren land. It's a physically beautiful place stewarded by a kind, loving, patient person and her family and friends where children and adults can learn something about reality."

- "I like this farm because I get to see animals and I get to learn to be calm with animals and not to be afraid of my fears and other emotions and how to interact with other people." Their parent expressed: "… deep love of the animals, calming atmosphere, nature and pure relaxation you feel at the farm."

DOI: http://dx.doi.org/10.5772/intechopen.1002513

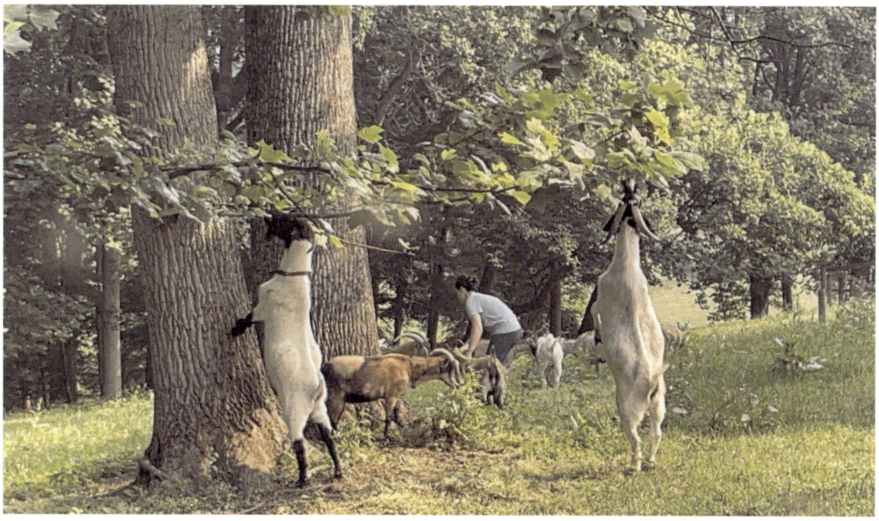

Figure 32.
Forest bathing with goats.

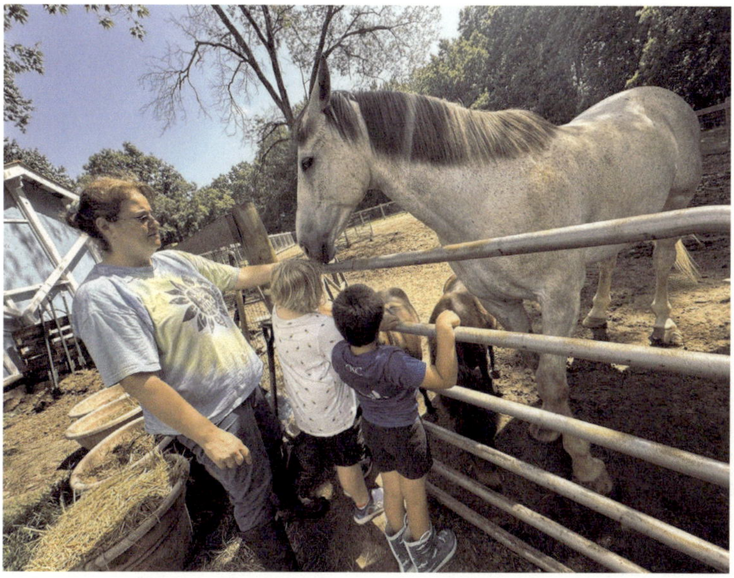

Figure 33.
Interacting with the horses.

- "I love how I can be with the animals and all my friends and have fun at the same time." Their parent added: "Coming to the farm is her happy place. Taking care of the animals has taught her how to understand responsibility at home."

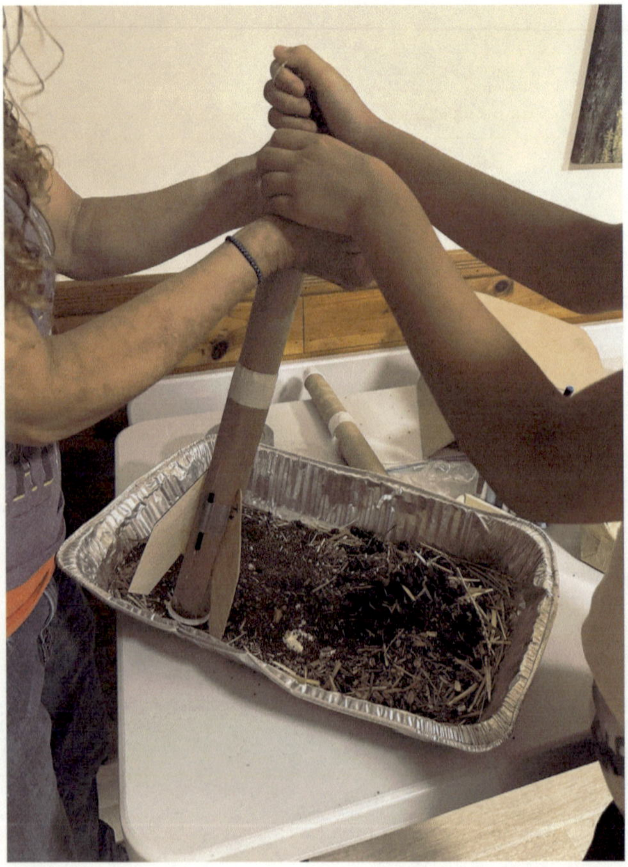

Figure 34.
Filling rocket with goat poo and seeds.

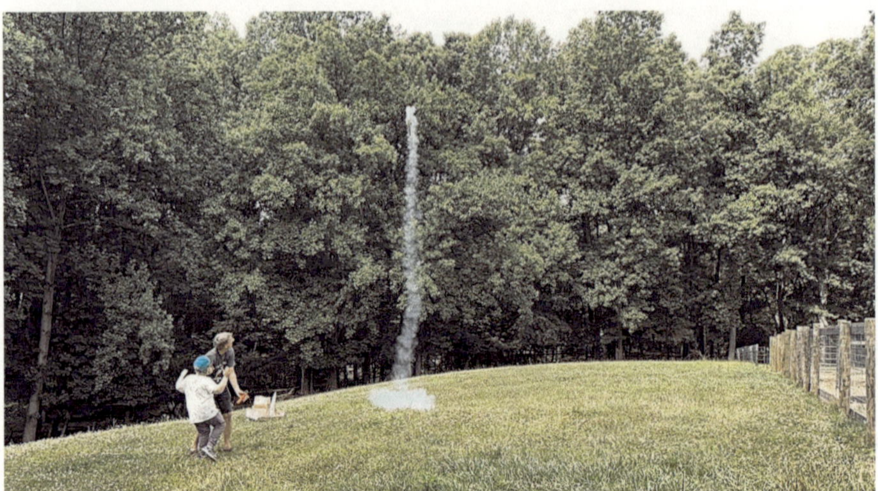

Figure 35.
Shooting a homemade rocket.

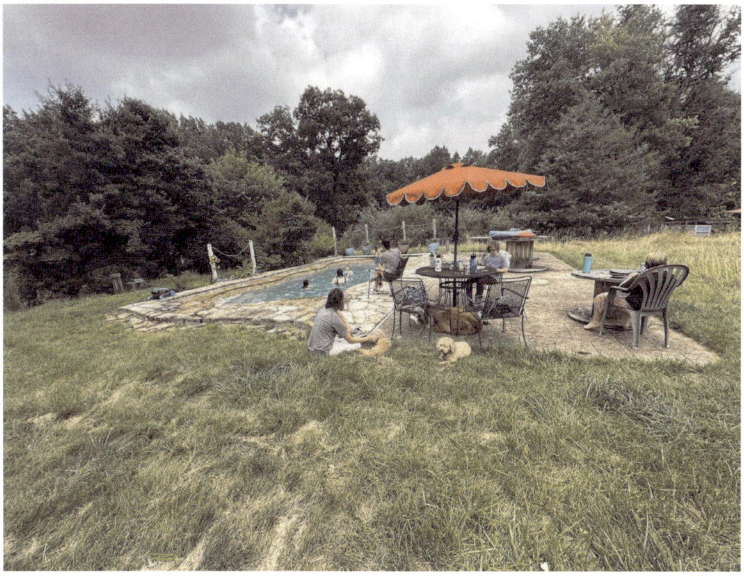

Figure 36.
Pool time.

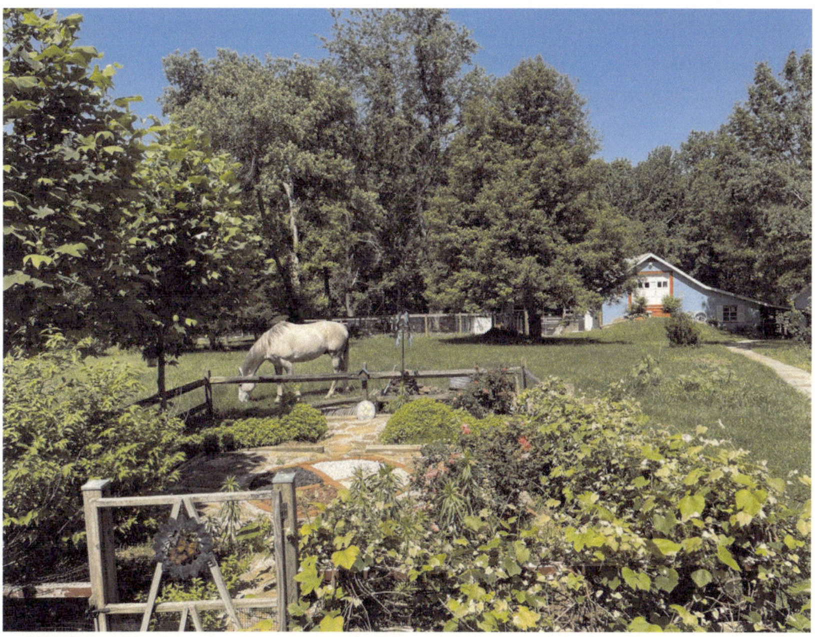

Figure 37.
Medicine wheel garden.

6. Conclusions

Children and adolescents with neurodiverse conditions and trauma histories can benefit from neurotherapy licensed mental health professional interacting with gently raised farm animals. The green care farm at Dream Catcher Meadows combines a sanctuary for rescued, injured, orphaned, unwanted, and birth defected farm animals with social, recreational and agriculture educational opportunities for both atypical and neurotypical youth. The nonprofit green care farm is a mileu for group activities, like Earthkeepers, to provide a third place to find a sense of belonging and purpose. The farm is also an adjunct individual therapy site for experiential therapy with a licensed, board-certified child/adolescent psychiatrist. By linking with local farmers, 4-H programs, farm animal veterinary centers, and/or leasing space on a smaller hobby farm, psychiatrists and mental health professionals can improve their ability to connect with and treat a wider variety of patients who may not respond as well to typical mental health treatment. Community-based farm animal assisted therapy and green care farms may ultimately reduce the economic cost of residential care and/or mental illness for complex patients with neurodevelopmental histories and adverse childhood experiences. Future funding opportunities to research and collaborate with other mental health networks and public sector agencies may help extend the practice of farm animal-assisted neurotherapy into other communities and global regions.

Acknowledgements

The authors would like to acknowledge Katie Thompson and Alicia Rose for sharing their photos, listening to the ideas and the initial conceptualization of the chapter, providing a reference for "entrainment," and including their perspectives about the history of psychiatric institutional farms.

Conflict of interest

The authors declare no conflict of interest.

Notes/thanks/other declarations

Special thank you to our Earthkeepers and their parents for contributing your perspectives about the farm and allowing some of your photos to be used in the article; to my 2-legged teens for putting up with my journal writing, farming, and neurodiverse perspective; to our small dedicated army of Earthkeeper ambassadors for helping with farm operations and groups, and to our furry and feathered friends who make the farm such a special "third place" for kids, teens and volunteers in our community. We would also like to thank all the Boy Scouts of America who have completed their Eagle Scout projects for the betterment of the farm and Dr. Rocket for envisioning, creating and facilitating our successful rocket launches of soil conditioner into the pastures. We are also grateful for Jeremy Fedors, MS and Eliane Ferreria, MSPH for giving of their time, energy, love and generosity to build, improve, care for, and ensure the sustainability of Dream Catcher Meadows and 7th Generation Foundation, Inc. We also would like to acknowledge the State of Maryland for a very generous $50,000 bond bill in 2018 for capital improvements toward our 5.63 acre pasture and paddock fencing and 2018 and 2019 community grants in matching funds of $50,000 from Montgomery County, MD for new roofs, gutters, painting and repairs to our barn and outbuildings.

Author details

Susan D. Rich[1*], Briana R. Hickey[2] and Elizabeth K. Kaprielian[3]

1 Therapeutic and Learning Centers, P-LLC.; Potomac, USA

2 7th Generation Foundation, Inc.; Potomac, USA

3 Goucher College; Towson, USA

*Address all correspondence to: dr.sdrich@gmail.com

References

[1] American Psychiatric Association. Diagnostic and Statistical Manual. 5th ed. The American Psychiatric Association; 2013. pp. 86 and 798

[2] Weir K. A hidden epidemic of fetal alcohol syndrome: New legislation could help bring awareness and resources to prevention, diagnosis, and treatment of fetal alcohol spectrum disorders. Monitor on Psychology. 2022; **53**(5):24

[3] Frye RE. A personalized multidisciplinary approach to evaluating and treating autism spectrum disorder. Journal of Personalized Medicine. 2022;**12**(3):464. DOI: 10.3390/jpm12030464

[4] Available from: https://www.niaaa.nih.gov/international-fetal-alcohol-spectrum-disorders-awareness-day-september-9

[5] Rich SD. Perspective chapter: Autism spectrum disorder neurophenotype with preconceptional and prenatal alcohol exposure – A call for industry responsibility in prevention. In: Autism Spectrum Disorders - Recent Advances and New Perspectives. December 2nd, 2022. London: IntechOpen; 2023. DOI: 10.5772/intechopen.108820

[6] Flannigan K, Pei J, McLachlan K, Harding K, Mela M, Cook J, et al. Responding to the unique complexities of fetal alcohol spectrum disorder. Frontiers in Psychology, 25 January 2022. Sec. Psychology for Clinical Settings. 2021;**12**:1-8. DOI: 10.3389/fpsyg.2021.778471

[7] Rosen TE, Mazefsky CA, Vasa RA, Lerner MD. Co-occurring psychiatric conditions in autism spectrum disorder. International Review of Psychiatry. 2018;**30**(1):40-61. DOI: 10.1080/09540261.2018.1450229

[8] DiLalla LF, McCrary M, Diaz E. A review of endophenotypes in schizophrenia and autism: The next phase for understanding genetic etiologies. American Journal of Medical Genetics. Part C, Seminars in Medical Genetics. 2017;**175**(3):354-361. DOI: 10.1002/ajmg.c.31566 Epub 2017 Jun 29

[9] Gillett G, Leeves L, Patel A, Prisecaru A, Spain D, Happé F. The prevalence of autism spectrum disorder traits and diagnosis in adults and young people with personality disorders: A systematic review. The Australian and New Zealand Journal of Psychiatry. 2023;**57**(2):181-196. DOI: 10.1177/00048674221114603 Epub 2022 Aug 19

[10] Pillay J, Boylan K, Newton A, Hartling L, Vandermeer B, Nuspl M, et al. Harms of antipsychotics in children and young adults: A systematic review update. Canadian Journal of Psychiatry. 2018;**63**(10):661-678. DOI: 10.1177/0706743718779950 Epub 2018 Jun 4

[11] Fattorusso A, Di Genova L, Dell'Isola GB, Mencaroni E, Esposito S. Autism spectrum disorders and the gut microbiota. Nutrients. 2019;**11**(3):521. DOI: 10.3390/nu11030521

[12] Lord C, Brugha TS, Charman T, Cusack J, Dumas G, Frazier T, et al. Autism spectrum disorder. Nature Reviews. Disease Primers. 2020;**6**(1):5. DOI: 10.1038/s41572-019-0138-4

[13] Lipinski S, Boegl K, Blanke ES, Suenkel U, Dziobek I. A blind spot in mental healthcare? Psychotherapists lack education and expertise for the support

of adults on the autism spectrum. Autism. 2022;**26**(6):1509-1521. DOI: 10.1177/13623613211057973 Epub 2021 Nov 26

[14] Charlson F, Ali S, Benmarhnia T, Pearl M, Massazza A, Augustinavicius J, et al. Climate change and mental health: A scoping review. International Journal of Environmental Research and Public Health. 2021;**18**(9):4486. DOI: 10.3390/ijerph18094486

[15] Hassink J, van Dijk M. Farming for health: Green-care farming across Europe and the United States of America. In: The First Product of the European Community of Practice. Part of the Book Series: Wageningen UR Frontis Series (WURF, Vol. 13). Springer. 2006

[16] Available from: https://health.maryland.gov/springgrove/phototours/Pages/history.aspx

[17] Boo K. Forest Haven Is Gone, but the Agony Remains. The Washington Post: Nash Holdings; March 14, 1999. Available from: https://www.washingtonpost.com/archive/politics/1999/03/14/forest-haven-is-gone-but-the-agony-remains/c2e3340a-08c6-4745-abdb-badb334648eb/

[18] Maurer P. Abandoned D.C.: Inside the ruins of the forest Haven Asylum. DCist. November 18, 2013. Archived from the original on October 7, 2015.

[19] Available from: https://www.historicwarfield.com/history/

[20] McMillen FM, Kane JS. Institutional memory: The Records of St. Elizabeths Hospital at the National Archives. Prologue Magazine. 2010;**42**(2). Available from: https://www.archives.gov/publications/prologue/2010/summer/institutional.html

[21] Dalzell-Ward AJ. Community as doctor: New perspectives on a therapeutic community, by Robert N. Rapoport. (Tavistock publications. 1960. Pp. 325. Price 42s.). Health Education Journal. 1961;**19**(2):113-114. DOI: 10.1177/001789696101900213

[22] Rapoport RN. What is a Therapeutic Milieu?. In: Greenblatt M, Levinson DJ and Willis RH, editors. The Patient and the Mental Hospital. 1st ed. Arno Press; 1980. p. 20. The Free Press; January 1, 1957. Available from: https://www.google.com/books/edition/Community_as_Doctor/IXRHAQAAQBAJ?hl=en&gbpv=1&dq=Schwartz,+Morris:+What+is+a+Therapeutic+Milieu%3F+In+Greenblatt,+Milton,+et+al.:+The+Patient+and+the+Mental+Hospital,&pg=PA33&printsec=frontcover

[23] Maslow AH. Hierarchy of Needs: A Theory of Human Motivation. CreateSpace Independent Publishing Platform. 2023. Republished by David Webb on Kindle Books at Available from: http://www.all-about-psychology.com/

[24] Bazis L. The Frightful Forest Haven Asylum. Mainstream: The Student Newspaper for Paint Branch High School. Paint Branch High School, Montgomery County Public Schools. Available from: https://pbmainstream.com/3473/features/the-frightful-forest-haven-asylum/; [Retrieved 07/25/2023]

[25] Forest Haven Asylum: Abandoned Home for the Abandoned. Sometimes Interesting. 04/12/2014. Available from: https://sometimes-interesting.com/forest-haven-asylum/ [Retrieved 07/25/2023]

[26] Peele R. A personal conversation over lunch with Rich S. October 2019

[27] Koyanagi C, Bazelon DL. Learning from History: Deinstitutionalization of

People with Mental Illness As Precursor to Long Term Care Reform. Henry J. Kaiser Family Foundation Commission on Medicaid and the Uninsured, Center for Mental Health Law; August 2007

[28] Torrey EF. The Insanity Offense: How America's Failure to Treat the Seriously Mentally Ill Endangers its Citizens. Reprint ed. WW Norton and Company; January 2, 2012

[29] Clay RA. A renaissance for humanistic psychology: The field explores new niches while building on its past. Monitor on Psychology. 2002;**33**(8) Available from: https://www.apa.org/monitor/sep02/renaissance

[30] Hassnik J, Van Dijk M. Farming for Health, Green-Care Farming across Europe and the United States of America. Oct 2006

[31] Elsey H, Murray J, Bragg R. Green fingers and clear minds: Prescribing 'care farming' for mental illness. The British Journal of General Practice. 2016; **66**(643):99-100. DOI: 10.3399/bjgp16X683749 [Erratum in: Br J Gen Pract. 2016 Jul;66(648):352]

[32] de Bruin S, de Boer B, Beerens H, Buist Y, Verbeek H. Rethinking dementia care: The value of green care farming. Journal of the American Medical Directors Association. 2017;**18**(3):200-203. DOI: 10.1016/j.jamda.2016.11.018 Epub 2017 Jan 31

[33] Ura C, Okamura T, Yamazaki S, Shimmei M, Torishima K, Eboshida A, et al. Rice farming care as a novel method of green care farm in east Asian context: An implementation research. BMC Geriatrics. 2021;**21**(1):237. DOI: 10.1186/s12877-021-02181-2

[34] Cacciatore J, Gorman R, Thieleman K. Evaluating care farming as a means to care for those in trauma and grief. Health & Place. 2020;**62**:102281. DOI: 10.1016/j.healthplace.2019.102281 Epub 2020 Feb 13

[35] Lee AY, Kim SO, Gim GM, Kim DS, Park SA. Care farming program for family health: A pilot study with mothers and children. International Journal of Environmental Research and Public Health. 2019;**17**(1):27. DOI: 10.3390/ijerph17010027

[36] Kay BR. Bittersweet farms. Journal of Autism and Developmental Disorders. 1990;**20**(3):309-321. DOI: 10.1007/BF02206544

[37] Anderson KA, Chapin KP, Reimer Z, Siffri G. On fertile ground: An initial evaluation of green care farms in the United States. Home Health Care Services Quarterly. 2017;**36**(1):1-15. DOI: 10.1080/01621424.2017.1291390 Epub 2017 Feb 7

[38] Artz B, Bitler DD. Green care: A review of the benefits and potential of animal-assisted care farming globally and in rural America. Animals (Basel). 2017;7(4):31. DOI: 10.3390/ani7040031

[39] Mandrell P. Introduction to Equine-Assisted Psychotherapy: A Comprehensive Overview. 2nd ed. Self-published; 2014

[40] Siu AMH, Kam M, Mok I. Horticultural therapy program for people with mental illness: A mixed-method evaluation. International Journal of Environmental Research and Public Health. 2020;**17**(3):711. DOI: 10.3390/ijerph17030711

[41] Lampert T, Costa J, Santos O, Sousa J, Ribeiro T, Freire E. Evidence on the contribution of community gardens to promote physical and mental health and well-being of non-institutionalized

individuals: A systematic review. PLoS One. 2021;**16**(8):e0255621. DOI: 10.1371/journal.pone.0255621

[42] Jared S. Hope Grows Here. University Gazette; July 12th 2019

[43] Available from: https://www.nourishinghearts.ca/

[44] Available from: https://www.med.unc.edu/psych/cecmh/services/recovery-services/farm-at-penny-lane/

[45] London MD, Mackenzie L, Lovarini M, Dickson C, Alvarez-Campos A. Animal assisted therapy for children and adolescents with autism Spectrum disorder: Parent perspectives. Journal of Autism and Developmental Disorders. 2020;**50**(12):4492-4503. DOI: 10.1007/s10803-020-04512-5

[46] Fine AH, Mackintosh TH. Animal-assisted interventions: Entering a crossroads of explaining an instinctive bond under the scrutiny of scientific inquiry. In: Encyclopedia of Mental Health. Friedman HS, editor. Second ed. 2016. Academic Press. pp. 68-73. DOI: 10.1016/B978-0-12-397045-9.00120-8. ISBN 9780123977533

[47] O'Malley K, Rich SD. Clinical implications of a link between fetal alcohol spectrum disorders (FASD) and autism or asperger's disorder – A neurodevelopmental frame for helping understanding and management. In: Fitzgerald M, editor. Recent Advances in Autism Spectrum Disorders. Vol. I. March 6, 2013 Chapter 20

[48] Ancona D and Leong Chong C. Entrainment; cycles and synergy in organizational behavior. Working paper 3443-92-BPS. July 1992

[49] Connolly B. Get your next 'natural high' from sound healing therapy. 12/06/16. Available from: https://observer.com/2016/12/get-your-next-natural-high-from-sound-healing-therapy/

[50] Available from: https://brain.ieee.org/topics/neurotherapy-treating-disorders-by-retraining-the-brain/

[51] Diagnostic and Statistical Manual. 5th ed. American Psychiatric Association; 2013. p. 86

[52] West NS. Chickens Provide a New Form of Animal Assisted Therapy for Memory Loss Patients. Boston Globe; June 27, 2013

[53] Available from: https://www.greatandsmallride.org/

[54] Butler SM, Diaz C. 'Third Places' as Community Builders. Brookings Institute Commentary; September 14, 2016 Available from: https://www.brookings.edu/articles/third-places-as-community-builders/

[55] Available from: https://onehealthinitiative.com/

[56] Sasso JM, Ammar RM, Tenchov R, Lemmel S, Kelber O, Grieswelle M, et al. Gut microbiome-brain Alliance: A landscape view into mental and gastrointestinal health and disorders. ACS Chemical Neuroscience. 2023; **14**(10):1717-1763. DOI: 10.1021/acschemneuro.3c00127 Epub 2023 May 8

[57] Sorboni SG, Moghaddam HS, Jafarzadeh-Esfehani R, Soleimanpour S. A comprehensive review on the role of the gut microbiome in human neurological disorders. Clinical Microbiology Reviews. 2022;**35**(1): e0033820. DOI: 10.1128/CMR.00338-20 Epub 2022 Jan 5

[58] Bicknell B, Liebert A, Borody T, Herkes G, McLachlan C, Kiat H.

Neurodegenerative and neurodevelopmental diseases and the gut-brain axis: The potential of therapeutic targeting of the microbiome. International Journal of Molecular Sciences. 2023;**24**(11):9577. DOI: 10.3390/ijms24119577

[59] The Microbiome Connecting Thread: From Farm to Food to Human Health. Illinois Regenerative Agriculture Initiative, iSEE Research News. Feb 20, 2023.

[60] Blum WEH, Zechmeister-Boltenstern S, Keiblinger KM. Does soil contribute to the human gut microbiome? Microorganisms. 2019; 7(9):287. DOI: 10.3390/microorganisms7090287

[61] Chen Y, Xu J, Chen Y. Regulation of neurotransmitters by the gut microbiota and effects on cognition in neurological disorders. Nutrients. 2021;**13**(6):2099. DOI: 10.3390/nu13062099

Chapter 8

Early Trauma, Brain Development, and a Novel Therapeutic Approach

Hagit Friedman

Abstract

Trauma can result from an event that is perceived as life-threatening or as having the potential of seriously harming oneself or others. Such experiences, often accompanied by intense fear, terror, and helplessness, can lead to the development of PTSS and PTSD. Response to trauma depends on trauma feature characteristics and specific personal factors. In clinical literature, PTSD is often accompanied by severe functional impairment and includes well-described symptoms. These create behavior that limits the person and causes functional damage over time. Moreover, PTSS in early age may lead to adverse structural and functional changes in the development of brain neural circuits. PTSD has been one of the most investigated themes in medicine, psychiatry, neurophysiology, and rehabilitation over the last years. HPA axis, neural inflammation, and the neural mitochondrial oxidative stress are involved in the molecular mechanism of PTSD, reducing neuroplasticity and synapse proliferation. Here, current data on PTSD causes and symptoms, and the mechanisms and functions of the mitochondrial stress response, are reviewed, leading to 3LT novel scientifically and clinically based therapeutic approach. 3LT tool, aimed to the neural molecular mechanism of PTSS, targets mitochondrial dysfunction for the prevention and correction of neural lesions associated with PTSD.

Keywords: early trauma, neural development, brain insult, 3LT, low-level laser therapy, mitochondrial therapy, PTSD, neural rehabilitation, neuroplasticity, synaptic plasticity, developmental neurology, neuropediatrics, auricular therapy

1. Introduction

The risk of PTSD after a traumatic incident is between 1% to above 50% [1]. Worldwide, about 8% of all people encounter PTSD, with a lifetime incidence of PTSD between 1.3–12.2% [2]. Yet, the ICD defines PTSD as a psychiatric syndrome, linked with several others having resembling symptoms.

As a major public health problem, post-traumatic stress disorder (PTSD) has a substantial impact on individuals and society. The total excess economic burden of PTSD in the US is estimated to be more than $232.2 billion a year [3].

Early/child trauma is universally widespread with high prevalence, and more than 2/3 of the children report at least one traumatic event by the age of 16. Traumatic events involve: Psychological, physical, or sexual abuse; community/school violence; witnessing/experiencing national violence; national disasters/terrorism; commercial sexual abuse; unexpected/violent loss of a dear one; refugee/war experiences; military family-related stressors (deployment, parent loss/injury); Physical/sexual attack; negligence; serious accidents/life-threatening disease.

The main symptoms of trauma may change from one child to another and depend a lot on the child's age, and young kids may respond differently from older ones.

Preschool children are very vulnerable to traumatic events, and they usually show fear of being separated from their parent/caregiver; cry/yell a lot; eat poorly/lose weight; and have bad dreams. Elementary school children mainly become worried/fearful; feel guilt/shame; have a hard time concentrating, and have difficulty to sleep. Middle and high school children usually report feeling depressed/lonely; develop eating disorders/self-hurting actions; begin abusing alcohol/drugs; and become involved in risky sexual behavior.

According to the DSM-5 childhood trauma is defined as: "exposure to actual or threatened death, injury, or sexual violence" [4]. These may include direct experience, witnessing trauma, or learning about trauma that happened to an acquaintance.

When signs are present for more than a month after the traumatic event, the main symptom categorization that creates PTSD diagnosis is [5–7]:

a. flashbacks, intrusive thoughts, and nightmares.

b. hyperarousal, insomnia, restlessness, irritability, impulsivity, and anger.

c. Numbness, avoidance, withdrawal, confusion, dissociation, and depression.

Each of these reactions is a diagnostic criterion and is related to alterations in physiological routes and brain circuits, which contribute to neurodevelopmental deficits and cognitive–emotional dysregulation in children with early trauma [8].

PTSD is often correlated with certain physiologic biomarkers, and these include elevated blood glucose, insulin, and creatinine; elevated activity levels of certain genes, metabolites involved in energy processing, circulating microRNAs, and blood key proteins [9]. In addition, decreased plasma levels of fatty acids involved in neuroprotection were observed in PTSD patients [10]. These fatty acids block the action of the NFκB transcription factor (NFκB – Nuclear Factor-kappa B) and decrease production of reactive oxygen species (ROS) [11, 12] (hence, lower levels of fatty acids in PTSD lead to high ROS). Additional, PTSD biomarkers include high expression of mitochondrial nuclear gene chaperones, proteases, and antioxidant enzymes to repair mitochondria damaged organelles and restore functional activity in defective mitochondria [13]. Indeed, these biomarkers reflect intrinsic multilevel pathophysiologic process, including cellular metabolic changes that will chronically influence body and brain development and function.

Concerning PTSD outcomes, trauma is a risk factor for nearly all behavioral health and substance use disorders. Early trauma has difficult outcomes for the child, and for his family, as childhood trauma may develop into failure of mental processes [14–16], and various pathologies (i.e., distress, depression, disruptive behaviors, suicidality, substance use disorders, and more) [17–22]. Yet, only recently, we learn about trauma's physiologic effects in children's brains, and how these processes lie behind trauma's immediate and longstanding mental health outcomes.

2. Etiology of early trauma: enhanced neuroendocrine, and immune-inflammatory activity

HPA axis is strongly influenced by PTSD, causing neuroendocrine functional changes, structural abnormalities, and neurochemical alterations. These pathological changes negatively feedback on the brain activity *via* lateral amygdala, prefrontal cortex, and hippocampus.

Specifically, glucocorticoid activity inhibits lymphocyte proliferation, as a result, levels of pro-inflammatory cytokines IL-6, IL-12, IFN-γ, and TNF-α are significantly increased [23]. Additionally, rise in hypothalamic CRH (corticotrophin-releasing hormone) and pituitary ACTH (adreno corticotrophin hormone) hormone in PTSD were linked to severity of PTSD, psychosis, destructive personality disorders, and even suicide. Parallel to activity changes of HPA axis in PTSD, there is hyperactivity in the sympathetic noradrenergic and cholinergic neural circuits.

Research showed additional changes in immune system activity: higher levels of pro-inflammatory cytokines (IL-1β, TNFα, IL-2, IL-6, IL-17), interferon-gamma (INF-γ), C-reactive protein (CRP), and reduction in IL-4 concentration damage normal immune activity [24]. Such inflammatory processes are strongly correlated with mitochondria function: mitochondrial abnormalities result in ROS overproduction, causing broken mitochondrial DNA. Pro-inflammatory cytokines may also downregulate ATP (adenosine triphosphate) synthesis by IL-1β, TNFα, and IL-6. IL-6 enhanced activity causes amygdala and anterior cingulate cortex neuroinflammation [25, 26] and elevates amygdala and hippocampal dopamine concentration, resulting in dysregulation of normal HPA axis activity and stimulating the development of PTSD.

Altogether, PTSD is characterized by an increase in inflammatory neurohormones (corticosteroids, prostaglandins, etc.), and NFκB, which damage mitochondrial function and plasticity [12, 27, 28], decreased cellular energy production, and further neural deterioration.

3. Brain development and downregulation of neural plasticity due to early trauma

Until recently, the specific brain circuits, that make persons who experienced a trauma vulnerable to permanent clinical signs, were not clear. New studies showed that under stressful conditions Amygdala neural circuits release norepinephrine, that increase heart rate and interfere with regulation of emotions [29]. Moreover, high cortisol levels during trauma, are known to harm hippocampal cells neural activity [30], and typically cause reduction in hippocampal size and function [31].

Additionally, cortical thinning in brain areas correlated with surviving attempts, and resistance has an important function in PTSD signs. It was found that cortical thinning in the superior frontal cortex (SFC), insula, superior temporal cortex, dorsolateral prefrontal cortex, superior parietal cortex, and precuneus, correlated with persistent PTSD [32]. Specifically, they found that in people who experienced trauma, cortical thinning in the SFC was correlated with maladaptive coping approach, and thinner insula layers are linked with lower resistance ability. These findings are especially important in the context of cortex neural proliferation and synapse formation during brain development.

4. Neural components of early emotional trauma: mitochondria and oxidative stress

A lot of energy is required for brain cells daily vitality, survival, and functioning. Mitochondria are cellular organelles, which are the cellular "powerhouses," i.e. mitochondria are responsible for supplying energy for function and growth in the living cell. In addition to energy supply, the mitochondria participate in the cellular iron metabolism and in cellular calcium balance. Moreover, mitochondria are associated with normal and defective cell proliferation and participate in "programmed cell death." Each eukaryotic cell may have hundreds to tens of thousands of mitochondria, depending on cellular function and its energy consumption.

Mitochondria are inherited from the mother through the ovum, may develop mutations as they reproduce, and have almost no repair mechanisms. Most of the proteins that make up the mitochondria are encoded in the cell nucleus, and since the mitochondria are inherited from the mother, they have no "backup" from the father's genome when mutations or damage to the mitochondria occur. However, since the ovum contains a lot of mitochondria to begin with, some may be damaged without it being clinically apparent. This "hidden injury" may exist over several generations until a stage is achieved when there are only very few normal mitochondria, and then a neural problem may be revealed in the form of a defect or a strong tendency to emotional or mental injury.

Genetic changes in mitochondria may be caused not only by maternal inheritance (when cells divide to form the embryo) but also by a coding change called a "*de novo* mutation" (a new mutation in the mitochondria in fetal cells), which may happen due to an environmental/epigenetic cause.

Mitochondria are an important source of ROS in mammalian cells. Mitochondrial response to early emotional trauma consists of several continuous pathways: first – the HPA axis, which is a most important neuroendocrine rout implicated in stress response through release of hormones and prohormones. At the end point of HPA axis, glucocorticoids, released by adrenal gland into bloodstream, regulate mitochondrial transcription in target tissues. Then, mitochondrial stress response includes changes in mitochondrial dynamics, retrograde signaling, mitochondrial unfolded protein response, mitochondrial selective autophagy/apoptotic cell death. Finally, cellular stress response results in excitotoxicity when frequent and powerful membrane potential changes cause excessive synaptic release of glutamate, which binds to NMDA receptor, leading to excess calcium influx, failure of mitochondrial membrane potential, decreased ATP creation, and boosted ROS production.

As the genes involved in PTSD mechanism are shared by other prevalent mental syndromes (depression, anxiety, and more), it was believed until recently that several mental syndromes may be risk factors for PTSD. However, recently, the molecular mechanism of depression [33] and the molecular mechanism of PTSD focus us to basic molecular constituents of the eukaryote cell – the mitochondria.

Studies show that the etiology of PTSD involves processes of inflammation and stimulation of the immune system, which cause damage to the neural mitochondria [34–38], which, in turn, causes damage to the neural circuits – damage to the proliferation of contact points (= synapses) between neural cells and damage to neural circuits architecture plasticity.

Mitochondrial disorders include a decrease or increase in mitochondrial function, depending on the cause and the developmental time window, and may lead to neuronal damage. It was found that neurodevelopmental impairment, or susceptibility to mental–emotional injury, may be the result of mitochondrial disorder and abnormal mitochondrial physiology [39–42].

To summarize, an increase in inflammatory neurohormones in PTSD may damage mitochondrial function, causing decreased cellular energy production, and further neural deterioration. This is especially significant for the cells of the nervous system – neurons and glial cells as it has been found that impaired neural mitochondrial function in stress is linked to the development of diverse brain mental and emotional pathologies [43–45].

Mitochondrial function is greatly affected by environmental factors, and impaired mitochondrial function is linked to environmental triggers [46–52]. Therefore, it is important to focus PTSD therapy on improving patient's mitochondrial function, using a safe and noninvasive tool that has been scientifically proven to overcome the environmental impact.

5. Novel therapeutic tool

An important factor for children's recovery is having access to effective therapy.

Today, first-line healing approaches for PTSD include psychotherapy and pharmacotherapy. In psychotherapy, we include mainly CBT (cognitive behavioral therapy), CRT (cognitive remediation therapy), and EMDR (eye movement desensitization and reprocessing). In pharmacotherapy, we mainly refer to the drugs paroxetine, sertraline, and venlafaxine, which are FDA-approved for PTSD [53, 54]. However, it was shown that these approaches either have only partial effectiveness or have a mechanism, which is not clear. Furthermore, data show that psychological treatment is primarily dependent on the patient's psychological tolerance and is likely to cause secondary harm to the patient [55].

In recent years, the use of additional therapeutic tools has increased, including therapies based on East Asian ancient knowledge combined with modern clinical empirical scientific knowledge [56–60].

Employing 3LT, we use an innovative and well-known scientific therapeutic approach to solve the neural damage caused by early trauma.

Our 3LT therapeutic protocol consists of: A. specific physical properties of laser energy chosen according to the patient's clinical picture (including clinically proven specific wavelength and frequency). B. specific skin points over, which the laser is activated. These skin points are chosen according to western clinically proven auricular therapy and according to Traditional Chinese Korean and Japanese Medicine and our knowledge and experience in neuroanatomy and neurophysiology, relating to the patient's clinical picture.

5.1 Physical characteristics of low power/cold laser tool

Low-power laser therapy has evolved in recent years into a clinical procedure used for three main purposes: (1) To reduce inflammation, edema, and chronic injuries; (2) To promote healing of wounds, deep tissues, and nerves; (3) To treat neurological injuries and pain.

Our goal is to alleviate the trauma, utilizing low-level laser therapy (3LT = Low-Level Laser Therapy) tool. This approach is aimed at the injury mechanism following a traumatic experience and is based on research and clinical evidence.

Low-power laser heals neurological injuries, including PTSD by reducing the activity of the HPA axis, lowering the concentration of inflammatory proteins, regulating the energy-yielding activity of mitochondria, and increasing the production of ATP and nerve growth factors.

LASERs (Light Amplification by Excitation of Radiation emission) are electromagnetic radiation producing devices. LASER radiation has uniform wavelength, phase, and polarization. A low-power laser device (Low-Level Laser = 3 L) is a special type of laser that affects living tissues and biological systems by nonthermal means [61]. Our low-power laser system uses wavelengths in the range of red and blue light. Studies have found that red to NIR (near-infrared) light has a healing effect on local and systemic injuries and can affect the functioning of the brain and other organs.

Low-power laser therapy applies a noninvasive therapeutic laser for stimulation over specific skin body points. This technique is safe and noninvasive and has become an important tool for the treatment of patients at risk, including premature newborns [62–64]. For example, stimulation of Specific skin body points for pain relief using a low-power laser creates a local photochemical effect [65] that causes specific changes in brain neuron activity [66, 67], which are perceived by the patient as a reduction in pain intensity. These changes can be measured and quantified by brain imaging [68, 69].

A "photochemical effect" means that when the right parameters are employed (power, wavelength, frequency, duration, and location), the laser beam reduces tissue oxidative stress and increases ATP levels in cells, improves cell metabolism, and reduces inflammation [70–72].

Because 3LT is targeted at the very basic building blocks of eukaryote cells, it has shown beneficial effects for various clinical conditions and processes, i.e.:

It was found that 3LT improves the healing of soft tissues, reduces inflammation, and relieves chronic and acute physical and mental pain [73–80].

3LT has been shown to alter axonal conduction, opioid receptor binding, and endorphin production [81–83].

In clinical studies, it was found that 3LT causes an immediate decrease in acute and chronic pain perception and functional enhancement [84–86].

3LT showed promising results for myocardial function [87], mesenchymal stem cell regeneration [88], skin injuries [89–92], brain trauma, TBI [93–96], diabetic retinopathy [97], oncology [98], and more.

We employ a combination of specific scientifically proven skin points/locations, frequencies, and wavelengths according to the patient's characteristics.

3LT is a noninvasive tool that involves the projection of specific wavelengths, over the surface of the skin, at selected points. Infrared waves can produce diverse biological reactions in the body such as increasing the formation of ATP, the release of NO (nitric oxide) and CCO (cytochrome c oxidase), regulation and reduction of ROS, a change in membrane activity of intracellular organelles, (mainly the mitochondria), a change in transmembrane calcium flux, in the production of stress proteins, and more [57, 70, 99–102].

In eukaryote cells, 3LT creates a shift toward higher oxidation in the total redox potential of the mitochondria [103] and briefly increases the level of ROS [90]. This change in the redox state of the mitochondria regulates several cellular proteins and protein genes. As a result, ATP levels and blood flow increase, and the availability of oxygen in damaged areas of the brain is improved [104].

Our laser device has three therapeutically proven wavelength ranges, 670 nm, 808 nm, and 915 nm. These wavelengths are within the "optical window" that allows optimal tissue penetration depth (lowest absorption of water, hemoglobin, and melanin).

The treatment reaches all relevant tissue layers because the visible red spectrum wavelength range penetrates the upper tissue layers, and the infrared wavelength range (not visible to the human eye) penetrates deeper tissue layers. As a result of the activity of these laser wavelengths, ATP synthesis, (which is the main cause of cell excitation and energetic activity increase), through the wavelengths of cytochrome-C-oxidase, is perfectly activated. In particular, the wavelengths of 670 nm, 808–830 nm, and 905–915 nm were found to be suitable for photobiomodulation and are now available at high power in the therapeutic laser device.

In addition, our 3LT device includes a laser source with a blue range wavelength because it was found that despite its low tissue penetration ability, involvement of a blue wavelength laser source brings the best results in terms of energy. A blue wavelength is absorbed by NADH (nicotinamide adenine dinucleotide + hydrogen) – the first complex of the cellular respiratory chain; blue and red laser wavelengths are absorbed by the complex of cytochrome C, with a blue wavelength (405 nm) showing five times higher absorption compared to red laser wavelength [105, 106]. Hence, it was found that bichromate laser radiation (red and blue wavelength range) yields a bigger change in the mitochondria redox potential by increased oxidation of NADH. This way, the proton-motive force increases (the force that drives the flow of protons into the mitochondrial matrix), and thereby ATP cycle is enhanced [107]. In addition, electron transfer is accelerated, and both effects cause an increase of ATP synthesis. This change at the cellular-molecular level is manifested clinically and functionally.

5.2 Clinical considerations – skin points over which the laser is activated

Acupuncture, an ancient therapy, has been long employed all over the world for the treatment of chronic and acute medical situations [108, 109], using invasive metal needles. World Health Organization advocated acupuncture for at least 20 pathologies [110], including for coping with pain in elder people [111, 112], children [113–117], and neonates [118–122]. For example, it was found that acupuncture increases the secretion of the natural neuromodulator adenosine, also known as anti-inflammatory and pain relief substance [123, 124]. In addition, acupuncture has been shown to have potential benefits for a variety of mental disorders [125, 126], and acupuncture for PTSD in adults was found to help with core symptoms [127, 128]; it was found that acupuncture can alleviate the anxiety behavior, as well as the recognition and memory ability of PTSD rats [129].

However, recent studies show that the main efficient acupuncture points for mature patients with PTSD [129], or earthquake survivors with major psychiatric disorder (MPD) [130], are near vertex skull points, located on fontanels (Fonticuli cranii) cranial suture lines (Suturae cranii). These acupuncture points named – Baihui, Sishencong, and Shenting, were punctured to depth of 20–25 mm obliquely [131] for a duration of 20 min per session [132]. Such a protocol, even after necessary adjustment, would not be appliable for children, toddlers, or infants. With young age patients, we should avoid skull acupuncture points and keep away from open suture fontanels. Using 3LT tool, we may combine suitable distal acupuncture skin points with selected auricular points and under-knee or under-tung laser applicator instead of over-fontanelle skull direct needle acupuncture points.

Auriculotherapy is an ancient technique initially used to treat pain. It was rediscovered in the 1940s and developed by French physician Dr. Paul Nogier and his colleagues. He showed that the ear contains a representation map of the body so that any pathology will be associated with a compatible modification of specific ear points. The therapeutic technique involves modifying of the dysfunctional ear point activity, which generates an impulse that is transmitted to the brain. Specific parts of the ear are innervated by specific branches of four cranial nerves and plexus (V, VII, IX, X). These nerves carry impulses between the body the brain and the ear. The ear point map is validated using fMRI [133, 134].

In low-Level Laser therapy, we employ an accurate laser beam, over suitable skin/ear points, to regulate mitochondrial function and create the required therapeutic effect according to specific clinical considerations.

6. Conclusion and recommendation

3LT is a suitable therapeutic tool for all populations without exclusion. 3LT is noninvasive, flexible, and diverse, yet always based on the physical characteristics of the laser beam and its therapeutic effects on human body cells through specific somatotopic skin points. Hence, even patients at risk, including old and sick or fragile babies with childhood trauma, may be suitable for laser therapy, using evidence-based protocols tailored for their needs.

Patients with childhood trauma usually have an already challenged immune system (because of trauma path physiology) and already exhibit a lot of stress. Using real needles (as with needle-based auricular therapy, or needle acupuncture), in repetitive ~20-minute sessions, with old patients having health complications or young patients in trauma may be dangerous, not efficient, and not practical.

Employing 3LT therapeutic tool, which we know exactly its molecular and cellular mechanism and has been proven to cause no damage or pain, is the most efficient and kind therapy we may offer these patients.

We recommend to further amplify the assimilation of evidence-based 3LT in medical training and to further encourage clinical studies to identify additional pathologies for which 3LT may be suitable, especially for the benefit of high-risk patients.

Author details

Hagit Friedman
Simaney-Derech Institute and Haifa, Zichron-Yaakov, Isreal

*Address all correspondence to: drhagitfriedman@gmail.com

References

[1] Spoont MR, Williams JW, Kehle-Forbes S, Nieuwsma JA, Mann-Wrobel MC, Gross R. Does this patient have post-traumatic stress disorder?: Rational clinical examination systematic review. Journal of the American Medical Association. 2015;**314**:501-510

[2] Karam EG, Friedman MJ, Hill ED, Kessler RC, McLaughlin KA, Petukhova M, et al. Cumulative traumas, and risk thresholds: 12-month PTSD in the world mental health (WMH) surveys. Depression and Anxiety. 2014;**31**:130-142

[3] Davis LL, Schein J, Cloutier M, et al. The economic burden of posttraumatic stress disorder in the United States from a societal perspective. The Journal of Clinical Psychiatry. 2022;**83**(3):21m14116

[4] American Psychiatric Association. Trauma- and Stressor-Related Disorders, in Diagnostic and Statistical Manual of Mental Disorders. Fifth ed. Arlington, VA: American Psychiatric Publishing; 2013

[5] Van der Meer CA, Bakker A, Smit AS, van Buschbach S, Den Dekker M, Westerveld GJ, et al. Gender and age differences in trauma and PTSD among dutch treatment-seeking police officers. The Journal of Nervous and Mental Disease. 2017;**205**:87-92

[6] Mann SK, Marwaha R. Post-traumatic stress disorder. In: StatPearls. Treasure Island (FL): StatPearls Publishing; 2022

[7] Shalev A et al. Post-traumatic stress disorder. The New England Journal of Medicine. 2017;**376**:2459-2469

[8] De Bellis MD. Developmental traumatology: A contributory mechanism for alcohol and substance use disorders. Special Review in Psycho-neuroendocrinology. 2001;**27**:155-170

[9] Michopoulos V, Vester A, Neigh G. Post-traumatic stress disorder: A metabolic disorder in disguise? Experimental Neurology. 2016;**284**:220-229

[10] Konjevod M, Tudor L, Svob Strac D, Nedic Erjavec G, Barbas C, Zarkovic N, et al. Metabolomic and glycomic findings in post-traumatic stress disorder. Progress in Neuro-Psychopharmacology & Biological Psychiatry. 2019;**88**:181-193

[11] Mocking RJT, Assies J, Ruhé HG, Schene AH. Focus on fatty acids in the neurometabolic pathophysiology of psychiatric disorders. Journal of Inherited Metabolic Disease. 2018;**41**:597-611

[12] Gupta S, Guleria RS. Involvement of nuclear factor-κB in inflammation and neuronal plasticity associated with post-traumatic stress disorder. Cell. 2022;**11**:2034

[13] Suomalainen L, Haravuori H, Berg N, Kiviruusu O, Marttunen M. A controlled follow-up study of adolescents exposed to a school shooting – Psychological consequences after four months. European Psychiatry. 2011;**26**(8):490-497

[14] Ford JD, Stockton P, Kaltman S, Green BL. Disorders of extreme stress (DESNOS) symptoms are associated with type and severity of interpersonal trauma exposure in a sample of healthy young women. Journal of Interpersonal Violence. 2006;**21**(11):1399-1416

[15] Carrion VG, Weems CF, Ray RD, Reiss AL. Toward an empirical

definition of pediatric PTSD: The phenomenology of PTSD symptoms in youth. Journal of the American Academy of Child and Adolescent Psychiatry. 2001;**41**:166-173

[16] Widom CS, DuMont K, Czaja SJ. A prospective investigation of major depressive disorder and comorbidity in abused and neglected children grown up. Archives of General Psychiatry. 2007;**64**:49-56

[17] Widom CS. Posttraumatic stress disorder in abused and neglected children grown up. American Journal of Psychiatry. 1999;**156**:1223-1229

[18] Copeland W, Keeler G, Angold A, Costello E. Traumatic events and posttraumatic stress in childhood. Archives of General Psychiatry. 2007;**64**:577-584

[19] Luntz BK, Widom CS. Antisocial personality disorder in abused and neglected children grown up. American Journal of Psychiatry. 1994;**151**:670-674

[20] Clark DB, Lesnick L, Hegedus A. Trauma and other stressors in adolescent alcohol dependence and abuse. Journal of the American Academy of Child and Adolescent Psychiatry. 1997:1744-1751

[21] Dube SR, Miller JW, Brown DW, Giles WH, Felitti VJ, Dong M, et al. Adverse childhood experiences and the association with ever using alcohol and initiating alcohol use during adolescence. Journal of Adolescent Health. 2006;**38**(4):444e1-10

[22] Dube SR, Felitti VJ, Dong M, Chapman DP, Giles WH, Anda RF. Childhood abuse, neglect, household dysfunction and the risk of illicit drug use: The adverse childhood experiences study. Pediatrics. 2003;**111**(3):564-572

[23] Kim TD, Lee S, Yoon S. Inflammation in post-traumatic stress disorder (PTSD): A review of potential correlates of PTSD with a neurological perspective. Antioxidants (Basel). 2020;**9**:107

[24] López-Armada MJ, Riveiro-Naveira R, Vaamonde-García C, Valcárcel-Ares MN. Mitochondrial dysfunction and the inflammatory response. Mitochondrion. 2013;**13**(2):106-118

[25] Ventrano VA. Histologic Analysis of Cortical Tissue from Patients with Post-Traumatic Stress Disorder and Chronic Traumatic Encephalopathy. OpenBU. Boston University Libraries; 2017

[26] Eslinger PJ et al. The neuroscience of social feelings: Mechanisms of adaptive social functioning. Neuroscience & Biobehavioral Reviews. 2021;**128**:592-620

[27] Speer KE et al. HPA axis function and diurnal cortisol in post-traumatic stress disorder: A systematic review. Neurobiology of Stress. 2019;**11**:100180

[28] Dunlop BW et al. The hypothalamic-pituitary-adrenal axis in PTSD: Pathophysiology and treatment interventions. Progress in Neuro-Psychopharmacology & Biological Psychiatry. 2019;**89**:361-379

[29] Ousdal OT, Milde AM, Hafstad GS, Hodneland E, Dyb G, Craven AR, et al. The association of PTSD symptom severity with amygdala nuclei volumes in traumatized youths. Translational Psychiatry. 2020;**10**:288

[30] Schmidt SCE, Gnam JP, Kopf M, Rathgeber T, Woll A. The influence of cortisol, flow, and anxiety on performance in E-sports: A field study. BioMed Research International. 2020;**2020**:9651245

[31] Tull MT, Vidaña AG, Betts JE. Emotion regulation difficulties in PTSD. In: Tull MT, Kimbrel NA, editors. Emotion in post-traumatic stress disorder: Etiology, assessment, neurobiology, and treatment. Elsevier Academic Press; 2020. pp. 295-310

[32] Lee H et al. Cerebral cortical thinning in brain regions involved in emotional regulation relates to persistent symptoms in subjects with posttraumatic stress disorder. Psychiatry Research. 2023;**327**:115345

[33] Oved K, Morag A, Pasmanik-Chor M, Rehavi M, Shomron N, Gurwitz D. Genome-wide expression profiling of human lymphoblastoid cell lines implicates integrin beta-3 in the mode of action of antidepressants. Translational Psychiatry. 2013;**3**(10):e313

[34] Hori H, Kim Y. Inflammation and post-traumatic stress disorder. Psychiatry and Clinical Neurosciences. 2019;**73**:143-153

[35] Sumner JA, Nishimi KM, et al. Posttraumatic stress disorder and inflammation: Untangling issues of Bidirectionality. Biological Psychiatry. 2020;**87**:885-897

[36] Kaplan GB et al. Mitochondrial dysfunction in animal models of PTSD: Relationships between behavioral models, neural regions, and cellular maladaptation. Frontiers in Physiology. 2023;**14**:1105839

[37] Lushchak O et al. An orchestrating role of mitochondria in the origin and development of post-traumatic stress disorder. Frontiers in Physiology. 2023;**13**:1094076

[38] Reed EC et al. Defining the nuanced nature of redox biology in post-traumatic stress disorder. Frontiers in Physiology. 2023;**14**:1130861

[39] Friedman H. Autism Spectrum Disorder (ASD): From Molecular Mechanism to Novel Therapeutic Approach. In: Learning Disabilities – Neurobiology, Assessment, Clinical Features and Treatments. UK, London: IntechOpen; 2022

[40] Singh K et al. Developmental regression and mitochondrial function in children with autism. Annals of Clinical Translational Neurology. 2020;**7**:683-694

[41] Hassan H et al. Alterations in mitochondrial respiratory capacity and membrane potential: A link between mitochondrial dysregulation and autism. MitoFit Preprint Arch. Current Issues in Molecular Biology. 2021;**43**(3):2238-2252

[42] Nguyen A et al. Mechanisms of mitochondrial oxidative stress in brain injury: From pathophysiology to therapeutics. Oxygen. 2023;**3**(2):163-178

[43] Picard M et al. Psychological stress and mitochondria: A systematic review. Psychosomatic Medicine. 2018;**80**(2):141-153

[44] Daniels T et al. Stress and psychiatric disorders: The role of mitochondria. Annual Review of Clinical Psychology. 2020;**16**:165-186

[45] Shen X et al. Mitochondrial quality control in the brain: The physiological and pathological roles. Frontiers in Neuroscience. 2022;**16**:1075141

[46] Frye RE et al. Mitochondria may mediate prenatal environmental influences in autism Spectrum disorder. Journal of Personalized Medicine. 2021;**11**:218

[47] Byun HM, Baccarelli AA. Environmental exposure and mitochondrial epigenetics: Study design and analytical challenges. Human Genetics. 2014;**133**(3):247-257

[48] Meyer JN et al. Mitochondria as a target of environmental toxicants. Toxicological Sciences. 2013;**134**(1):1-17

[49] Reddam A et al. Environmental chemical exposures and mitochondrial dysfunction: A review of recent literature. Current Environmental Health Reports. 2022;**9**:631-649

[50] Duarte-Hospital C et al. Mitochondrial dysfunction as a Hallmark of environmental injury. Cell. 2022;**11**(1):110

[51] Jayasundara N. Ecological significance of mitochondrial toxicants. Toxicology. 2017;**391**(1):64-74

[52] Helley MP et al. Mitochondria: A common target for genetic mutations and environmental toxicants in Parkinson's disease. Frontiers in Genetics. 2017;**8**:177

[53] Kim YD, Heo I, Shin BC, et al. Acupuncture for posttraumatic stress disorder: A systematic review of randomized controlled trials and prospective clinical trials. Evidence-based Complementary and Alternative Medicine. 2013;**2013**:e615857

[54] Lee DJ, Schnitzlein CW, Wolf JP, et al. Psychotherapy versus pharmacotherapy for posttraumatic stress disorder: Systemic review and meta-analyses to determine first-line treatments. Depression and Anxiety. 2016;**33**:792-806

[55] Lv T, Wu Y. Research progress in the mechanism of acupuncture improving hippocampal injury in post-traumatic stress disorder. Journal of Nanjing University of traditional Chinese Medicine. 2022;**42**:147-153

[56] Wynn GH. Complementary and alternative medicine approaches in the treatment of PTSD. Current Psychiatry Reports. 2015;**17**:62

[57] Farivar S et al. Biological effects of low-level laser therapy. Journal of Lasers in Medical Sciences. 2014;**5**(2):58-62

[58] Nalamachu S. An overview of pain management: The clinical efficacy and value of treatment. The American Journal of Managed Care. 2013;**19**:s261-s266

[59] Yang QF, Ding JC, Qi ZZ, et al. Comparative research on intervention in anxiety behavior of PTSD-like rats by electro-acupuncture and repetitive transcranial magnetic stimulation and serum corticosterone. Journal of Nanjing University of traditional Chinese Medicine. 2012;**28**:357-359

[60] Hickey AH. Adding a Face and the Story to the Data: Acupuncture for PTSD in the Military. Cambridge: Springer International Publishing; 2015

[61] Zein R et al. Review of light parameters and photobiomodulation efficacy: Dive into complexity. Journal of Biomedical Optics. 2018;**23**(12):12090

[62] Kurath-Koller S et al. Changes of locoregional skin temperature in neonates undergoing laser needle acupuncture at the acupuncture point large intestine. Evidence-based Complementary and Alternative Medicine. eCAM; 2015;**2015**:571857

[63] Raith W et al. Thermographic measuring of the skin temperature using laser needle acupuncture in preterm neonates. Evidence-based Complementary and Alternative Medicine. eCAM; 2012;**2012**:614210

[64] Raith W et al. Near-infrared spectroscopy for objectifying cerebral effects of laser acupuncture in term and preterm neonates. Evidence-based Complementary and Alternative Medicine. eCAM; 2013;**2013**:346852

[65] Smith KC. The photobiological basis of low-level laser radiation therapy. Laser Therapy. 1991;**3**:19-24

[66] Walker J. Relief from chronic pain by low power laser irradiation. Neuroscience Letters. 1983;**43**:339-344

[67] Bischko JJ. Use of the laser beam in acupuncture. Acupuncture & Electro Therapeutics Research. 1980;**5**:29-24

[68] Siedentopf CM et al. fMRI detects activation of the visual association cortex during laser acupuncture of the foot in humans. Neuroscience Letters. 2002;**327**:53-56

[69] Litcher G et al. Acupuncture using laser needles modulates brain function: First evidence from functional transcranial Doppler sonography and fMRI. Lasers in Medical Science. 2004;**19**:6-11

[70] Ferraresi C et al. Time response of increases in ATP and muscle resistance to fatigue after low-level laser (light) therapy (LLLT) in mice. Lasers in Medical Science. 2015;**30**(4):1259-1267

[71] de Freitas LF et al. Proposed mechanisms of photobiomodulation or low-level light therapy. IEEE Journal of Selected Topics in Quantum Electronics. 2016;**22**(3):7000417

[72] Mussttaf RA et al. Assessing the impact of low-level laser therapy (LLLT) on biological systems: A review. International Journal of Radiation Biology. 2019;**95**(2):120-143

[73] Fulop AM et al. A meta-analysis of the efficacy of laser phototherapy on pain relief. The Clinical Journal of Pain. 2019;**26**:729-736

[74] Chow RT et al. 830 nm laser irradiation induces varicosity formation, reduces mitochondrial membrane potential, and blocks fast axonal flow in small and medium diameter rat dorsal root ganglion neurons: Implications for the analgesic effects of 830 nm laser. Journal of the Peripheral Nervous System. 2007;**12**:28-39

[75] Xu S, Wan B. Recent advances in low-level laser therapy on depression. Stress and Brain. 2022;**2**(4):123-138

[76] Ohno T. Pain suppressive effect of low power laser irradiation. A quantitative analysis of substance P in the rat spinal dorsal root ganglion. Nihon Ika Daigaku Zasshi. 1997;**64**(5):395-400

[77] Bjordal JM, Johnson MI, Iversen V, Aimbire F, Lopes-Martins RAB. Low-level laser therapy in acute pain: A systematic review of possible mechanisms of action and clinical effects in randomized placebo-controlled trials. Photomedicine and Laser Surgery. 2006;**24**(2):158-168

[78] Chow R, Armati P, Laakso EL, Bjorda JM, Baxter GD. Inhibitory effects of laser irradiation on peripheral mammalian nerves and relevance to analgesic effects: A systematic review. Photomedicine and Laser Surgery. 2011;**29**(6):365-381

[79] Yan W, Chow R, Armati PJ. Inhibitory effects of visible 650-nm and infrared 808 nm laser irradiation on somatosensory and compound muscle action potentials in rat sciatic nerve: Implications for laser-induced analgesia. Journal of the Peripheral Nervous System. 2011;**16**(2):130-135

[80] Masoumipoor M, Jameie S, Janzadeh A, Nasirinezhad F, Soleimani M, Kerdary M. Effects of 660-and 980-nm low-level laser therapy on neuropathic pain relief following chronic constriction injury in rat sciatic

nerve. Lasers in Medical Science. 2014;**29**(5):1593-1598

[81] Chow RT et al. Efficacy of low-level laser therapy in the management of neck pain: A systematic review and meta-analysis of randomized placebo or active treatment controlled trials. Lancet. 2009;**374**:1897-1908

[82] Cidral-Filho FJ et al. Light-emitting diode therapy induces analgesia in a mouse model of postoperative pain through activation of peripheral opioid receptors and the L-arginine/nitric oxide pathway. Lasers in Medical Science. 2014;**29**:695-702

[83] Yamamoto H et al. Antinociceptive effect of laser irradiaion on Hoku points in rats. Pain Clinic. 1988;**8**:43-48

[84] Isolan C et al. Photobiomodulation therapy reduces postoperative pain after third Olar extractions: A randomized clinical trial. Medicina Oral, Patología Oral y Cirugía Bucal. 2021;**26**(3):e341-e348

[85] Djavid GE. In chronic low back pain, low level laser therapy combined with exercise is more beneficial than exercise alone in the long term: A randomized trial. The Australian Journal of Physiotherapy. 2007;**53**:155-160

[86] Leal EC et al. Adjunctive use of combination of super-pulsed laser and light-emitting diodes phototherapy on nonspecific knee pain: Double-blinded randomized placebo-controlled trial. Lasers in Medical Science. 2014;**29**(6):1839-1184

[87] Gao X et al. Photobiomodulation regulation as one promising therapeutic approach for myocardial infarction. Oxidative Medicine and Cellular Longevity. 2021;**2021**:9962922

[88] Eroglu B et al. Photo biomodulation has rejuvenating effects on aged bone marrow mesenchymal stem cells. Scientific Reports. 2021;**11**(1):13067

[89] Avci P et al. Low-level laser (light) therapy (LLLT) in skin: Stimulating, healing, restoring. Seminars in Cutaneous Medicine and Surgery. 2013;**32**(1):41-52

[90] Amaroli A et al. Photobiomodulation with 808-nm diode laser light promotes wound healing of human endothelial cells through increased reactive oxygen species production stimulating mitochondrial oxidative phosphorylation. Lasers in Medical Science. 2018;**34**(3):495-504

[91] Khan I et al. Accelerated burn wound healing with photobiomodulation therapy involves activation of endogenous latent TGF-β1. Scientific Reports. 2021;**11**:13371

[92] Amini A et al. The combined effect of photobiomodulation and curcumin on acute skin wound healing in rats. Journal of Lasers in Medical Sciences. 2021;**12**:e9

[93] Poiani G et al. Photobiomodulation using low-level laser therapy (LLLT) for patients with chronic traumatic brain injury: A randomized controlled trial study protocol. Trials. 2018;**19**(1):17

[94] Shah EJ et al. Inhibiting mitochondrial cytochrome c oxidase downregulates gene transcription after traumatic brain injury in drosophila. Frontiers in Physiology. 2021;**12**:628777

[95] Zhang Q et al. Study of near infrared technology for intracranial hematoma detection. Journal of Biomedical Optics. 2000;**5**:206-213

[96] Zhang Q et al. Low-level laser therapy effectively prevents secondary brain injury induced by immediate early responsive gene X-1 deficiency. Journal

of Cerebral Blood Flow and Metabolism. 2014;**34**(8):1391-1401

[97] Ahmed SA et al. Low-level laser therapy with 670 nm alleviates diabetic retinopathy in an experimental model. Journal of Current Ophthalmology. 2021;**33**(2):143-151

[98] Tam SY et al. Review on the cellular mechanisms of low-level laser therapy use in oncology. Frontiers in Oncology. 2020;**10**:1255

[99] Huang YY et al. Transcranial low-level laser (light) therapy for traumatic brain injury. Journal of Biophotonics. 2012;**5**:827-837

[100] Khuman J et al. Low level laser light therapy improves cognitive deficits and inhibits microglial activation after controlled cortical impact in mice. Journal of Neurotrauma. 2012;**29**:408-417

[101] Osipov AN et al. Effects of laser radiation on mitochondria and mitochondrial proteins subjected to nitric oxide. Frontiers in Medicine. 2018;**5**:112

[102] Antunes F et al. On the mechanism and biology of cytochrome oxidase inhibition by nitric oxide. Proceedings of the National Academy of Sciences of the United States of America. 2004;**101**:16774-16779

[103] Karu TI et al. Absorption measurements of a cell monolayer relevant to phototherapy: Reduction of cytochrome c oxidase under near IR radiation. Journal of Photochemistry and Photobiology B: Biology. 2005;**81**:98-106

[104] Thunshelle C, Hamblin MR. Transcranial low-level laser (light) therapy for brain injury. Photomedicine and Laser Surgery. 2016;**34**:587-598

[105] Sies H, Jones DP. Reactive oxygen species (ROS) as pleiotropic physiological signaling agents. Nature Reviews. Molecular Cell Biology. 2020;**21**:363-383

[106] Yu W, Naim JO, et al. Photomodulation of oxidative metabolism and electron chain enzymes in rat liver mitochondria. Photochemistry and Photobiology. 1997;**66**:866-871

[107] Berry BJ et al. Use the protonmotive force: Mitochondrial uncoupling and reactive oxygen species. Journal of Molecular Biology. 2018;**430**(21):3873-3891

[108] Wong IV, Cheuk DKL, Chu V. Acupuncture for hypoxic ischemic encephalopathy in neonates (protocol). Cochrane Database of Systematic Reviews. 2009;**3**:CD007968

[109] Morey SS. NIH issues consensus statement on acupuncture. American Family Physician. 1998;**57**(10):2545-2546

[110] Bonafede M, Dick A, Noyes K, Klein JD, Brown T. The effect of acupuncture utilization on healthcare utilization. Medical Care. 2008;**46**:41-48

[111] Ruth M et al. Laser acupuncture for chronic back pain. A Double-Blind Clinical Study. Schmerz. 2010;**24**(5):485-493

[112] Niemtzow RC. Battlefield acupuncture. Medical Acupuncture. 2007;**19**(4):225-228

[113] Reintal M, Andersson S, Gustafsson M, et al. Effects of minimal acupuncture in children with infantile colic – A prospective, quasi-randomised single blind controlled trial. Acupuncture in Medicine. 2008;**26**(3):171-182

[114] Schlager A et al. Laser stimulation of acupuncture point P6 reduces postoperative vomiting in children

undergoing strabismus surgery. British Journal of Anaesthesia. 1998;**81**:529-532

[115] Jindhal V et al. Safety and efficiency of acupuncture in children, a review of the evidence. Journal of Pediatric Hematology/Oncology. 2008;**30**(6):431-442

[116] Wu et al. Using acupuncture for acute pain in hospitalized children. Pediatric Critical Care Medicine. 2009;**10**(3):291-296

[117] Gottschling S et al. Laser acupuncture in children with headache: A double-blind, randomized, bicenter, placebo-controlled trial. Pain. 2008;**137**(2):405-412

[118] Stahler van Amerongen K et al. Ear acupuncture points in neonates. The Journal of Alternative and Complementary Medicine. 2008;**14**(1):47-52

[119] Ecevit A et al. Acupuncture in preterm babies during minor painful procedures. Journal of Traditional Chinese Medicine. 2011;**31**(4):308-310

[120] Landgren K, Kvorning N, Hallström I. Acupuncture reduces crying in infants with infantile colic: A randomized, controlled, blind clinical study. Acupuncture in Medicine. 2010;**28**(4):174-179

[121] Golianu et al. Non-pharmacological techniques for pain management in neonates. Seminars in Perinatology. 2007;**31**(5):318-322

[122] Raith W et al. Active ear acupuncture points in neonates with neonatal abstinence syndrome (NAS). The American Journal of Chinese Medicine. 2011;**39**:29

[123] Freitas AC et al. Assessment of anti-inflammatory effect of 830nm laser light using c-reactive protein levels. Brazilian Dental Journal. 2001;**12**(3):187-190

[124] Goldman N, Chen M, Fujita T, Xu Q, Peng W, Liu W, et al. Adenosine A1 receptors mediate local anti-nociceptive effects of acupuncture. Nature Neuroscience. 2010;**13**(7):883-888

[125] Errington-Evans N. Acupuncture for anxiety. CNS Neuroscience & Therapeutics. 2012;**18**(4):277-284

[126] Lee S, Kim S. The effects of acupuncture on sleep disorders and its underlying mechanism: A literature review of rodent studies. Frontiers in Neuroscience, Sec. Translational Neuroscience. 2023;**8**(17):1243029

[127] Grant S, Colaiaco B, Motala A, Shanman R, Sorbero M, Hempel S. Acupuncture for the treatment of adults with posttraumatic stress disorder: A systematic review and meta-analysis. Journal of Trauma & Dissociation. 2018;**19**(1):39-58

[128] Ding N, Li L, Song K, Huang A, Zhang H. Efficacy and safety of acupuncture in treating post-traumatic stress disorder: A protocol for systematic review and meta-analysis. Medicine. 2020;**99**(26):e20700

[129] Tang X, Lin S, Fang D, Lin B, Yao L, Wang L, et al. Efficacy and underlying mechanisms of acupuncture therapy for PTSD: Evidence from animal and clinical studies. Frontiers in Behavioral Neuroscience. 2023;**17**:1163718

[130] Kwon CY, Leem J, Kim DW, Kwon HJ, Park HS, Kim SH. Effects of acupuncture on earthquake survivors with major psychiatric disorders and related symptoms: A scoping review of clinical studies. PLoS One. 2023;**18**(6):e0286671

[131] Li H. A Study of Acupuncturing "Chou's Tiaoshen" Acupoints on Patients in Subacute Insomnia. ISRCTN Registry. BMC Part of Springer Nature; 2018. DOI: 10.1186/ISRCTN24323119

[132] Jialing Z, Zongshi Q, Tsz HS, et al. Electroacupuncture plus auricular acupressure for chemotherapy-associated insomnia in breast cancer patients: A pilot randomized controlled trial. Integrative Cancer Therapies. 2021;**20**:1-11

[133] Mercane B, Ginatempo F, Manca A, Francesco Melis F, Enrico P, Franca DF. Anatomo-physiologic basis for auricular stimulation. Acupunture in Medicine. 2018;**30**:141-150

[134] Alimi D, Chelly JE. New universal nomenclature in Auriculotherapy. Journal of Alternative and Complementary Medicine. 2018;**24**:7-14